USMLE ROAD MAP

PATHOLOGY

Edited by

GEORGE R. WETTACH, MD

THOMAS W. PALMROSE, MD

TERRY K. MORGAN, MD, PhD

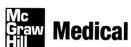 **Medical**

New York   Chicago   San Francisco   Lisbon   London   Madrid   Mexico City
Milan   New Delhi   San Juan   Seoul   Singapore   Sydney   Toronto

USMLE Road Map: Pathology

Copyright © 2009 by The McGraw-Hill Companies, Inc. All rights reserved. Printed in the United States of America. Except as permitted under the United States Copyright Act of 1976, no part of this publication may be reproduced or distributed in any form or by any means, or stored in a data base or retrieval system, without the prior written permission of the publisher.

1 2 3 4 5 6 7 8 9 0 DOC/DOC 12 11 10 9

ISBN 978-0-07-148267-7
MHID 0-07-148267-9
ISSN 1947-2315

Notice

Medicine is an ever-changing science. As new research and clinical experience broaden our knowledge, changes in treatment and drug therapy are required. The authors and the publisher of this work have checked with sources believed to be reliable in their efforts to provide information that is complete and generally in accord with the standards accepted at the time of publication. However, in view of the possibility of human error or changes in medical sciences, neither the authors nor the publisher nor any other party who has been involved in the preparation or publication of this work warrants that the information contained herein is in every respect accurate or complete, and they disclaim all responsibility for any errors or omissions or for the results obtained from use of the information contained in this work. Readers are encouraged to confirm the information contained herein with other sources. For example and in particular, readers are advised to check the product information sheet included in the package of each drug they plan to administer to be certain that the information contained in this work is accurate and that changes have not been made in the recommended dose or in the contraindications for administration. This recommendation is of particular importance in connection with new or infrequently used drugs.

This book was set in Adobe Garamond by Aptara®, Inc
The editors were Kirsten Funk and Harriet Lebowitz.
The production supervisor was Phil Galea.
Project Management was provided by Deepa Krishnan, Aptara Inc
The designer was Eve Siegel.
RR Donnelley was the printer and binder.

This book is printed on acid-free paper.

CONTENTS

USING THE USMLE ROAD MAP SERIES FOR SUCCESSFUL REVIEW

What is the Road Map Series?

Short of having your own personal tutor, the *USMLE Road Map* Series is the best source for efficient review of major concepts and information in the medical sciences.

Why do you need a Road Map?

It allows you to navigate quickly and easily through your pathology course notes and textbook and prepares you for USMLE and course examinations.

How does the Road Map Series work?

Outline Form: Connects the facts in a conceptual framework so that you understand the ideas and retain the information.

Color and Boldface: Highlights words and phrases that trigger quick retrieval of concepts and facts.

Clear Explanations: Are fine-tuned by years of student interaction. The material is written by authors selected for their excellence in teaching and their experience in preparing students for board examinations.

Illustrations (Photomicrographs and Clinical Images): Provide the vivid impressions that facilitate comprehension and recall.

Rapid Review Glossary: Defines common terms, diseases, signs, syndromes, and bodies for easy reference and efficient review at the end of the book

 Clinical Correlations: Link all topics to their clinical applications, promoting fuller understanding and memory retention.

 Developmental Insights: Identify relationships between developmental processes and subsequent pathology.

 Clinical Problems: Give you valuable practice for the clinical vignette-based USMLE questions.

 Explanations of Answers: Are learning tools that allow you to pinpoint your strengths and weaknesses.

CONTRIBUTORS

Antony Bakke, PhD, Director of Clinical Immunology Laboratory, Oregon Health and Sciences University, Portland, Oregon

Christopher L. Corless, MD, PhD, Director of Surgical Pathology, Oregon Health and Sciences University, Portland, Oregon

Jennifer Dunlap, MD, Resident, Oregon Health and Sciences University, Portland, Oregon

Ken Gatter, MD, JD, Hematopathologist and Director of Anatomic Pathology, Oregon Health and Sciences University, Portland, Oregon

Eric A. Goranson, MD, Resident, Oregon Health and Sciences University, Portland, Oregon

David Gray, MD, Hematopathology Fellow, Oregon Health and Sciences University, Portland, Oregon

Sakir H. Gultekin, MD, Director of Neuromuscular Pathology Laboratory, Oregon Health and Sciences University, Portland, Oregon

Michelle Jorden, MD, Medical Examiner, Cook County, Illinois

Julie Kingery, MD, Molecular Diagnostics Fellow, Oregon Health and Sciences University, Portland, Oregon

Atiya Mansoor, MD, Director of Consultation Service, Oregon Health and Sciences University, Portland, Oregon

Craig Midgen, MD, Resident, Oregon Health and Sciences University, Portland, Oregon

Terry K. Morgan, MD, PhD, Director of Cytopathology, Oregon Health and Sciences University, Portland, Oregon

Thomas W. Palmrose, MD, Cytopathology Fellow, Oregon Health and Sciences University, Portland, Oregon

Richard Press, MD, PhD, Director of Molecular Pathology, Oregon Health and Sciences University, Portland, Oregon

Reva Ricketts-Loriaux, DO, Cytopathology Fellow, Oregon Health and Sciences University, Portland, Oregon

Sarah J. Rollin, MD, Staff Pediatrician, Providence Medical Group, Portland, Oregon

Richard Scanlan, MD, Director of Transfusion Medicine Service, Oregon Health and Sciences University, Portland, Oregon

Dustin V. Shackleton, MD, Resident, Oregon Health and Sciences University, Portland, Oregon

Jeffery Stewart, DDS, School of Dentistry, Oregon Health and Sciences University, Portland, Oregon

Michele Thompson, MD, Dermatopathology Fellow, Oregon Health and Sciences University, Portland, Oregon

Megan Troxell, MD, PhD, Director of Immunohistochemistry Laboratory, Oregon Health and Sciences University, Portland, Oregon

Douglas Weeks, MD, Pediatric Pathologist and Chairman, Oregon Health and Sciences University, Portland, Oregon

George R. Wettach, MD, Resident, Oregon Health and Sciences University, Portland, Oregon

Clifton R. White, Jr., MD, Director of Dermatopathology, Oregon Health and Sciences University, Portland, Oregon

Sandra L. White, MD, Surgical Pathology Fellow, Oregon Health and Sciences University, Portland, Oregon

Randy Woltjer, MD, PhD, Neuropathologist, Oregon Health and Sciences University, Portland, Oregon

PREFACE

Our goal is to provide an essential resource complementing the speed of online reviews (eg, *WebPath*) and the rich detail of Robbins & Cotran *Pathologic Basis of Disease.* We organized *USMLE Road Map: Pathology* like a routine physical examination, including the clinical presentation, diagnostic features, and prognostic indications of conditions encountered on the wards and on the boards. We hope you find this approach to pathology effective.

It takes a village to prepare a manuscript of this scope and depth. We are very grateful for the time and expertise provided by our contributing authors. Special thanks to Susan Carley Oliver for composing the images and figures. We thank Drs. Donald Houghton, David Sauer, Susan Sharp, and Shirley Welch, as well as Lisa Lee Pate, Sarah Blundell, Kay Larkin, Tera Jones, Katherine Krupela, Sherry Davis, and Jon Alexander for their photographic contributions and editorial comments. We also thank our pathology medical student fellows for reviewing early drafts of this manuscript and providing detailed comments.

Finally, we offer special thanks to Harriet Lebowitz, Kirsten Funk, and Jennifer Bernstein for their patience and hard work preparing this manuscript for publication.

George R. Wettach, MD
Thomas W. Palmrose, MD
Terry K. Morgan, MD, PhD

CHAPTER 1
AUTOPSY AND FORENSIC MEDICINE: CELLULAR INJURY AND REPAIR

That on the ashes of his youth doth lie . . .
Consumed with that which it was nourish'd by.
—Shakespeare, "Sonnet 73"

I. Environmental Pathology

A. Role of Forensic Medicine

1. Environmental pathology is most often encountered and diagnosed in a medical examiner's office where forensic pathologists conduct autopsies in order to determine a cause and manner of death.
2. There are five manners of death rendered in forensics:
   a. Natural (eg, myocardial infarction due to thrombosis)
   b. Accident (eg, motor vehicle trauma, falls)
   c. Homicide (eg, gunshot, strangulation, stabbing, assault)
   d. Suicide (eg, self-inflicted gunshot wound)
   e. Undetermined (eg, remains unclear after thorough crime scene investigation)
3. Only a forensic pathologist can determine a manner of death other than natural.

B. Accidents

1. Accidental deaths are considered unintentional injury.
2. The most common causes of accidental deaths are motor vehicle trauma, drug overdoses, and firearms (Figure 1–1).

C. Drugs and Toxins

1. Toxicology involves analyzing bodily fluids, such as blood, bile, and urine, for the presence of toxins or drugs.
2. Toxicology is an integral part of the autopsy and may provide the cause and manner of death (eg, cocaine overdose).
3. **Tobacco** use is the leading cause of lung disease.
   a. Tobacco smoke contains particulate matter (tar), irritants, **carbon monoxide,** and 43 known **carcinogens.**
   b. It inhibits respiratory mucosa cilia and is absorbed into the blood to exert its effects.
   c. Tobacco smoke is responsible for 30% of cancer deaths and 90% of all **lung cancer** deaths, including secondhand smoke.

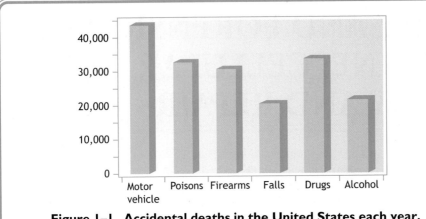

Figure 1–1. Accidental deaths in the United States each year.

d. Tobacco plays a role in causing ischemic heart disease, chronic obstructive pulmonary disease, asthma, bronchitis, and stroke (including women who are older than 35 years who take oral contraceptive pills), low birth weight in infants, and sudden infant death syndrome (SIDS).

4. **Ethanol** is the most widely **abused** legal drug in the world.
   a. A blood alcohol level of **80 mg/dL** (0.08 grams%) is the legal definition for drunk driving.
   b. Ethanol is a central nervous system **depressant,** which causes a relaxed feeling that can progress to decreased inhibitions and movement abnormalities (ie, stumbling drunk).
   c. Chronic ethanol abuse leads to multiple organ pathology.
      (1) **Liver** changes include fatty change, acute hepatitis, and micronodular **cirrhosis** (Figure 1–2).
      (2) Brain effects include **Wernicke-Korsakoff syndrome** due to thiamine deficiency, which grossly presents as hemorrhage into the mamillary bodies and cerebellar degeneration.
         (a) Clinical manifestations of Wernicke syndrome are ataxia, ophthalmoplegia, and short-term memory loss.
         (b) Although on a continuum, Korsakoff syndrome is an irreversible form of Wernicke syndrome.
      (3) Heart effects include dilated **cardiomyopathy,** due to the direct toxic effect of the drug on the heart.
      (4) Ethanol causes **gastritis** and may cause **pancreatitis.**
      (5) Ethanol abuse may lead to **testicular atrophy** in men.
      (6) Ethanol consumption during pregnancy is not recommended because it may lead to **fetal alcohol syndrome.**
         (a) It appears that acetaldehyde (metabolite of ethanol) crosses the placenta and damages the fetus.
         (b) Fetal alcohol syndrome has characteristic facies: small head, epicanthal folds, low nasal bridge, small eye openings, flat midface, short nose, smooth philtrum, thin upper lip, and underdeveloped jaw.

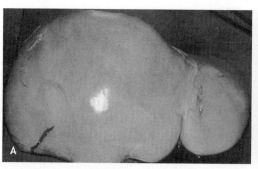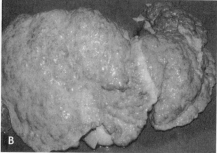

Figure 1–2. Ethanol causes liver damage. Alcohol causes reversible steatohepatitis (fatty liver, **A**), which if prolonged may lead to irreversible micronodular cirrhosis (**B**).

   (c) Fetal alcohol syndrome is the most common type of preventable **mental retardation.**
   (d) The amount of ethanol required to cause this syndrome is not well established; therefore women are advised to refrain from drinking during pregnancy.

ETHANOL AND ALDEHYDE DEHYDROGENASE

- *Ethanol is metabolized into acetaldehyde by **alcohol dehydrogenase** in the liver.*
- *Acetaldehyde is converted into acetic acid by **aldehyde dehydrogenase.***
- *Many people of Asian descent, as well as Native Americans, have a functional polymorphism in the aldehyde dehydrogenase gene that affects ethanol metabolism.*
- *The result is flushing of the skin and sensitivity to ethanol.*

5. **Acetaminophen** is a widely used analgesic and is generally regarded as a safe medication with a large therapeutic window.
   a. Toxicity may be seen in the setting of suicidal overdose.
   b. The toxic dose is greater than 15 g.
   c. Acetaminophen is metabolized in the liver, where its major metabolites include inactive sulfate and glucuronide conjugates; these are eventually excreted by the kidneys.
      (1) A small amount is processed by hepatic **cytochrome P-450,** resulting in the toxic metabolite (*N*-acetyl-*p*-benzoquinone imine [NAPQI]).
      (2) At usual doses, NAPQI is detoxified rapidly by the liver and excreted by the kidneys.
      (3) Toxic dose leads to excessive NAPQI accumulation.
         (a) Acute symptoms include vomiting and diarrhea.
         (b) The antidote (N-acetylcysteine; **NAC**) may be given within 10 hours of the overdose.
         (c) There is irreversible damage to the liver within 48 hours of overdose, including **centrilobular necrosis,** which causes a gross **nutmeg pattern** (Figure 1–3).
         (d) As the liver fails, the patient will exhibit **jaundice** and hepatic **encephalopathy.**

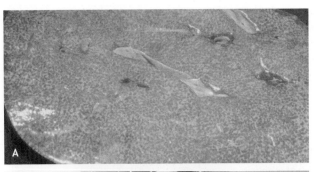

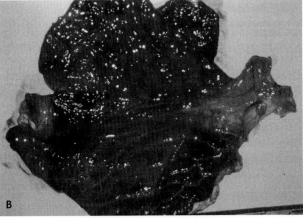

Figure 1–3. Acetaminophen and cyanide. An overdose of acetaminophen (>15 g) leads to centrilobular necrosis in the liver creating a "nutmeg" pattern **(A)**. If not rapidly treated, overdose is lethal. Cyanide poisoning has an almond smell (to some people) and causes hemorrhagic gastritis **(B)**.

6. **Arsenic** is still used on occasion as a homicidal **poison** and in some countries as chemotherapy for leukemia.
   a. It is a poison dating back to ancient times.
   b. Arsenic is found in wood preservatives and electronics.
   c. It is tasteless, odorless, and is absorbed by the gastrointestinal tract.
   d. The toxic dose is as little as 200 mg.
      (1) It inhibits sulfhydryl-containing enzymes.
      (2) **Death** is slow and painful.
      (3) In one large fatal dose, symptoms are gastrointestinal and can begin as little as 30 minutes after ingestion with vomiting, rice-water stool diarrhea, garlic breath, and dry mouth, possibly with a metallic taste.
      (4) Smaller doses over the long term lead to transverse white bands in the fingernails (**Mees lines**), **pancytopenia,** and **neuropathy.**
7. **Cyanide** causes deadly hypoxia by combining with the ferric iron atom of intracellular cytochrome oxidase.
   a. Cyanide may be found in most chemical laboratories.

b. The minimal lethal dose is 200 mg.

    c. There is a distinct **almond odor** during autopsy, which is only detected by a portion of the population.

    d. Other autopsy findings include bright cherry red lividity and hemorrhage into the stomach (Figure 1–3).

    e. When inhaled as a gas, it can take only minutes to cause death (eg, used in death camps during World War II).

8. Lead poisoning may arise from various sources, including lead paint, leaded gasoline, and lead plumbing.

    a. Lead is absorbed through the gastrointestinal tract in infants and children, who show greater absorption rates.

    b. Absorbed lead is taken up in bone, developing teeth in children (lead lines along gingival surfaces), and soft tissue.

    c. Toxicity causes **cognitive** retardation, **neuropathy**, renal toxicity, anemia, and fatigue.

9. The most widely used **pesticides (organophosphates)** are parathion and malathion.

    a. Excessive respiratory exposure causes irreversible inhibition of **cholinesterase.**

        (1) The SLUDGE syndrome may develop in cases of toxic exposure:

            Salivation

            Lacrimation

            Urination

            Defecation

            Gastrointestinal distress

            Emesis

        (2) Accumulating acetylcholine inhibits the intercostal muscles leading to respiratory failure and death.

    b. The antidote is **pralidoxime chloride.**

10. Paraquat is a commonly used **weed killer.**

    a. Excessive exposure causes pulmonary edema, hyaline membranes, and may cause interstitial fibrosis.

    b. End-stage disease is pulmonary fibrosis (**honeycomb lung**).

D. Trauma

1. Mechanical trauma includes blunt force, sharp force injury, strangulation, and firearm deaths.

2. Blunt force injury may arise from assaults, motor vehicle accidents, crushing accidents (eg, usually work related), and falls.

3. Characteristic features of blunt force trauma include the following:

    a. **Abrasions** (scrapes) are the denudation of the superficial epidermis (Figure 1–4) and usually do not cause scars.

    b. **Contusions** (bruises) are the damage of small blood vessels causing bleeding into soft tissue.

    c. **Lacerations** are caused by stretching of the skin, leading to irregular tearing with underlying soft tissue bridges.

    d. **Fractures** of the bones are a sign of forceful impact and may be simple (clean break) or compound (pierces the skin).

4. Sharp object injury includes stab wounds and **incisions.**

    a. A stab wound is deeper than it is wide.

    b. An incised wound is longer than it is deep.

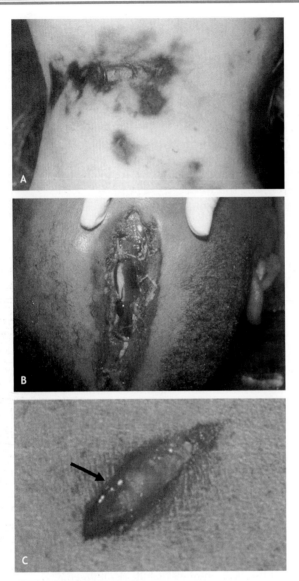

Figure 1–4. Skin trauma. A: Abrasions are caused by the superficial disruption of the epidermal layer, which may be caused by strangulation (as in this case). **B:** Lacerations are forceful tearing of skin leading to irregular borders with an abraded skin margin and underlying tissue bridging. In contrast, **C:** stab wounds have sharp borders (arrow) and no underlying tissue bridging.

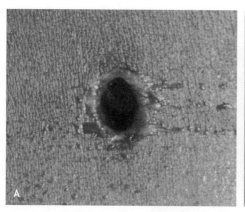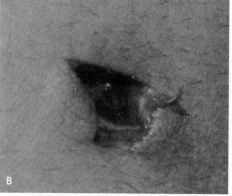

Figure 1–5. Gunshot wounds. A: Entrance wounds have a central oval defect, while the exit wound (**B**) is lacerated (torn).

5. **Strangulation** may be manual (hands) or by ligature and is caused by compression of the neck blood vessels, which causes cerebral hypoxia, leading to unconsciousness and death.
6. **Firearm** deaths are usually related to homicide or suicide.
   a. Entrance wounds tend to have an oval defect with a surrounding rim of abrasion (Figure 1–5).
   b. Exit wounds tend to have a lacerated appearance.
E. Burns
   1. Burns are categorized by the source.
      a. **Flame:** Direct contact with fire.
      b. **Contact:** Direct contact with a hot object (tea pot).
      c. **Radiant heat:** Indirect contact near a heat source (fire).
      d. **Scalding:** Contact with a hot liquid.
      e. **Chemical:** Contact with reagent that damages skin.
      f. **Electrical:** Contact with high voltage source.
      g. **Radiation:** Contact with radiation source (eg, sun).
   2. Burns can be partial or full thickness and are staged as follows:
      a. **First-degree burn:** Erythematous skin base without blister.
      b. **Second-degree burn:** Blister formation sparing the dermis.
      c. **Third-degree burn:** Destruction of the epidermis and dermis.
   3. Severity of burn depends on stage and body surface area involved.
      a. Greater than *50% involvement* portends a poor prognosis.
      b. Patients should seek medical attention if the burn is third degree (painless, charred), is larger than the palm of your hand, the patient has inhaled smoke, or is in shock.

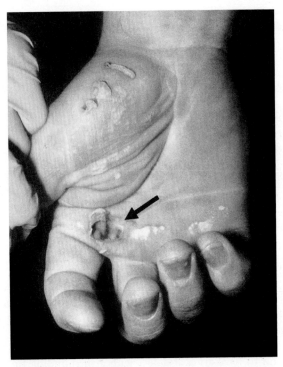

Figure 1–6. Burn from electrocution. This burn shows blistering (arrow) and skin destruction. If the burn is superficial (first degree) there is no blistering; second-degree burns show blistering, but no dermal damage; third-degree burns have underlying soft tissue destruction, including nerves, presenting as charred "painless" burn.

4. Inhalation injury (eg, resulting from inhalation of soot material) may lead to laryngeal edema.
5. People in fires may also suffer **carbon monoxide** poisoning, which can be fatal.
6. **Electrical** burns tend to appear as an erythematous lesion with blister formation or as a charred white lesion (Figure 1–6).
   a. Deaths by electrocution are rare and are usually accidental.
   b. Ventricular fibrillation occurs at 75–100 milliamps.
   c. To determine amperage, the following equation can be used: **Amperage = Volts/Resistance.**
   d. Histologic examination reveals **vacuolization** of the **stratum corneum** and **streaming** of the nuclei.
   e. Forensic pathologists suspect a diagnosis of electrocution if a person suddenly collapses "yelling profanity" and is found next to electrical equipment.
   f. High intensity current, such as lightening, can produce an arborescent pattern on the skin (**Lichtenberg sign**).

7. **Radiation** may cause hyperthermia and burns.
   a. Infants and the elderly are at greatest risk.
   b. **Ionizing radiation** causes DNA damage by cross-linking DNA strands and generating oxygen-derived free radicals, which lead to double-stranded DNA breaks.
      (1) Effects depend on the following:
         (a) **Dose rate**: A single dose can cause greater injury than fractionated doses because of widespread damage.
         (b) **Cell division**: Rapidly dividing cells are more radiosensitive (hematopoietic cells, gastrointestinal epithelium, endothelial cells, squamous cells, and lymphocytes).
         (c) **Radiation field**: A single dose to the whole body is more lethal than regional doses.
      (2) Complications include fibrosis and carcinogenesis.
         (a) **Fibrosis** leads to scarring and loss of function.
         (b) **Carcinogenesis** includes increased risk of skin cancer, leukemia, osteogenic sarcoma, and lung cancer.

HEAT STROKE

CLINICAL CORRELATION

- *Hyperthermia is defined as a rectal temperature > 40.5 °C.*
- *When the body cannot compensate by heat loss, heat stroke develops.*
- *Clinical manifestations include hot, dry skin; altered mental status; hypotension; tachycardia; and hyperventilation.*
- *Heat stroke is usually seen in the young or elderly after exertion in high temperatures.*

II. Cell Injury, Adaptation, and Death

A. **Reversible Injury**
   1. Reversible injury is the ability to heal without permanent damage.
   2. Cells can adapt to physiologic stress.
   3. Cells adapt by changing number, size, or differentiation.
      a. Hyperplasia is an increase in the number of cells.
      b. Hypertrophy is an increase in cell size.
      c. Atrophy is a decrease in cell size.
      d. Metaplasia is an alteration of cell differentiation.
      e. Intracellular accumulations are an altered metabolism.
   4. **Hyperplasia** can be physiologic or pathologic.
      a. **Hormones** may drive hyperplasia (eg, pregnant uterus or lactating breast).
      b. Compensatory hyperplasia may occur with **tissue damage** (eg, liver regeneration after partial hepatectomy, or wound repair).
      c. Initiation of cell proliferation includes induction of transcription factors and cell cycle proteins.
      d. Pathologic hyperplasia is a risk factor for neoplasia and is usually due to excessive hormonal stimulation (eg, polycystic ovary disease leading to excessive estrogen production), or the effects of growth factors.
   5. **Hypertrophy** is an increase in the **size** of the cell due to the synthesis of structural components rather than cellular swelling.
      a. It is usually a physiologic process due to increased **functional demands** placed on the cell (eg, hypertrophy of striated muscles from weight lifting, or cardiac myocyte hypertrophy secondary to systemic hypertension).

    b. There is expression of **embryonic genes** in hypertrophic cells, which appears to be triggered by both mechanical and trophic factors (stretch receptors, growth factors).

    c. The process can become pathologic when the limit of hypertrophy is exceeded and the cells can no longer compensate for the increased burden (eg, congestive heart failure).

6. Atrophy is the **reduction** of cell or organ size.

    a. Physiologic atrophy occurs during fetal development (eg, regression of the notochord) and throughout life (eg, muscle).

    b. Common causes of atrophy include:

        (1) Decreased workload or **denervation** (eg, paralysis).

        (2) Diminished blood supply (eg, atherosclerosis).

        (3) Inadequate nutrition (eg, **marasmus** "muscle wasting").

        (4) Loss of hormone stimulation (eg, menopause).

        (5) Aging (build up of cellular waste and DNA damage).

        (6) Compression (eg, organ compression by expanding tumor).

    c. The mechanism is incompletely understood, but it is thought to be an imbalance of synthesis and degradation.

    d. Increased number of **autophagic vacuoles** is seen.

7. Metaplasia is differentiation from one mature cell type to another (eg, squamous metaplasia of glandular respiratory epithelium).

    a. Metaplasia is an adaptive response to a hostile environment.

    b. Metaplasia is usually a change from glandular mucosa to keratin rich **squamous** mucosa (eg, squamous metaplasia of ciliated respiratory mucosa because of **smoking**) or mitochondria rich **oncocytic** cells (eg, apocrine change in breast, Hürthle change in thyroid, oncocytic change in the salivary glands).

    c. Metaplasia from squamous to glandular mucosa is unusual but is a common consequence of chronic reflux esophagitis (heart burn) known as **Barrett esophagus**.

    d. The mechanism is thought to arise from reprogramming of stem cells (reserve cells) from the basal layer (eg, squamous metaplasia at the cervical transformation zone).

    e. Metaplasia increases the patient's risk for carcinoma (eg, lung cancer from smoking, esophageal cancer from reflux).

8. Intracellular accumulations represent metabolic derangement.

    a. Endogenous substances may accumulate.

        (1) **Steatosis** (fatty change) develops in the liver because of metabolic changes associated with toxins (**ethanol** and certain drugs), diabetes mellitus, **obesity**, and pregnancy.

        (2) **Atherosclerosis** (cholesterol deposition and intimal damage) develops because of endothelial damage and elevated cholesterol levels.

        (3) **Immunoglobulin** produced in excess in chronically active plasma cells produce round red **Russell bodies.**

        (4) **Lipofuscin** is brown pigment derived from lipid peroxidation and is commonly seen in **aged** organs.

        (5) **Melanin** is a dark brown pigment made in skin, hair, and eye (iris and choroid layer). In skin, pigment production increases with **UV exposure,** which protects the underlying layers from damage.

(*6*) **Hemosiderin** is a granular brown pigment composed of **ferric oxide**, resulting from the breakdown of hemoglobin, which may be a sign of hemolysis, or disturbed iron metabolism (eg, hemochromatosis).

THE PROBLEM WITH AGING

- *Cellular aging is currently an irreversible "injury."*
- *It is thought to be programmed senescence and accumulated damage.*
- *Telomere shortening seems to play a key role in senescence.*
- *Replication of the chromosome caps appears to be incomplete with each cell division, causing shortening and final maturation.*
- *Cellular damage is caused by reactive oxygen species, which are usually a consequence of radiation, or toxins.*
- *Neoplastic cells express telomerase that lengthens chromosome caps, thereby immortalizing the tumor clone.*

    B. **Irreversible Injury**

       1. **Cell death** is irreversible and presents as **necrosis** or **apoptosis** (Table 1–1).

       2. Cell death has a long list of causes, but basically it is a consequence of cytoplasmic damage, DNA damage, or both.

       3. Necrosis is fundamentally a cytoplasmic driven process.

          a. It is a pathologic process resulting from the swelling and denaturation of the cell (eg, hypoxia leading to depleted ATP reserves and opening of ion channels leading to cellular swelling and enzyme release from digestive lysozymes).

          b. The release of cellular breakdown products and cytokines incites an inflammatory reaction and wound healing.

Table 1–1. Distinguishing necrosis from apoptosis.

Necrosis	Apoptosis
Cellular swelling	Cellular shrinkage
Nuclear swelling and lysis	Chromatin condensation and fragmentation (apoptotic bodies)
Death of many cells	Death of single cells
Lysosome breakdown	Lysosomes intact
Inflammation	No inflammation
Calcification	No calcification
Cessation of protein synthesis	Requires protein synthesis
Energy not required	Energy dependent

c. There is a well described and reproducible temporal sequence observed after necrotic cell death (eg, myocardial infarction):

        (1) **Hours** after the insult there are no clear features.

        (2) **1 day** after there are microscopic changes (waviness).

        (3) **1–3 days** after there is gross necrosis and a microscopic infiltration by neutrophils (Figure 1–7).

        (4) **3–7 days** after there is disintegration of the dead tissue and accumulation of macrophages.

        (5) **1–2 weeks** after there is granulation tissue (fibroblast and blood vessel proliferation).

        (6) **2–8 weeks** after there is increasing collagen deposition.

        (7) **>2 months** after there is a dense fibrous scar.

    d. **Liquefactive necrosis** affects soft organs (eg, brain infarction from stroke) (Figure 1–8).

    e. **Hemorrhagic necrosis** affects highly vascular organs (eg, pulmonary infarction from embolism).

    f. **Caseous necrosis** is the cheesy white center of granulomas (eg, tuberculosis).

    g. **Fat necrosis** is dead adipose tissue (eg, trauma to breast, or enzyme release in pancreatitis).

    h. Areas of necrosis may **calcify** (breast microcalcifications associated with necrosis from fibrocystic change or carcinoma).

  4. Apoptosis is fundamentally a DNA driven process.

    a. It is **programmed cell death** without an inflammatory response.

    b. There are two primary pathways:

        (1) **Extrinsic pathway** is through the death receptors (members of tumor necrosis factor (**TNF**) family), which deliver the apoptotic signal.

        (2) **Intrinsic pathway** works by increasing mitochondrial permeability and releasing pro-apoptotic molecules into the cytoplasm (eg, **BCL-2**).

    c. Both primary pathways lead to the execution phase, which uses specific proteases (eg, **caspase**) to shrink and breakdown the cell.

    d. Classic examples of apoptosis include:

        (1) Cells deprived of growth factors trigger apoptosis.

        (2) Radiation induces DNA damage and apoptosis.

p53 AND TUMOR SUPPRESSOR GENES

• *p53 is a tumor suppressor gene because it induces apoptosis in cells with DNA damage (source of mutation and uncontrolled cell growth).*

• *As people age, there is a progressive risk that these tumor suppressor genes will mutate, leading to uncontrolled mutation and cancer.*

III. Inflammation and Repair

  A. Acute Inflammation

    1. This is a rapid response to offending stimuli (eg, trauma, necrosis, infection, and toxins) that occurs within minutes and usually only lasts a few days.

    2. The cardinal features of acute inflammation include:

    a. **Rubor** (redness from vasodilation).

    b. **Tumor** (swelling from permeability and edema).

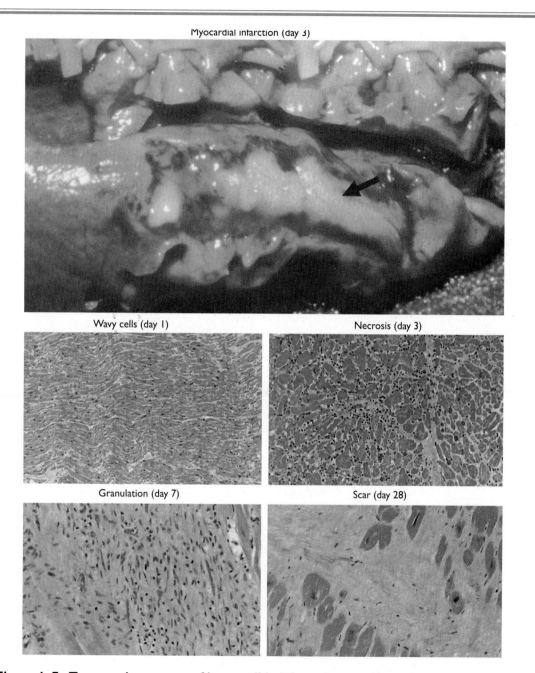

Figure 1–7. Temporal sequence of irreversible injury. Autopsied heart from a patient who died 3–7 days after a myocardial infarction. Representative photomicrographs show the classic temporal sequence of injury and repair.

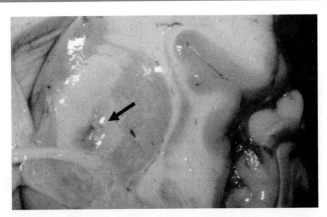

Figure 1–8. Liquefactive necrosis in the brain of a patient who died after a stroke. Ischemia of the basal ganglia led to infarction and necrosis.

    c. **Calor** (heat from fever caused by necrosis and cytokines).
    d. **Dolor** (pain from prostaglandins).
    e. Loss of function (**functio laesa**).
  3. The process begins with **endothelial cell activation** (Figure 1–9).
    a. Vasodilation and increased permeability stimulated by **nitric oxide** (endothelial cells), **histamine** (mast cells), and **bradykinin** (plasma) increases overall blood flow but slows the speed of blood across the endothelial surface.
    b. **Integrins** on leukocytes attach to endothelial **selectins**.
    c. Endothelial **intracellular adhesion molecule-1** (**ICAM-1**) and **vascular cell adhesion molecule** (**VCAM**) guides leukocytes through this barrier into surrounding tissue (**diapedesis**).
  4. **Chemotaxis** is cellular locomotion across a chemical gradient.
    a. Exogenous stimuli attract neutrophils (eg, bacterial antigens attract leukocytes).
    b. Endogenous stimuli attract and activate neutrophils (eg, **C5a complement**, **leukotriene B4**, cytokines **IL-1** and **TNF**).
  5. Acute inflammation can be exudative (serous), fibrinous (extravasation), and suppurative (neutrophils = pus).
  6. When neutrophils cannot neutralize the causative agent, or if there is tissue necrosis, a chronic inflammatory reaction develops.

 B. Complement Pathway
  1. The complement system is composed of precursor proteins and their active cleavage products that are predominantly found in the **plasma**.
  2. The **classic pathway** is triggered by C1 binding an **antigen: antibody complex** culminating in C3a and then C5a activation.

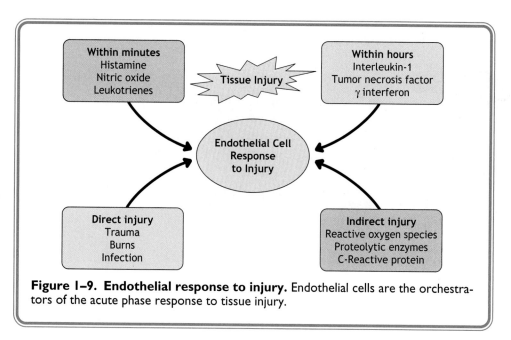

Figure 1–9. Endothelial response to injury. Endothelial cells are the orchestrators of the acute phase response to tissue injury.

3. The **alternative pathway** activates C3a and then C5a via bacterial surface polysaccharides (eg, lipopolysaccharide (**LPS**) (Figure 1–10).

COMPLEMENT SYSTEM IN HEALTH AND DISEASE

- *Escherichia coli infection leads to LPS release and C3 activation.*
- *Bacteria are also coated by C3b opsonization, which binds the CR3 receptor on neutrophils activating them for phagocytosis.*
- *Phagosomes containing E coli fuse with lyzosomal granules leading to reactive oxygen species burst (O_2-; H_2O_2, $OH-$).*
- *Defects in C3 lead to fatal infections if untreated.*
- *Defects in C2 and C4 are associated with autoimmune disease (lupus).*
- *Defects in the membrane attack complex lead to Neisseria infections.*

    C. **Chronic Inflammation**
       1. Chronic inflammation is a prolonged response (at least weeks in duration) to stimuli, which may be *de novo.*
       2. Many insidious human diseases are related to chronic inflammation.
       3. Primary causes include the following:
         a. Exposure to **toxins** (eg, cholesterol and atherosclerosis).
         b. **Foreign bodies** (eg, asbestos, silica, suture material).
         c. **Autoimmunity** (eg, systemic lupus erythematosus, rheumatoid arthritis).
         d. Persistent **infections** (tuberculosis, fungi, viruses).
       4. Chronic inflammation is characterized by **mononuclear** cell infiltration (eg, macrophages, lymphocytes, plasma cells, and histiocytes), **architectural** changes (eg, gland dropout in inflammatory bowel disease), and **fibrosis.**

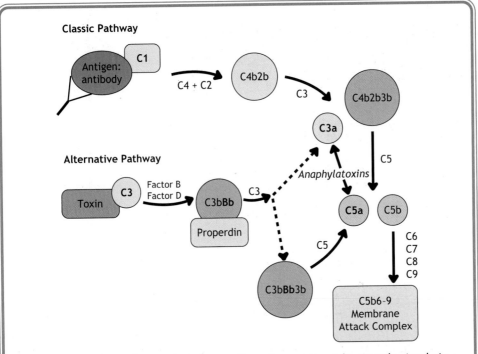

Figure 1–10. Complement pathway. Complement is predominantly circulating plasma proteins that marshal a response to antigen : antibody complexes (classic pathway) or by the alternative pathway, which is activated by bacterial toxins (eg, LPS), or venom. Either way, the result is production of anaphylatoxins (C3a, C5a) and the membrane attach complex.

   a. **Macrophages** are the demolition crew of the body.
      (1) C5a recruits monocytes from the bloodstream and activates them into macrophages.
      (2) Macrophages also release a number of cytokines and proteases that lead to tissue destruction.
   b. **Lymphocytes** (B-cells and T-cells) are attracted to the site by integrins and chemokines.
      (1) **B-cells** proliferate in reactive germinal centers and eventually mature into plasma cells to make polyclonal **antibodies** (kappa and lambda light chains).
      (2) **T-cells** produce cytokines, including gamma interferon (**IFN**), which is a major activator of macrophages.
5. **Granulation tissue** is a well-orchestrated process to clean up the dead tissue and replace the area with fibrous connective tissue that will provide maximal strength.
   a. Preexisting capillaries in surrounding undamaged tissue form new capillaries in the damaged area.

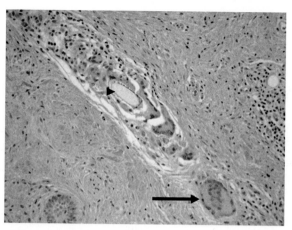

Figure 1–11. Chronic inflammation. Example of chronic inflammatory response to ruptured hair follicle. The offending keratinized fragment of hair (arrowhead) incites a response composed of lymphocytes, plasma cells, eosinophils, and multinucleated histiocytic giant cells (arrow).

    b. Basic fibroblast growth factor (bFGF) stimulates angiogenesis and fibroblast proliferation.

    c. **Tumor growth factor-β** stimulates fibroblasts and collagen synthesis.

    d. Vitamin C and zinc are also needed for wound healing

    e. Ironically, although strong, the resulting scar is non-functional and may lead to significant clinical sequelae (ie, myocardial scar decreases heart contractility leading to congestive heart failure).

    f. Scars may also be hypertrophic (**keloid**).

6. **Granulomatous inflammation** is a specific type of chronic inflammatory response characterized by nodules of activated macrophages (**histiocytes**) with a plump red epithelioid morphology and **multinucleated giant cells** (fused histiocytes) (Figure 1–11).

    a. **Foreign body** granulomas are most common and arise around inert foreign material (eg, suture, silica).

    b. **Noncaseating granulomas** may also be seen in autoimmune disease (eg, **sarcoid**) and **Hodgkin lymphoma.**

    c. **Caseating granulomas** are necrotic in the center and are almost always due to infection (eg, tuberculosis, fungi).

        (1) Organisms may be identified by culture (microbiology).

        (2) In tissue sections, organisms may be identified by special stains (eg, Fite stain for acid-fast bacteria; Gomori methenamine silver (GMS) stain for fungi).

        (3) Molecular testing (eg, polymerase chain reaction, [PCR]) is becoming more widely used to detect subtle infections.

CLINICAL PROBLEMS

1. Which of the following statements regarding smoking is **CORRECT?**

   A. It is a stimulant that increases the ciliary actions of the respiratory epithelial lining.

   B. It inhibits the ciliary actions of the respiratory lining and contributes to obstructive pulmonary disease.

   C. It causes lung cancer, but not bladder cancer.

   D. It contains particulate matter and irritants, the most dangerous being carbon dioxide.

   E. It is recommended for pregnant women.

2. Ethanol is metabolized by:

   A. Alcohol dehydrogenase into acetaldehyde

   B. Alcohol dehydrogenase into acetate

   C. Aldehyde dehydrogenase into acetaldehyde

   D. Aldehyde dehydrogenase into acetate

   E. None of the above

3. The polymorphism associated with an increased sensitivity to ethanol is in which gene:

   A. Aldehyde dehydrogenase

   B. Acetate

   C. Cytochrome P-450

   D. Alcohol dehydrogenase

   E. None of the above

4. A 19-year-old woman was admitted to the hospital after ingesting a full bottle of acetaminophen. Laboratory tests revealed markedly elevated liver enzymes. What metabolite contributed to her now life-threatening liver damage?

   A. Depletion of cytochrome P-450 enzyme system

   B. Glucuronide conjugates

   C. N-acetyl-p-benzoquinone imine (NAPQI)

   D. Sulfate conjugates

   E. N-acetylcysteine (NAC)

5. Acetaminophen intoxication specifically causes:

   A. Diffuse liver necrosis

   B. Periportal liver necrosis

   C. Lobular necrosis

D. Centrilobular necrosis

    E. None of the above

6. Some of the clinical manifestations of organophosphate poisoning include the following:

    A. Lacrimation, salivation, and defecation

    B. Lacrimation, dry mouth, and defecation

    C. Emesis, urinary retention, and constipation

    D. Salivation, urination, and dry eyes

    E. Salivation, emesis, and constipation

7. Reversible injury encompasses:

    A. Metaplasia, hypertrophy, atrophy, and fibrosis

    B. Hyperplasia, hypertrophy, and necrosis

    C. Hyperplasia, hypertrophy, apoptosis

    D. Hyperplasia, metaplasia, hypertrophy, atrophy, and necrosis

    E. Hyperplasia, hypertrophy, atrophy, and metaplasia

8. The difference between the classic and alternate complement pathway is:

    A. The alternate pathway needs antibody

    B. The classic pathway needs antibody

    C. The classic pathway needs C5

    D. The alternate pathway needs C5

    E. The classic pathway needs Factors B and D

9. During the acute inflammatory process, integrins attach to:

    A. Receptors on neighboring leukocytes

    B. Molecules within the lipoxygenase pathway

    C. Antigens on leukocytes

    D. Selectins on endothelial cells

    E. Cytokines (IL-8)

10. Which of the following statements are **FALSE:**

    A. Necrosis is programmed cell death and causes cell shrinkage

    B. Apoptosis results in nuclear swelling and lysis

    C. Necrosis is energy dependent

    D. A myocardial infarct is considered apoptosis

    E. All of the above

ANSWERS

1. The answer is B. Smoking inhibits the mucociliary actions of the respiratory epithelial lining causing mucus to accumulate in the airway and causing symptoms of chronic bronchitis. Although smoking contains nicotine and is a stimulant, it does not stimulate clearance of mucus secretions. Although smoking is responsible for a large number of lung cancers, it also causes bladder cancer, oral cancers, and is a risk factor for many other cancers. Smoking leads to **carbon monoxide** accumulation, which inhibits red blood cell oxygenation. Smoking is not recommended for pregnant women.

2. The answer is A. Ethanol is metabolized in the liver to acetaldehyde by alcohol dehydrogenase. The liver is the primary route of elimination. Acetaldehyde is then converted to acetic acid by aldehyde dehydrogenase.

3. The answer is A. Approximately 50% of the Asian population has a genetic polymorphism in aldehyde dehydrogenase that affects alcohol metabolism.

4. The answer is C. Acetaminophen is metabolized in the liver, where its major metabolites include inactive sulfate and glucuronide conjugates, which are eventually excreted by the kidneys. Only a small amount is metabolized via the hepatic cytochrome P-450 enzyme system (its CYP2E1 and CYP1A2 isoenzymes), resulting in an alkylating metabolite (*N*-acetyl-*p*-benzoquinone imine), abbreviated as NAPQI. At usual doses, the toxic metabolite NAPQI is quickly detoxified by combining irreversibly with the sulfhydryl groups of glutathione to produce a nontoxic conjugate that is excreted by the kidneys. N-acetylcysteine (NAC) can be used as an antidote within 8–10 hours of an acetaminophen overdose.

5. The answer is D. Acetaminophen intoxication produces a gross nutmeg pattern in the liver diagnostic of centrilobular necrosis. Although there can be diffuse necrosis in some fulminant cases of acetaminophen intoxication, most cases show centrilobular necrosis. The necrosis is centered around central veins and is not confined to only the lobules. Periportal hemorrhage and necrosis are seen in women with eclampsia.

6. The answer is A. Organophosphates cause *irreversible* inhibition of cholinesterase causing accumulation of acetylcholine leading to bradycardia and the "massive runs." The effects may be recalled as the SLUDGE syndrome: **S**alivation, **L**acrimation, **U**rination, **D**efecation, **G**astrointestinal distress, **E**mesis.

7. The answer is E. Reversible changes include hyperplasia, hypertrophy, metaplasia, atrophy, and fatty metamorphosis. Irreversible injury can best be thought of in terms of changes that cannot be reversed such as fibrosis (ie, cirrhosis of the liver, fibrosis replacing a myocardial infarct), necrosis and apoptosis (dead tissue).

8. The answer is B. The main difference between the classic and alternate pathway is that the classic pathway requires C1 activation by antibody complexed with an antigen. The alternate pathway does not require an antibody and instead uses microbial surface antigens.

9. The answer is D. Acute inflammation is a vascular process. Leukocytes start to tumble across the endothelium and transiently adhere. Sialyl-Lewis-X modified glycoprotein and integrins are present on the surface of the leukocytes attaching to P-selectin and E-selectin on endothelial cells. Products of the lipoxygenase pathway are involved in chemotaxis.

10. The answer is E. All the statements are false.

CHAPTER 2
MOLECULAR DIAGNOSTICS

The best research tool is an H&E stained slide and the brain.
—Hans Popper, MD, PhD

I. Immunohistochemistry

A. Methods

1. As cells differentiate into different tissues like skin, lymphoid cells, and muscle, they specialize and express specific proteins, which may be detected by purified antibodies against those antigens.
2. Immunohistochemistry begins with hybridizing an antibody solution with the tissue (eg, anti-cytokeratin with section of lymph node).
3. It is then hybridized with a secondary anti-antibody conjugated to a reporter enzyme that precipitates a signal in cells that are positive for the antigen (eg, carcinoma is positive, lymphocytes are negative) (Figure 2–1).
4. Immunostaining may be done using frozen tissue sections, formalin fixed sections (routine pathology), or fresh suspended cells (flow cytometry) using either enzyme reporters or fluorescence.
5. A growing array of antibodies are routinely used (Table 2–1).

B. Interpretation

1. Despite its potential, immunohistochemical results must be interpreted with care.
2. The expression pattern of antigens may change as individual tumor cells dedifferentiate and begin to express an antigenic profile unlike their original cellular lineage.
3. The specificity of a particular marker varies significantly from one tumor type to another.
4. The location of immunoreactivity (nuclear, cytoplasmic, membranous, or extracellular) must be considered. For example, the antibody to TTF-1 stains the nuclei of small cell carcinoma (specific), but it stains the cytoplasm of hepatocellular carcinoma (not specific).

II. Assays Using In Situ Chromosomes

A. Cytogenetics

1. Cytogenetics is the study of individual chromosomes, their structure, and inheritance patterns.

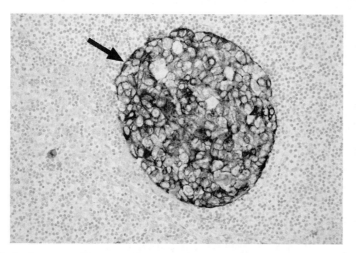

Figure 2–1. Immunohistochemical staining may be used to characterize cellular differentiation, like cytokeratin staining (arrow) of metastatic carcinoma to an axillary lymph node.

2. After white blood cells or single-cell suspensions of tumor cells are cultured in media, they are stimulated to divide with mitogens then arrested in cell cycle metaphase.
3. The chromosomes are then released from the nucleus, fixed, and spread onto slides for staining and microscopic examination.
4. The individual chromosomes are identified and categorized (morphologically) based on their staining characteristics and centromere placement (Figure 2–2).
   a. **Acrocentric** chromosomes have their centromere near one end of the chromosome and have satellite short arms encoding ribosomal RNA (rRNA).
   b. **Metacentric** chromosomes have a centrally placed centromere.
5. Chromosome studies are indicated for the following reasons:
   a. Cases of developmental delay
   b. Presence of dysmorphic features, neoplasia, or fertility issues
   c. Family history of chromosome disorders
   d. Pregnancy in women who are older than 36 years
6. Chromosomal abnormalities include incorrect numbers of chromosome (aneuploidy) and structural rearrangements.
   a. **Aneuploidy** refers to any number of chromosomes more or less than the expected 46 (eg, 47 in trisomy 21).
   b. **Structural** rearrangements occur when chromosomes break and the constituent pieces reassemble abnormally (translocations).

Table 2–1. Commonly used immunohistochemical stains.

Marker	Classic Use for Diagnosis
AFP	Yolk sac tumor and hepatocellular carcinoma
BCL-2	Follicular lymphoma
CD3	T-cells
CD20	B-cells
CD30	Hodgkin disease
CD31	Vascular tumors
CD45	White blood cells
CDX2	Gastrointestinal tract, especially colon
Cytokeratins	Epithelial cells, carcinoma
Desmin	Smooth and striated muscle differentiation
E-cadherin	Favors ductal over lobular breast carcinoma
Estrogen Receptor	Breast carcinoma prognostic and therapeutic marker
GFAP	Atrocytes; neural tumors
HCG-beta	Choriocarcinoma
HepPar-1	Hepatocellular carcinoma
HER2/neu	Breast carcinoma prognostic and therapeutic marker
HMB-45	Melanoma
Ki-67	Mitotic activity
Melan-A (MART-1)	Melanoma
p63	Epithelial cells (squamous, transitional)
PLAP	Seminoma
PR	Breast carcinoma prognostic marker
PSA	Prostatic carcinoma
S100	Melanoma or neural differentiation
Chromogranin	Neuroendocrine differentiation (carcinoid)
TTF-1	Thyroid and lung carcinomas
Vimentin	Mesenchymal marker to confirm antigenicity

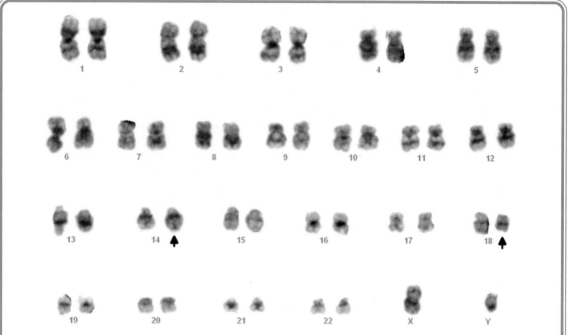

Figure 2–2. Cytogenetics is used to screen for chromosomal anomalies in many neoplasms, including lymphoma (shown here and in Table 2–2), sarcomas (see Chapter 15), brain tumors (see Chapter 16), and pediatric small round blue cell tumors (see Chapter 19). Arrows show t(14;18) translocation.

          (1) Balanced rearrangements may not be clinically evident because all the chromosomal material is present.

          (2) However, balanced translocations may result in aberrant expression of fused genes leading to neoplasia (eg, common in various lymphomas) (Table 2–2).

   B. Fluorescence In Situ Hybridization (FISH)

      1. FISH is the use of DNA probes labeled with fluorescent dyes to hybridize with chromosomal DNA fixed on slides.

         a. The fluorescent staining pattern is then viewed at the appropriate wavelength of light to localize specific genes or chromosomes (eg, to highlight red or green labels).

         b. Interphase FISH uses probes while cells are in interphase, allowing for a large number of nuclei to be tested.

         c. Metaphase FISH allows for specific localization of the probe-binding region within a specific chromosome.

      2. Each probe is intended to detect a unique sequence (eg, *HER2/neu*) or specific portion of a chromosome (eg, chromosome 17 centromere) (Figure 2–3).

      3. Sequence-specific DNA probes permit unique DNA sequences to be tested for DNA insertions, deletions, and translocations.

Table 2–2. Common translocations in hematopoietic malignancies.

Mutation	Genes	Disease
t(15;17)	PML-RARa	Acute promyelocytic leukemia
t(8;21)	ETO-AML1	Acute myelocytic leukemia
t(9;22)	BCR-ABL	Chronic myelocytic leukemia
t(12;21)	CBFa-ETV6	Acute lymphocytic leukemia
t(8;14)	c-myc-IgH	Burkitt lymphoma
t(14;18)	BCL2-IgH	Follicular lymphoma
t(11;14)	BCL1-IgH	Mantle cell lymphoma

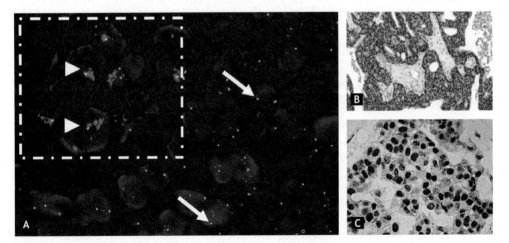

Figure 2–3. A: Fluorescent in situ hybridization (FISH) may be used to test for gene amplifications, or gene fusions (arrows, chromosome 17 reference). Routine breast cancer molecular studies include immunostaining for ER **(B)**, PR, providing a mitotic index with Ki-67 **(C)**, and testing for *HER2/neu* amplification (arrowheads) by FISH.

4. Chromosomal paints are DNA probes for a mix of DNA from all or part of a chromosome to visually inspect the chromosome for translocated fragments.

5. Multiple chromosomal paints may be used simultaneously to identify each metaphase chromosome with a unique color in a process known as **spectral karyotyping.**

III. Assays Using Extracted DNA

A. Southern Blot

1. Southern blot has been used for decades to identify mutations and polymorphisms.

2. It is now being replaced by faster and cheaper polymerase chain reaction (PCR) assays, or direct DNA sequencing platforms.

3. Southern blots require large amounts of high quality, high molecular weight genomic DNA.

   a. DNA is digested with one or more **restriction enzymes**, which are specific for each individual (eg, used for paternity testing), or gene (eg, β-globin chain in sickle cell anemia).

   b. The variably sized DNA fragments are resolved by **agarose gel electrophoresis**, transferred to a membrane, hybridized with a labeled probe, washed, and detected.

4. Southern blot may be used to detect deletions, insertions, or duplications too small to be detected by conventional cytogenetics. For example, deletions in the dystrophin gene (muscular dystrophy) are detected by Southern blot analysis.

5. Trinucleotide repeat diseases (repetitive duplication of three nucleotides of DNA) such as **myotonic dystrophy** and **Fragile X syndrome** can also be diagnosed by Southern blot.

B. Polymerase Chain Reaction

1. PCR revolutionized DNA diagnostics in the 1990s.

2. Small quantities of genomic DNA (or RNA) of a gene of interest can be amplified (copied) using short sequence specific primers, a mixture of the four deoxynucleotides (dNTPs), and a thermostable DNA polymerase (eg, *Taq polymerase*).

3. The process begins by denaturing the nucleic acid sample (heating to 94 °C) and allowing the primers to anneal to the sample near their most specific "melting" temperature (eg, 55–65 °C).

4. The temperature is then raised to 72 °C, which allows the polymerase to extend the primers into a full length product, extending from the forward primer to the reverse primer sequence; thereby copying the sequence of interest.

5. This three-temperature cycle is repeated 25–45 times, each time geometrically doubling the template, providing millions of copies, which may then be visualized by gel electrophoresis, sequenced, or cloned into vectors for further analysis.

6. The speed and high throughput of PCR has ensured its role in several applications.

   a. Since relatively sparse amounts of genetic material are required, PCR is used to identify tissue remains in **forensics.**

   b. It is useful for detecting small insertions/deletions, as in the 3-base pair deletion (delta F508) of the cystic fibrosis transmembrane regulator (*CFTR)* gene in CF.

7. Real-time PCR is a further modification that allows for quantitative measurement of the target sequence by incorporating a fluorescent probe into the PCR reaction.

a. This is especially useful in monitoring viral load for several infectious diseases, including HIV, cytomegalovirus (CMV), and hepatitis C virus (HCV).

b. Cancer cell burden may also be measured with PCR, assuming there is a tumor-specific genetic marker.

8. **Reverse transcription PCR (RT-PCR)** converts RNA to DNA, which can then undergo amplification.

9. **Real-time reverse transcription PCR (real time RT-PCR)** allows for quantitation of a specific RNA transcript (eg, measuring aberrant BCR-ABL **mRNA** created by the t(9;22) translocation in chronic myelogenous leukemia).

C. DNA Sequencing

1. The specific nucleotide sequence of a particular gene is most commonly determined with the Sanger dideoxynucleotide method.

a. PCR generated DNA fragments are denatured and annealed with either of their sequence specific primers.

b. The primer is then extended in four separate reaction tubes, each containing a mixture of the four dNTPs, DNA polymerase, and one of four labeled dideoxynucleotides (each with a different fluorophore color), representing the four nucleotides (A, G, C, and T).

c. When a ddNTP is incorporated in a fragment, extension of that fragment stops thereby yielding a cocktail of extension lengths with specific colored labels for each length.

d. The fragments from all four reactions are separated by high-resolution capillary electrophoresis, which determines where each nucleotide resides within the DNA sequence.

2. The appearance of two different nucleotides at the same location indicates a heterozygous mutation.

3. Sequencing helps detect single-nucleotide mutations, deletions, and insertions.

D. Comparative Genomic Hybridization (CGH)

1. CGH is a whole genome analysis method that allows for the widespread screening of DNA for copy number (gene dosage) differences between a control sample and a test sample.

2. The control sample of DNA is labeled with green dye, while a test sample is labeled with red dye.

3. The two are then mixed together in equal amounts and hybridized to a microarray chip.

4. These chips are spotted with several thousand known short oligonucleotide sequences representing all the chromosomes.

5. After hybridization to the oligonucleotides, a red to green ratio at each spot is evidence of DNA content in the sample versus control.

a. Increased red signal indicates a gain of DNA (insertion).

b. Increased green signal indicates a loss of DNA (deletion).

6. CGH has multiple applications.

a. It is used clinically to screen for deletions or insertions.

b. It is also used to test for gene amplifications.

IV. **Common Inherited Diseases**

A. Trisomy (discussed in detail in Chapter 19).

B. Monosomy (discussed in detail in Chapter 19).

C. Huntington Disease

1. Huntington disease is a devastating adult-onset neurodegenerative disease that leads to progressive motor dysfunction, personality changes, and gradual cognitive loss.
2. It is caused by an autosomal dominant **trinucleotide expansion** (CAG repeats) within the *Huntington* gene.
3. Fortunately, it is rare (prevalence 3-7/100,000).
4. Clinical expression varies with the length of the CAG repeats.
   a. Normally, individuals have between nine and 35 repeats.
   b. 36-41 repeats have reduced penetrance, meaning that the disease may never develop or that it may develop later in life.
   c. 40 or more repeats carries a high risk of disease.
   d. PCR analysis can assess the size of the CAG repeat.
5. CAG expansion lengthens during paternal spermatogenesis.
   a. This leads to more repeats with each successive generation in a process called, **"anticipation."**
   b. Therefore, the disease may become more frequent, severe, and present earlier in the patient's life in later generations.

D. Fragile X Syndrome

1. This is the most common hereditary cause of **mental retardation,** occurring in 16-25/100,000 births.
2. It results from an X-linked trinucleotide expansion (**CGG repeats** in the 5′-untranslated region of the *FMR1* gene).
3. Patients present with developmental delay and behavioral difficulties and may have mildly dysmorphic facies.
   a. Males may have macro-orchidism (**large testicles**).
   b. Carrier females are at increased risk for **ovarian failure.**
4. As with Huntington disease, the effects are related to the length of the expansion.
   a. Unaffected individuals have 60 or fewer CGG repeats.
   b. Patients with Fragile X syndrome have more than 200 repeats.
   c. Maternal expansions between 60 and 200 are unstable and are considered to be pre-mutations since they have the possibility of expanding during gametogenesis.
5. The term "fragile X" is derived from the appearance of the tips of the long arms of the X chromosome, which fail to condense properly for **cytogenetic** examination under conditions of **folate starvation.**
6. The size of the CGG expansion is measured by PCR on Southern blot.

E. Duchenne Muscular Dystrophy

1. Duchenne muscular dystrophy is a progressive myopathy caused by an X-linked mutation of the **dystrophin gene** present in 1/3500 male births.
2. Typically, it presents in children between the ages of 3–5 years.
3. Manifestations include the following:
   a. Difficulty walking
   b. **Pseudohypertrophy of the calves**
   c. **Gowers sign** (to stand from supine position)
4. The dystrophin protein is expressed in smooth, cardiac, and skeletal muscle and is dysfunctional or absent in these patients.

a. Dystrophin gene mutations can be large deletions or duplications and are diagnosed by Southern blot analysis.

    b. Skeletal muscle biopsy with immunohistochemical staining for dystrophin expression is also used for diagnosis.

F. **Cystic Fibrosis**

  1. Cystic fibrosis shows autosomal recessive inheritance.

  2. It is most common in Northern Europeans > Africans > Asians.

  3. There are approximately 1400 reported mutations in the *CFTR* gene, which encodes a chloride channel that regulates secretion viscosity.

  4. Most available genetic tests, for both prenatal diagnosis and carrier testing, consist of a panel of at least 25 of the most frequent mutations to identify nearly 90% of the cases.

  5. Full *CFTR* gene sequencing or other mutation-scanning methods can be used to identify the remaining rare mutations.

G. **Hereditary Breast and Ovarian Cancer**

  1. Approximately 5–10% of breast cancers are associated with alterations in the breast cancer 1 and 2 (*BRCA1* and *BRCA2*) genes.

    a. The **BRCA1** and **BRCA2** genes encode for nuclear proteins (tumor suppressors) that are responsible for DNA repair.

    b. A loss of function mutation leads to cancer.

    c. Carriers of a heterozygous *BRCA1* or *BRCA2* mutation have a significantly increased risk (45–60%) of breast cancer.

  2. There are multiple conditions associated with an increased likelihood of carrying a *BRCA1* or *BRCA2* mutation, such as multiple family members with cancer (eg, breast, ovarian, and prostatic carcinoma), a history of cancer in young adults, and a personal or family history of more extensive bilateral disease.

  3. The estimated prevalence for *BRCA1* mutations is 1/500–1/1000.

  4. According to **Knudsen hypothesis**, tumor formation most likely requires "two-hits," the presence of the mutation as well as a secondary event that results in the loss of the other allele.

  5. Diagnosis of a *BRCA1* or *BRCA2* mutation is usually done with full gene sequencing, because of the large spectrum of mutations.

  6. Known carriers are monitored closely.

    a. Women receive more frequent breast and pelvic examinations.

    b. Some carriers choose to undergo a prophylactic surgery.

    c. Men have earlier prostate examinations and serum prostate-specific antigen (PSA) screens.

H. **Hemochromatosis**

  1. Hereditary hemochromatosis is an autosomal recessive disorder of iron overload, frequently caused by a missense mutation in the **HFE gene** located on the short arm of chromosome 6.

  2. Transmembrane iron uptake is regulated by several proteins, including the hemochromatosis (*HFE*) gene product, transferrin, transferrin receptor, and ferroportin.

    a. The *HFE* gene product is homologous to major histocompatibility complex (MHC) class I proteins.

    b. It ordinarily forms a heterodimer with beta$_2$-microglobulin.

3. Mutations in HFE cause increased iron uptake by the gastrointestinal mucosa, leading to toxic iron stores in the liver (**cirrhosis**), heart (**arrhythmia**), pancreas (**diabetes**), skin (**pigmentation**), and thyroid (**hypothyroidism**).

4. Disease onset is variable, but it often occurs between 40–60 years of age in men and after menopause in women.

5. Hemochromatosis must be differentiated from secondary iron overload resulting from multiple transfusions, hemolytic anemia, hemodialysis, and ingested sources.

6. The diagnosis is made by clinical symptoms, family history, increased serum ferritin levels, liver biopsy with increased iron stores, and direct DNA testing for the C282Y and H63D mutations in the HFE gene.

    a. Approximately 1/400 people of **European** ancestry possess two mutant alleles with a carrier rate of approximately 1/10, making this the *most frequent* single-gene disorder in this population.

    b. C282Y mutation accounts for 80–90% of symptomatic patients.

    c. H63D is a minor mutation, accounting for 3–8% of patients.

V. Hematologic Disease

A. Factor V Leiden Mutation

1. Factor V Leiden is a common hereditary hypercoagulable syndrome resulting from a single point mutation in the factor V gene.

2. The point mutation involves replacing an arginine (R) with a glutamine (Q) at amino acid 506 (R506Q).

    a. Ordinarily, activated factor V protein is cleaved and subsequently inactivated by protein C at arginine 506.

    b. The presence of glutamine slows inactivation considerably.

    c. This cleavage-resistant variant has a longer half-life and leads to hypercoagulability.

    d. It is the *most common* inherited **thrombophilia** in Europeans.

3. Patients are at an increased risk for deep venous **thrombosis** and pulmonary embolism.

    a. Recurrent thrombotic episodes, **thrombosis** among patients younger than 50 years, thrombosis of unusual sites, pregnancy-related thrombosis, and family history suggest a hereditary hypercoagulable syndrome (eg, factor V Leiden).

    b. Additional risk factors such as immobility, hormone therapy, trauma, and neoplasm, synergistically increase the risk.

    c. Thrombosis likely requires at least "two hits" (eg, factor V mutation and additional risk factors).

    d. Clinical manifestations vary by gene dosage.

        (1) **Heterozygotes** show a 4- to 10-fold increased risk of thrombosis.

        (2) **Homozygotes** have an ~80-fold increased risk.

    e. Mutations are found in 50–60% of patients with recurrent or estrogen-related thrombosis.

4. DNA testing is used to confirm the R506Q mutation.

5. It must be differentiated from other thrombophilias caused by the prothrombin G20210A mutation, and protein C, protein S, or antithrombin deficiency.

B. Prothrombin G20210A Mutation

1. This is another hereditary thrombophilia resulting from a single point mutation (G20210A) in the factor II (prothrombin) gene.

2. The mutation stabilizes the mRNA transcript of prothrombin, resulting in higher serum levels and a hypercoagulable state.

3. G20210A appears to be synergistic with factor V Leiden mutation for hypercoagulability.

4. The mutation is not unusual (1% of patients are heterozygous); **heterozygotes** have a 3- to 5-fold increased risk.

5. DNA testing is used to confirm the G20210A mutation.

C. Philadelphia Chromosome

1. This is a tumor-specific chromosome translocation **t(9;22)** that leads to aberrant expression of a **BCR-ABL** fusion protein with enhanced tyrosine kinase activity that is characteristic of chronic myeloid leukemia.

2. The ABL tyrosine kinase proto-oncogene on 9q34 and the BCR (break point cluster region) on 22q11 are involved.

3. The translocation can be detected by routine cytogenetic evaluation, FISH, Southern blot analysis, or RT-PCR.

   a. RT-PCR for the BCR-ABL mRNA is the most sensitive method.

   b. Serial RT-PCR assays are typically used during targeted therapy of **chronic myelogenous leukemia (CML)** with a tyrosine kinase inhibitor (eg, imatinib) to monitor tumor response.

4. Nearly all cases of **CML** are positive for the Philadelphia chromosome t(9;22).

5. t(9;22) may also be identified in a minority of cases of B lineage acute lymphoblastic leukemia (**ALL**) and predicts a poor prognosis.

VI. Infectious Disease

A. Hepatitis C Virus

1. Hepatitis C is a member of the Flavivirus family of RNA virus.

2. It is spread through blood and vertical transmission.

3. Infection carries a significant risk of chronic hepatitis, cirrhosis, and hepatocellular carcinoma.

4. Seroconversion occurs 11–12 weeks after exposure; symptoms and increasing transaminases are often present after only 6–8 weeks.

5. Diagnosis is by serologic or RT-PCR testing.

   a. During the window of seronegativity (6–11 weeks after infection) the patient will have a negative HCV-antibody test.

   b. RT-PCR is the only method at this time to detect the virus.

   c. RT-PCR quantifies viral load, allowing the clinician to follow a patient's response to treatment.

   d. Antiviral therapy is tailored to virus genotype which is determined by genotype specific probes or sequencing.

B. Cytomegalovirus

1. CMV is one of the Herpesviridae, neurotropic, DNA viruses capable of latent infection, which may emerge during immune compromise.

2. The majority of the US population is seropositive but remain asymptomatic if they are immunocompetent.

3. Characteristic "owl eye" inclusions are seen in the nucleus or cytoplasm of infected cells.

4. Diagnosis is possible with serologic tests, viral culture, or direct PCR testing for viral DNA load.

a. PCR testing is useful for situations when there is concern for viral reactivation during immunosuppression.

    b. Results of serial CMV quantitative PCR testing can help guide antiviral therapy.

CLINICAL PROBLEMS

For questions 1–3: Routine screening mammography of an otherwise healthy 51-year-old woman reveals several small dense lesions within her right breast. Results of a follow-up biopsy indicate ductal carcinoma in situ with high nuclear grade, comedo necrosis, and microcalcifications.

1. The best specific immunohistochemical marker to rule out invasive carcinoma would be:

   A. Ki-67

   B. HER2/neu

   C. p63

   D. Desmin

   E. Estrogen receptor

2. Which immunohistochemical stain would best distinguish between ductal and lobular carcinoma of the breast?

   A. E-cadherin

   B. CEA

   C. TTF-1

   D. SMA

   E. Progesterone receptor

3. Which stain is used to predict response to hormonal therapy?

   A. E-cadherin

   B. CEA

   C. TTF-1

   D. SMA

   E. ER/PR

4. Cystic fibrosis is diagnosed in a child. The parents were quite surprised, since no one in either family had ever been diagnosed with this disease. What is the risk of cystic fibrosis in their next child?

   A. Essentially no recurrence risk

   B. 1 in 4 chance with each child

   C. 1 in 2 chance with each male

D. 1 in 2 chance with each child

   E. The couple should avoid having additional children

5. Which translocation is associated with both chronic myelogenous leukemia and acute lymphoblastic leukemia?

   A. t(8;21)

   B. t(14;18)

   C. t(9;22)

   D. t(11;14)

   E. t(8;14)

ANSWERS

1. The answer is C. Ductal carcinoma is considered invasive when neoplastic cells are identified outside the myoepithelial layer that surrounds the ducts. Both p63 and SMA stain for these myoepithelial smooth muscle cells, but p63 is more specific for myoepithelial cells in breast, thyroid, and prostate tissue.

2. The answer is A. E-cadherin binds a cell adhesion molecule expressed by epithelial cells and is used to identify ductal carcinoma of the breast. The loss of E-cadherin is common to lobular carcinomas.

3. The answer is E. Neoplastic cells that retain hormone receptors are more easily managed with chemotherapy. For example, tamoxifen, a modulator of estrogen receptors, antagonizes estrogen receptors in the breast, depriving ER-positive carcinomas of a critical metabolic signal.

4. The answer is B. Because cystic fibrosis is inherited in an autosomal recessive manner, each child they conceive has 1 in 4 (25%) chance of acquiring the disease. Since the *CFTR* mutation is not associated with a sex chromosome, the gender of the child in this case is irrelevant.

5. The answer is C. The presence of a reciprocal translocation between chromosomes 9 and 22, known as the Philadelphia chromosome, is a highly sensitive marker for chronic myelogenous leukemia (CML), identified in nearly 95% of CML cases. It is also found in a subset of patients in whom acute lymphoblastic leukemia and acute myelogenous leukemia are diagnosed. The specificity of t(9;22) is not as high as its sensitivity.

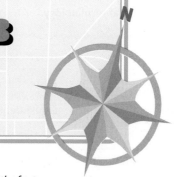

CHAPTER 3
SKIN

What spirit is so empty and blind, that it cannot recognize the foot
is more noble than the shoe, and skin more beautiful than the garment?
—Michelangelo

I. Normal Skin

A. The Epidermis

1. The epidermis is composed of the basal, spinous, granular, and cornified layers.
   a. The **basal layer** is considered the germinative layer of the epidermis.
   b. Keratinocytes of the **spinous layer** produce keratin, the major component of the stratum corneum. It is called the stratum spinosum because of the intercellular bridges, or "spines," between the keratinocytes.
   c. In the **stratum granulosum,** or granular layer, cells flatten and acquire dark keratohyalin granules.
   d. The **stratum corneum** is the major physical barrier of the skin and is composed of corneocytes that are large, flat, plate-like cells filled with keratin stacked in vertical layers; they are bound together by a lipid-rich cement like "bricks and mortar."

2. **Melanocytes** are dendritic pigment-producing cells located in the basal layer.

B. The Dermis and Subcutaneous Tissue

1. The dermis is a strong and elastic support structure that contains blood vessels and nerves.
2. The structural components of the dermis include collagen fibers, elastic fibers, and ground substance.
3. The dermis and subcutaneous tissue contain four types of cutaneous adnexa: hair follicles, sebaceous, eccrine, and apocrine glands.

C. Terminology

1. Table 3–1 describes the clinical terminology used to describe skin lesions.
2. Table 3–2 lists the dermatopathic terminology that is used to describe the histologic characteristics of a lesion.

Table 3–1. Clinical terminology.

Term	Description
Bulla	Blister filled with clear fluid, >1 cm
Crust	Liquid debris (serum or pus) that has dried on the skin
Induration	Firmness to palpation
Lichenification	Palpable, visibly thickened skin with accentuated skin markings
Macule	Flat skin lesion recognized by discoloration, <1 cm
Nodule	Elevated lesion, "marble-like," >1 cm in width and depth
Papule	Smaller palpable skin lesion, <1 cm
Patch	Flat skin lesion recognized by discoloration, >1 cm
Plaque	Larger palpable skin lesion, >1 cm Coalescent papules
Scale	Visibly altered stratum corneum Scales are dry and whitish
Vesicle	Blister filled with clear fluid, <1 cm

II. Inflammatory Diseases

  A. **Spongiotic Dermatitis**

  1. Spongiotic dermatitis is the histologic term for inflammatory skin diseases clinically characterized as "eczema," such as atopic dermatitis, contact dermatitis, and nummular dermatitis.

  2. Patients with eczema (spongiotic dermatitis) complain of pruritus (itching).

  a. Skin examination reveals papules and plaques with indistinct borders and epidermal changes, such as vesicles, scales, weeping, crusts, and **lichenification** (thickening of the skin in response to persistent rubbing).

  b. Histologically, edema is present between the keratinocytes throughout the spinous layer of the epidermis, so-called spongiosis.

  c. If severe, spongiosis results in **vesicle** formation.

  d. In chronic eczema, there is lichenification; i/e. acanthosis, a thickening of the epidermis and hyperkeratosis, a thickening of the stratum corneum. In the superficial dermis, there is a perivascular inflammation of lymphocytes and sometimes, **eosinophils.**

  B. **Seborrheic Dermatitis**

  1. Seborrheic dermatitis, one example of spongiotic dermatitis, is a persistent inflammatory eruption that affects the **scalp (dandruff), face,** and **upper chest** of adults.

Table 3–2. Dermatopathology terminology.

Term	Description
Acantholysis	Loss of keratinocyte cell-cell adhesion resulting in round rather than polygonal appearing cells
Acanthosis	Hyperplasia of the epidermis
Atrophic	Thinning; reduction in size or amount
Dyskeratosis	Abnormal cornification occurring (prematurely) in keratinocytes of the spinous layer
Hypergranulosis	Hyperplasia of the stratum granulosum
Hyperkeratosis	Increased thickness of stratum corneum
Lichenification	Hyperkeratosis, hypergranulosis, acanthosis and fibrosis of the papillary dermis corresponding to clinical skin thickening
Lichenoid	A band-like inflammatory infiltrate (usually lymphocytes) below the dermal-epidermal junction
Orthokeratosis	Stratum corneum without retention of nuclei
Parakeratosis	Retention of nuclei within the cornified cells of the stratum corneum
Pedunculated	A papule connected to the skin by a stalk thinner than the lesion itself
Psoriasiform	Inflammatory pattern: epidermis with thickening and elongation of rete ridges
Spongiosis	Intercellular edema between the keratinocytes of the spinous layer
Vacuolar alteration	Alteration including vacuole formation in cells of the basal layer

2. Seborrheic dermatitis is common, affecting 3–5% of the population and may represent an inflammatory reaction to the **yeast *Pityrosporum.***
3. The lesions are well-demarcated, salmon-colored, erythematous plaques with greasy scale in the hair-bearing, sebum-rich areas of the body, especially the scalp, face, ears, and chest.
4. It is commonly known as "dandruff" on the scalp of adults and "cradle cap" on the scalp of infants.
5. Severs forms develop for unknown reasons in immunodeficiency syndromes and in some neurologic diseases.

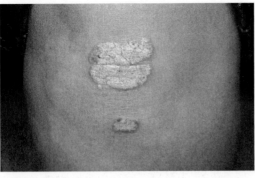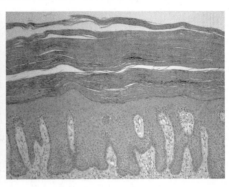

Figure 3–1. Gross photograph of silvery scale plaque on the knee. Biopsy shows psoriasiform dermatitis with hyperkeratosis and parakeratosis overlying elongated epidermal rete and increased upper dermal vascularity.

     6. Histologically there is a thickened epidermis, called psoriasiform change, with focal spongiosis and scale-crust.

C. **Lichen Simplex Chronicus**
     1. Lichen simplex chronicus (LSC) is a scaly, erythematous, at times hyperpigmented plaque that represents thickened, or lichenified, skin due to chronic rubbing or irritation.
     2. LSC results from incessant pruritic (itchy) conditions such as eczema, insect bites or psoriasis, that lead to persistent scratching or rubbing.
     3. Histologically, LSC shows hyperkeratosis, hypergranulosis, a hyperplastic epidermis and a thickened papillary dermis.
     4. Treatment is challenging and aimed at interrupting the patient's itch/scratch cycle, often with topical corticosteroids.

D. **Psoriasis**
     1. Psoriasis is a common, chronic inflammatory skin disease that affects 1–3% of the population.
     2. A **family history** of psoriasis exists in approximately one-third of patients.
     3. Psoriasis commonly presents as thick well-demarcated plaques, with a heavy **silvery scale** on the elbows, knees, scalp, buttocks, and trunk (Figure 3–1).
     4. Biopsy shows psoriasiform epidermal change (epidermal hyperplasia), elongated rete ridges, and parakeratosis (retention of nuclei in the stratum corneum). Often, neutrophils are present in the stratum corneum (**Munro microabscesses**) and in the spinous layer (**spongiform pustule of Kogoj**). There is usually a perivascular infiltrate of lymphocytes.

E. **Pityriasis Rosea**
     1. Pityriasis rosea is a common, acute, self-limited dermatitis that affects **adolescents** and young adults mostly.
     2. Recent studies suggest human herpes virus 6 and 7 may have a role.

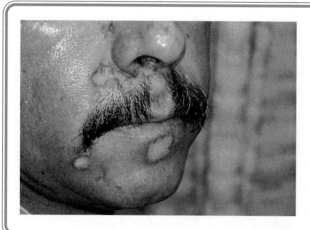

Figure 3–2. Discoid lupus erythematosus is characterized by disk-shaped hypopigmented plaques. Most cases are not associated with systemic lupus erythematosus.

3. It presents with asymptomatic, oval, thin, scaling papules and plaques on the trunk.
- **a.** The oval plaques are often oriented along the skin's relaxed tension lines.
- **b.** This characteristic pattern has been compared to the orientation of boughs of a **Christmas tree.**

4. A single larger lesion, called the **herald patch,** often appears several days before the generalized eruption.

5. Biopsy shows spongiosis, focal parakeratosis, perivascular lymphocytes, and extravasated red blood cells.

F. Discoid Lupus Erythematosus

1. Discoid lupus erythematosus (DLE) may be limited to the skin or may be one of the many manifestations of systemic lupus erythematosus (SLE); however, patients presenting with cutaneous DLE rarely develop systemic lupus erythematosus.

2. It appears on sun-exposed areas as disk-shaped, red to purple plaques with white adherent scale (Figure 3–2).

3. Biopsy shows a thin epidermis with hyperkeratosis involving follicular openings termed "follicular plugging." Vacuolar alteration of the epidermal-dermal interface (basal layer) is present with a perivascular and periadnexal lymphoplasmacytic infiltrate.

G. Lichen Planus

1. Lichen planus is a common, idiopathic eruption of polygonal, planar (flat topped), pruritic, purple papules (the five "p"s) distributed on the wrists, hands, trunk, legs, and the mouth.

2. Fine reticulated (lacy) scale is often present over the surface and is known as **Wickham striae.**

3. Approximately 10% of cases are associated with **hepatitis C.**

4. Histologically, there is hyperkeratosis, hypergranulosis (thickened stratum granulosum) in a wedge-shaped pattern, irregular acanthosis (termed "**saw-toothed**" rete ridges), and a **lichenoid** (or band-like) lymphocytic infiltrate in the upper dermis.

H. Bullous Pemphigoid

1. Bullous pemphigoid is an **autoimmune disorder** usually seen in **older** patients and is characterized by **subepidermal vesicles.**
2. It often starts in the groin, axilla, and flexural areas.
3. The blisters are large and tense and can occur on normal or erythematous skin.
4. The lesions may begin as urticarial hive-like papules and plaques that are intensely pruritic.
5. Bullous pemphigoid is caused by autoantibodies directed against the bullous pemphigoid antigen 1 (**BPA1**) in the hemidesmosome of the keratinocyte and bullous pemphigoid antigen 2 (**BPA2**), a transmembrane protein that connects part of the hemidesmosome in the basal keratinocyte to the lamina densa of the basement membrane.
6. Biopsy shows a subepidermal vesicle (blister) with perivascular lymphocytes and eosinophils.
7. Direct **immunofluorescence** of perilesional skin reveals linear **IgG** and complement deposition at the **basement membrane** zone.

I. Pemphigus Vulgaris

1. Pemphigus vulgaris is an **autoimmune** disorder of middle-aged adults and is characterized by an **intraepidermal vesicle**.
2. It often involves the mucous membranes (eg, oral mucosa) and skin with flaccid superficial bullae that rupture easily leaving large denuded bleeding and weeping painful erosions.
3. It is caused by autoantibodies against desmoglein 1 and desmoglein 3 proteins, which are keratinocyte adhesion molecules.
4. Biopsy shows an intraepidermal vesicle with acantholysis of the keratinocytes. Acantholysis results when keratinocytes lose cell to cell adhesions (desmosomes).
5. Direct **immunofluorescence** reveals epidermal staining of **IgG** and complement between the keratinocytes of the entire **spinous layer.**

J. Dermatitis Herpetiformis

1. Dermatitis herpetiformis is a chronic, intensely pruritic vesicular disease characterized by grouped vesicles, which are considered "herpetiform" or herpes-like, and uticarial plaques.
2. Lesions are often distributed symmetrically on the elbows, knees, buttocks, low back, and shoulders.
3. Patients have **gluten-sensitive enteropathy** (often asymtomatic) with small bowel villous atrophy; dermatitis herpetiformis may improve with a gluten-free diet.
4. Biopsy shows a subepidermal vesicle with collections of neutrophils in the dermal papilla.
5. Direct **immunofluorescence** reveals **IgA** deposition in the dermal papilla.

K. Erythema Nodosum

1. Erythema nodosum is a skin disease with painful, red, **bruise-like** nodules on the **shins**, usually in **young adults.**
2. It is often a reaction to **birth control pills,** other drugs, inflammatory bowel disease, streptococcal pharyngitis, sarcoidosis, yersiniosis and other infections.
3. Erythema nodosum is a septal **panniculitis** with inflammation located in the fibrous fat septae of the subcutaneous fat. Fat septae are thickened and inflamed with lymphocytes, histiocytes, neutrophils and multinucleated giant cells.

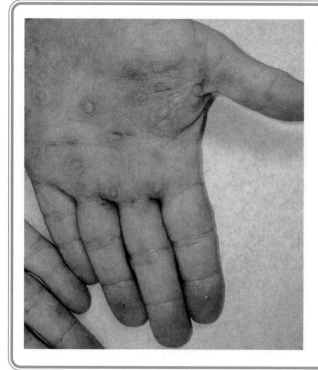

Figure 3–3. "Targetoid lesions" of erythema multiforme appear in the palm with dark centers surrounded by red and pale rings.

L. Urticaria
1. Urticaria is commonly known as **hives,** welts, or wheals.
2. It is a common condition that occurs in 20% of the population and is characterized by very **pruritic,** transient wheals that change shape and location during a 24-hour period.
3. It is an IgE-mediated type I hypersensitivity reaction to foods, drugs, or infection as well as multiple other factors, although in many cases a cause may not be found.
4. In the most severe cases, airway obstruction due to laryngeal edema may occur.
5. Biopsy shows a scant perivascular and interstitial infiltrate of lymphocytes, eosinophils, and neutrophils.

M. Erythema Multiforme
1. Erythema multiforme (EM) is an acute eruption in children and young adults often involving the palms, feet, and occasionally the mucous membranes.
2. EM is commonly caused by **herpes simplex virus,** other viruses, and drugs.
3. The classic EM papule is a "target" or "iris" **lesion** has three zones of color: 1) the central dark blister is surrounded by 2) a pale edematous zone with 3) a peripheral rim of erythema (Figure 3–3).
4. Biopsy reveals necrotic keratinocytes, perivascular lymphocytes, and vacuolar change at the dermal-epidermal junction.
5. Wide spread involvement by EM of two or more mucosal surfaced with more epidermal necrosis is **Stevens-Johnson syndrome.**

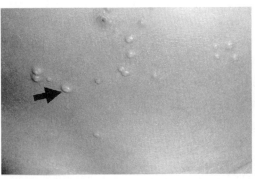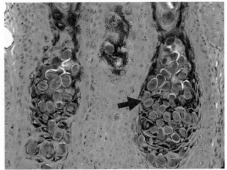

Figure 3–4. Molluscum contagiosum is a poxvirus transmitted by direct contact with skin or fomites. It is most commonly spread in children and sexually active adults. It presents as skin colored papules (arrow). Biopsy reveals bright red viral filled packets in the epidermis.

      6. Extensive full-thickness epidermal necrosis and sloughing of the skin is called **toxic epidermal necrolysis.**

  N. Acne
      1. Acne is a very common disorder affecting the pilosebaceous units of the skin.
      2. Patients with acne have open comedones (blackheads), closed comedones (whiteheads), red papules, pustules, cysts (ruptured inflamed follicles) and nodules.
      3. Acne can be seen on the face and trunk in all ages but more often in teenagers and young adults.
      4. Suspect exacerbating factors include increased keratinization of the infundibulum of the follicle, increased sebum production, hormones, secondary normal flora bacteria overgrowth and inflammation related to bacterial products and lipids.
      5. Biopsy reveals a dilated follicle, often ruptured, with perifollicular mixed infiltrated of neutrophils, lymphocytes, plasma cells, and multinucleated giant cells.
      6. Follicular plugging with cornified cells is often present, as are pustules within or adjacent to follicles.

III. Infections

  A. Molluscum Contagiosum
      1. Molluscum contagiosum is a very common self-limited viral infection (poxvirus) spread by direct contact.
      2. It is clinically characterized by multiple 1–4 mm skin colored umbilicated papules on the arms, legs, face, and axilla of children (Figure 3–4).
      3. It is more common and extensive in children with atopic dermatitis.
      4. It is sometimes seen on the penis, vulva, inguinal areas and buttock in adults. Molluscus contagiosum is considered a sexually transmitted disease in this setting.
      5. Biopsy reveals a very distinct appearance, a central dilated follicle is filled with molluscum bodies (Henderson-Patterson bodies), large viral intracytoplasmic inclusions appearing as glassy eosinophilic spheres (Figure 3–4).

B. **Herpes Simplex Virus (types 1 and 2) and Varicella-Zoster Virus**
  1. Herpes simplex virus (HSV) and Varicella-zoster virus (VZV) are common infections that present as painful **grouped vesicles** on an erythematous base, later becoming crusted or ulcerated.
      a. After initial infection, the herpes virus resides in a latent state in nerve ganglion cells.
      b. Herpes simplex clinically develops at the sites of a common human/human contact including lips, face, penis, vulva or buttocks.
  2. **Varicella** (known commonly as "**chickenpox**") spreads via the respiratory route and presents in childhood as an acute febrile illness with pharyngitis and generalized vesicles.
      a. Typically, the virus then remains dormant for years.
      b. A single recurrence may occur years later as herpes zoster ("**shingles**") with unilateral vesicles in a **dermatomal** distribution.
  3. Diagnosis of both types of herpes may be made clinically, with cultures, fluorescent antibody smears, or with a **Tzanck smear** (a cytologic preparation taken from a ruptured cutaneous vesicle that reveals characteristic multinucleated giant cells).
  4. Histologically, the HSV and VZV viruses are indistinguishable with intra-epidermal vesicles or ulceration, epidermal necrosis, and herpetic changes in the keratinocytes, which include enlarged and pale cells, margination of chromatin at the edge of the nucleus, pink intranuclear inclusions, and multinucleated keratinocytes – the so-called three Ms (*m*ultinucleation, nuclear *m*olding, and *m*argination of the chromatin).

C. **Verruca Vulgaris**
  1. Commonly known as **warts,** verrucae vulgares are benign neoplasms caused by infection of keratinocytes by human papillomavirus (HPV).
  2. They present as skin colored, scaly, verrucous papules with interrupted skin lines, often with black dots (which are thrombosed capillaries in the dermal papillae).
  3. Biopsy reveals acanthosis and hyperkeratosis with columns of parakeratosis over digitate (finger-like) projections of epidermis containing scattered koilocytes, which are vacuolated keratinocytes with pyknotic nuclei in the stratum granulosum (HPV infected cells).

D. **Dermatophytosis (Tinea)**
  1. Dermatophytosis is a very common intracorneal fungal infection caused by one of three general fungi: *Microsporum, Epidermophyton,* or *Trichophyton.*
  2. Some of the most common dermatophytoses are better known as "**athlete's foot**" (tinea pedis) or "**jock itch**" (tinea cruris).
  3. On examination, dermatophytoses cause scaly, erythematous plaques that often have an annular (ring-like) configuration leading to the name "**ringworm.**"
  4. Potassium hydroxide (KOH) preparation shows branching septate fungal hyphae.
  5. Biopsy reveals compact orthokeratosis, parakeratosis with neutrophils and hyphae in the stratum corneum highlighted by silver stains.

E. **Syphilis**
  1. Syphilis is a now rarely seen, but historically important, venereal infection of the spirochete *Treponema pallidum.*

2. It evolves through three stages with the primary stage occurring as a **painless ulcer** on the genitals or lip (**chancre**).
   a. **Secondary syphilis** has variable clinical features and has thus been called "the great imitator". It often is associated with red-brown or yellow plaques in a general distribution and on the palms and soles.
   b. **Tertiary syphilis** is very rare and may present with solitary or multiple plaques or ulcers.
3. Biopsy of secondary syphilis reveals psoriasiform epidermal hyperplasia with hyperkeratosis, parakeratosis, and neutrophils, as well as a perivascular infiltrate with lymphocytes and **plasma cells.**
4. **Spirochetes** are highlighted by Warthin-Starry silver stain.
5. While nearly eradicated over the past half century with the development of **penicillin** in the mid 1940s, there has been a resurgence of syphilis in **HIV-infected** patients.

IV. Benign Neoplasms

A. Seborrheic Keratosis

1. Seborrheic keratoses are a very common benign, often pigmented, neoplasm of keratinocytes that presents as a scaly, "pasted on," papule or plaque (Figure 3–5).

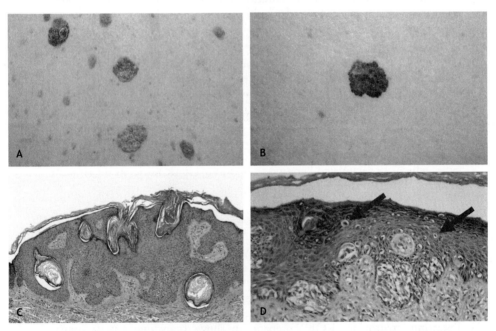

Figure 3–5. Pigmented skin lesions are common and may represent benign seborrheic keratosis, which has a scaly "stuck on" appearance **(A)**, or nodular plaque **(B)**, which is concerning for melanocytic neoplasia (recall ABCs of melanoma). Biopsy shows keratin horns in a seborrheic keratosis **(C)**. In contrast, an atypical melanocytic proliferation is seen in melanoma **(D)** with "pagetoid" spread of the tumor cells into the epidermis (arrows).

   2. They appear in older adults anywhere except the palms and soles.
   3. Biopsy reveals acanthosis and often papillomatosis with basket weave hyper-keratosis and pseudo-horn cysts (circular spaces filled with basket weave hyperkeratosis.

B. Solar Lentigo
   1. A solar lentigo is a common brown macule that appears on the exposed face and dorsal hands of sun damaged adults.
   2. Solar lentigo may eventuate in seborrheic keratosis, a benign neoplasm of keratinocytes.
   3. Histologically, there is a hyperpigmented basal layer often with hyperplastic, elongated rete ridges.

C. Simple Lentigo
   1. Simple lentigo is a common brown macule usually less than 5 mm in diameter that occurs in children and young adults and is unrelated to sun exposure.
   2. It is the precursor to a junctional nevus.
   3. It is benign neoplasm of melanocytes and histologically one sees increased melanocytes along the dermal epidermal junction and along elongated rete ridges.
   4. There is often significant pigmentation throughout the keratinocytes and in the stratum corneum.
   5. There are no nests of melanocytes and there is rarely solar elastosis.

D. Melanocytic Nevus
   1. Melanocytic nevus is a common benign neoplasm with variable clinical presentation depending on the specific type of nevus and the patient's age.
   2. Commonly, it is referred to as a "mole."
   3. Clinically, it is a hyperpigmented macule or papule, which is usually small and **symmetric** with one or two colors of pigmentation.
   4. Histologically it is characterized by collections of melanocytes, called nests, strands of melanocytes and single melanocytes at the dermal epidermal junction and/or in the dermis.

E. Hemangioma
   1. Hemangiomas are benign proliferations of blood vessels in the dermis.
   2. See Chapters 6 and 19 for detailed discussions.

F. Dermatofibroma
   1. A dermatofibroma is an area of focal dermal fibrosis with overlying epidermal thickening (acanthosis) and hyperpigmentation.
   2. It appears most commonly on the legs of women, but is also seen on the arms and trunk, rarely on the head or neck.
   3. The etiology is unknown.
   4. Clinically these can be diagnosed with the "dimple sign," where squeezing the lesion between the thumb and forefinger results in a depression or dimple.

V. Malignant Neoplasms

A. Mycosis Fungoides
   1. Mycosis fungoides is a cutaneous **T-cell lymphoma.**
   2. Despite its name, it is *not* caused by or related to a fungal infection.
   3. It is uncommon and accounts for less than 1% of all lymphomas.
   4. It presents as thin erythematous to violaceous scaly patches and plaques.

a. These are poorly demarcated during the early stages of disease and may resemble spongiotic dermatitis.
   b. It is often pruritic and usually presents in older patients, commonly in the hip girdle area.
   c. As the lesions evolve they may become elevated, indurated, and nodular.
5. Biopsy reveals a bandlike lymphocytic infiltrate in the superficial dermis with **atypical lymphocytes** within the basal layer and epidermis.
   a. The atypical lymphocytes have markedly irregular nuclear membranes, the so-called "**cerebriform.**"
   b. They also have a characteristic immunohistochemical phenotype by immuno staining or flow cytometry.
6. In the early stages, it can be managed with topical therapies and is only rarely fatal, resulting in less than 200 deaths each year.

B. **Actinic Keratosis (AK)**
   1. Also known as solar keratosis, AK is an ill-defined white to red, scaly papule that appears in sun damaged areas in older patients. These lesions exist singly or clustered. Actinic keratoses are an early stage of squamous cell carcinoma.
   2. Actinic keratosis is characterized histologically by atypical keratinocytes in the lower epidermis. The stratum corneum has an alternating pink and blue pattern.
   3. Actinic keratoses are treated with liquid nitrogen (cryotherapy) or topical chemotherapy agents such as 5-fluorouracil or imiquimod.

C. **Basal Cell Carcinoma (BCC)**
   1. BCC is the most common type of skin cancer; it is slow growing and occurs in one of six Americans.
   2. It presents as a pearly, red papule, nodule, or plaque commonly found on sun-exposed skin (Figure 3–6).

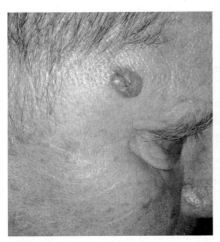
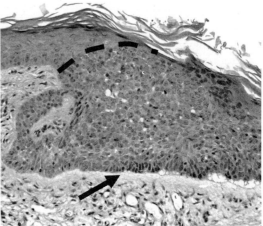

Figure 3–6. Basal cell carcinoma (BCC) may be nodular, superficial, or infiltrative. Biopsy shows a superficial BCC composed of high N:C ratio cells (demarcated from normal epidermis by dotted line) with peripheral palisading of tumor nuclei and clefting away from the dermis (arrow).

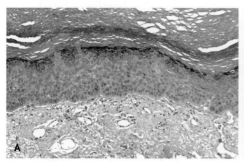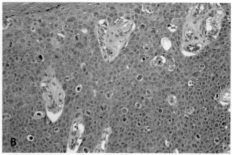

Figure 3–7. A: Sun damaged skin may develop low-grade dysplasia, so-called actinic keratosis with hyperkertotic horns overlying mildly atypical epidermal cells and elastosis of the dermis. **B:** In contrast, squamous cell carcinoma has malignant nuclei, conspicuous mitotic figures, and may invade into the underlying dermis.

    3. Metastases are exceedingly rare, but if BCC is left untreated, it may become locally destructive.

    4. Biopsy findings reveal an upper dermal proliferation of monomorphic epithelial cells with increased nuclear:cytoplasmic ratios and characteristic peripheral palisading with clefting (retraction artifact) between tumor cells and the surrounding collagen stroma (Figure 3–6).

  D. Squamous Cell Carcinoma

    1. Squamous cell carcinoma is the second most common type of skin cancer and presents as a red papule, nodule, plaque, or ulcer (Figure 3–7).

    2. It is usually found on **sun-damaged** skin, or is associated with **immunosuppression** (eg, organ transplant patient).

    3. Biopsy reveals atypical keratinocytes throughout the full thickness of the epidermis and often extension into the dermis; this gives the neoplasm a very pink appearance.

    4. Atypical keratinocytes cause parakeratosis in the corneal layers that results in the scaly, hyperkeratotic texture of these neoplasms, clinically.

    5. Abnormal patterns of cornification called keratin pearls can be seen within the neoplasm where atypical keratinocytes surround islands of parakeratosis.

    6. Even when invasive, it rarely **metastasizes** (<1% of cases).

  E. Melanoma

    1. Melanoma is the third most common type of skin cancer.

    2. The lifetime incidence of melanoma is increasing and affects approximately 1% of Americans, but the five year survival rate has improved from previous years.

    3. Melanoma most commonly presents as an asymmetric macule, papule, plaque, or nodule with irregular borders, varied colors (including black, red, white, and blue), and a diameter of more than **6 mm** (so-called "ABCD criteria").

    4. Approximately 25–33% of melanomas arise in preexisting melanocytic nevi but most develop de novo.

5. The histologic presentation of melanoma varies but is usually a large, **asymmetric** and poorly circumscribed proliferation of melanocytes. The melanocytes are often atypical, of varying sizes, and present above the epidermal basal layer (**pagetoid** melanocytes) (Figure 3–5).

6. Prognosis (5-year survival) depends on the stage of disease.
   a. **Stage 1:** Depth of invasion less than 2 mm (90% survival).
   b. **Stage 2:** No metastases to lymph nodes (70% survival).
   c. **Stage 3:** Positive lymph node metastases (50% survival).
   d. **Stage 4:** Distant metastases (eg, brain) (10% survival).

F. **Dermatofibrosarcoma Protuberans**

1. Dermatofibrosarcoma protuberans is a soft tissue malignancy of fibrocytes.

2. It is a rare slow growing neoplasm found on the trunk of young to middle aged adults; it is unrelated to sun damage.

3. Biopsy reveals densely cellular proliferation of thin spindled fibroblasts arranged in a storiform pattern within the dermis and usually invade into the subcutaneous fat, leaving islands of fat within the neoplasm, so-called "fat trapping."

4. Dermatofibrosarcoma protuberans often recurs after excision but rarely metastasizes.

G. **Merkel Cell Carcinoma**

1. This rare cutaneous neoplasm often presents in the head and neck of older adults.

2. It is a neural-crest derived neuroendocrine carcinoma that shows characteristic perinuclear cytokeratin 20 dot-like staining.

3. Biopsy reveals characteristic small cell carcinoma features, including delicate salt-and-pepper chromatin, increased nuclear:cytoplasmic ratios, high mitotic index, and necrosis (Figure 3–8).

4. Merkel cell carcinoma is capable of metastasis and is potentially lethal, although not nearly as malignant as small cell carcinoma of the lung.

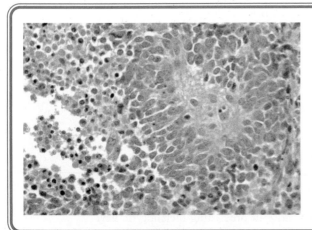

Figure 3–8. Merkel cell carcinoma is a type of neuroendocrine carcinoma (small round blue cell tumor) that presents in the skin. Although it has metastatic potential, the prognosis is significantly better than small cell carcinoma of the lung.

CLINICAL PROBLEMS

1. A biopsy of herpes simplex virus lesion demonstrates which of the following diagnostic findings?

    A. Spongiosis

    B. Multinucleated keratinocytes

    C. Lichenification

    D. Vasculitis

    E. Panniculitis

2. Molluscum contagiosum is caused by which type of virus?

    A. Pox

    B. Herpes

    C. Epstein-Barr

    D. Variola

    E. Vaccinia

3. In what percentage of patients with discoid lupus erythematosus does systemic lupus erythematosus develop?

    A. <5%

    B. 20%

    C. 50%

    D. 75%

    E. 100%

4. Spongiotic dermatitis is the histologic pattern for which of the following dermatoses?

    A. Discoid lupus erythematosus

    B. Contact dermatitis

    C. Psoriasis

    D. Erythema nodosum

    E. Erythema multiforme

5. A benign neoplasm characterized by nests of melanocytes along the epidermal basal layer and in the papillary dermis is diagnostic of which of the following?

    A. Melanoma

    B. Solar lentigo

    C. Seborrheic keratosis

    D. Compound nevus

    E. Junctional nevus

6. Lichen simplex chronicus is a thickened, scaly, and hyperpigmented plaque caused by which of the following?

   A. Infection

   B. Rubbing

   C. Allergy

   D. Autoantibodies

   E. Sun exposure

7. Which of the following layers is **NOT** part of the epidermis?

   A. Granular

   B. Spinous

   C. Subcutaneous

   D. Basal

   E. Cornified

8. Which of the following best describes mycosis fungoides?

   A. Dermatophyte infection

   B. Lymphoma

   C. Carcinoma

   D. Viral infection

   E. Autoimmune disease

9. Seborrheic keratosis is

   A. Benign

   B. Premalignant

   C. Malignant

   D. Hyperkeratosis

   E. Caused by trauma

10. An adult man has a nodule on the parietal scalp. Biopsy reveals a neuroendocrine appearing small round blue cell tumor with delicate chromatin, increased N:C ratios, and conspicuous mitoses, resembling oat cell carcinoma of the lung. Antibody staining for S100 is negative and cytokeratin 20 shows perinuclear dot-like staining. Which of the following is the best diagnosis?

   A. Melanoma

   B. Basal cell carcinoma

   C. Squamous cell carcinoma

   D. Merkel cell carcinoma

   E. Unknown, cytogenetic studies are required

ANSWERS

1. The answer is B. Herpes simplex infection causes keratinocyte *m*ultinucleation, nuclear *m*olding, and chromatin *m*argination.

2. The answer is A. Molluscum contagiosum is a type of poxvirus.

3. The answer is A. Systemic lupus erythematosus is rarely seen in patients with discoid lupus.

4. The answer is B. Contact dermatitis is a type of spongiotic dermatitis with edema and perivascular lymphocytic infiltrate.

5. The answer is D. A compound nevus is a benign melanocytic neoplasm with both a junctional and dermal component.

6. The answer is B. Lichen simplex chronicus is caused by chronic trauma, eg, rubbing (common in the vulva).

7. The answer is C. Subcutaneous tissue is deep to the epidermis.

8. The answer is B. Mycosis fungoides is a type of T-cell lymphoma.

9. The answer is A. Seborrheic keratosis is a benign epidermal neoplasm characterized by acanthosis and keratinous horn pseudo cysts. It may be pigmented, and it presents on the face and trunk of older adults.

10. The answer is D. The findings support Merkel cell carcinoma.

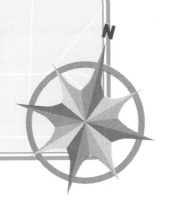

CHAPTER 4
HEAD AND NECK

*Experts consider the head [and neck] to be one
of the most important parts of the body.*
—Anonymous

I. Ears

A. External Ear

1. **Actinic keratosis** is a precursor lesion to carcinoma caused by ultraviolet radiation exposure leading to disordered and dysplastic epithelial growth (see Chapter 3 for additional details).
2. **Squamous cell carcinoma** is a malignant neoplasm of squamous epithelium commonly involving the outer rim of the ear (pinna).
3. **Basal cell carcinoma** is another common skin cancer.
4. **Auricular chondritis** may be localized like "wrestler's ear" or represent a systemic inflammatory condition like **polychondritis,** which can also involve the tracheal rings.
5. **Gout** can result in urate deposits involving the pinna.
   a. Tophaceous gout involving the ear is a chronic form of gout.
   b. It should not be confused with the acute form, which presents with podagra (acute monoarticular arthritis).

B. Ear Canal

1. **Otitis externa** is a common infection of the external ear canal, also called "swimmer's ear."
   a. The most frequently implicated pathogens are *Pseudomonas aeruginosa*, *Staphylococcus aureus*, then other **gram-negative organisms,** and occasionally, fungi, such as *Candida* or *Aspergillus* species.
   b. Entrapped moisture can macerate the skin that in turn provides an effective growth medium for bacteria and fungi.
   c. Patients may complain of a combination of otalgia, itchiness, discharge, changes in hearing, and tinnitus.
   d. Treatment often involves an astringent and an antibiotic.
   e. Chronic otitis is usually due to seborrheic dermatitis.
2. **Malignant otitis externa** is most often seen in patients with diabetes, AIDS, or in those who are otherwise immunosuppressed.

a. *Pseudomonas aeruginosa* is the most common organism.

      b. Infection results in extensive destruction of tissues.

C. Inner Ear

    1. Cholesteatoma is a reactive process of keratinizing squamous epithelium with growth and rupture, sometimes leading to reactive granulation tissue and destruction of middle ear structures.

    2. Otosclerosis is a common condition in which the stapes are abnormally fixed, resulting in **low-frequency** conductive hearing loss.

    3. Hereditary hearing impairment results in over half of childhood hearing impairment.

      a. It can be part of a syndrome or non-syndromic.

      b. It is multifactorial with multiple associated genetic loci.

    4. Eustachian tube dysfunction is caused by persistent obstruction of the eustachian tube.

      a. Patients are predisposed to acute otitis media and tympanic membrane rupture.

      b. Persistent unilateral eustachian tube dysfunction should prompt a careful head and neck examination to look for an obstructing neoplasm.

    5. Presbycusis is the most common cause of hearing loss; it is an age-related sensorineural process that results in **high frequency** hearing loss (in contrast to otosclerosis).

D. Vestibular System

    1. Acoustic neuroma is a schwannoma.

      a. It is a benign nerve sheath tumor of the eighth cranial nerve, located at the cerebellopontine angle, and is derived from the Schwann cell.

      b. As it grows, it may affect hearing and balance and lead to tinnitus and vertigo.

      c. Surgery is usually curative.

    2. Meniere disease, or endolymphatic hydrops, presents as episodic vertigo, tinnitus, and hearing loss because of distention of the endolymphatic system leading to destruction of vestibular and cochlear hair cells.

VERTIGO VERSUS SYNCOPE

- *It is important to elicit the specific symptom of vertigo because it may be confused with syncope, near-syncope, or nonspecific symptoms.*
- *While syncope is caused by insufficient cerebral vascular flow impairing consciousness, vertigo is caused by dysfunction of the labyrinthine apparatus or cerebellum.*
- *Clarifying the patient's symptoms is extremely helpful in localizing the cause and avoiding unnecessary testing.*

II. Nasal Cavity and Sinuses

A. Inflammatory Disorders

    1. Acute sinusitis results from obstruction of the sinus ostia due to viruses or allergens resulting in bacterial infection, usually *Streptococcus pneumoniae*, *Haemophilus influenzae*, or *Moraxella catarrhalis*.

2. **Chronic sinusitis** is probably a hypersensitivity reaction to fungal allergens, not invasive fungal disease, and is usually associated with *Aspergillus* species.
   a. It is characterized by thick rubbery mucoid material with extensive eosinophilic inflammation and **Charcot-Leyden crystals**.
   b. Sometimes fungal organisms can be demonstrated with silver stains—the usual organism is *Aspergillus*.
3. **Reactive polyps** are seen in allergic sinusitis and retention polyps with large cystic glands containing inspissated secretions may be a characteristic feature of cystic fibrosis.
4. **Invasive fungal sinusitis** occurs in diabetic and immunocompromised patients and represents a **medical emergency**.
   a. It is caused by *Mucor* and *Aspergillus* species.
   b. Diagnosis is made by biopsy followed by emergent surgery.
5. **Mucocele** is a complication of chronic sinusitis where inflammatory exudate and mucin separates epithelium and periosteum away from underlying bone resulting in a mass lesion and bone destruction.
6. **Wegener granulomatosis** is a necrotizing, granulomatous vasculitis with sinonasal, pulmonary, and renal involvement.
   a. It is associated with **c-ANCA** autoantibodies.
   b. It presents in the fourth or fifth decade of life.
   c. It is more common in men than women.
   d. Sinonasal involvement presents with nasal discharge, epistaxis, perforated septum, or anosmia.
   e. It can be difficult to diagnose on biopsy due to extensive areas of necrosis.
   f. The key to diagnosis is identifying vasculitis in a background of granulomatous inflammation (Figure 4–1).

B. Neoplasia
   1. **Sinonasal papillomas** are usually benign neoplasms of respiratory mucosa presenting with symptoms of nasal obstruction.
      a. Papillomas may present on the **nasal septum** where they grow in an exophytic pattern (Figure 4–2A).

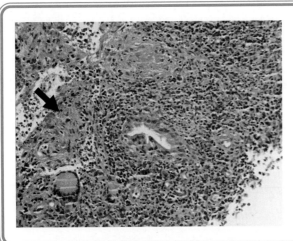

Figure 4–1. Wegener granulomatosis is characterized by neutrophils invading and destroying the arterial wall (vasculitis, arrow) in a background of granulomatous inflammation. It is associated with c-ANCA autoantibodies and presents with sinonasal, pulmonary, and renal involvement.

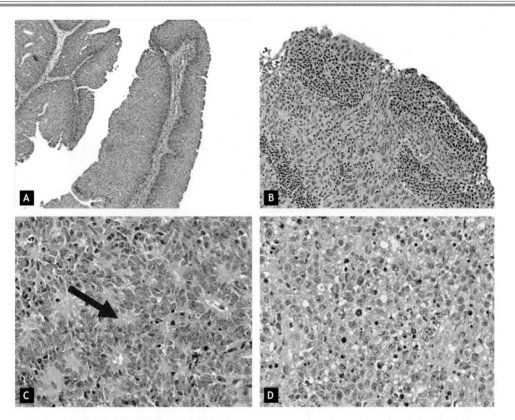

Figure 4–2. Sinonasal neoplasia. A: Schneiderian papillomas may be exophytic (usually septal) or inverted (usually lateral sinus). They may be squamous or oncocytic and may develop invasive carcinoma. **B:** Nasopharyngeal carcinoma is associated with Epstein-Barr virus (EBV) and if nonkeratinizing (as shown here) responds well to radiotherapy. **C:** Olfactory neuroblastoma has characteristic Homer-Wright rosettes (arrows) to distinguish it from sinonasal undifferentiated carcinoma (SNUC). **D:** T-cell lymphoma is more common in the sinonasal area than the usually more predominant B-cell lymphomas. NK/T-cell lymphoma (shown here) is associated with EBV and is very destructive, mimicking Wegener granulomatosis.

b. Papillomas involving the lateral nasal sidewall grow in an endophytic or inverted fashion (**inverted papilloma**), which is often destructive and has increased recurrent potential if incompletely excised.

c. Papillomas may transform into squamous cell carcinoma.

2. **Nasopharyngeal carcinoma** is an **Epstein-Barr virus (EBV)** associated malignancy of the nasopharyngeal epithelium, which is more common in patients of asiatic decent, including Native Americans.

a. It is either keratinizing or non-keratinizing (Figure 4–2B).

b. The keratinizing form appears similar to other squamous cell carcinomas, is less likely to stain for EBV, and is not sensitive to radiotherapy.

c. The nonkeratinizing form, including "undifferentiated" carcinoma, is significant because it is associated with EBV and more importantly is sensitive to radiotherapy, leading to markedly improved 5-year survival (60% rather than 10%).

3. **Sinonasal undifferentiated carcinoma** (SNUC) is distinguished from nonkeratinizing nasopharyngeal carcinoma because it is usually negative for EBV and has a poor prognosis.

4. **Olfactory neuroblastomas** (esthesioneuroblastoma) arise from the neuroepithelial elements of the olfactory membrane.

   a. It resembles a SNUC histologically (Figure 4–2C) but is significantly less malignant with an improved prognosis.

   b. A classic distinguishing feature is the **Homer-Wright rosette**, which is a tubule of tumor cells surrounding a central core of neuroglial fibers.

5. **NK/T-cell lymphoma**, which is also known as angiocentric T-cell lymphoma, is a destructive lymphoma that more often affects the sinonasal area and is more common in Asians.

   a. The most common presentation is a destructive nasal tumor, the so-called **lethal midline granuloma**.

   b. The differential diagnosis includes Wegener granulomatosis.

   c. It is an EBV-associated lymphoma (Figure 4–2D).

   d. Treatment is radiation and chemotherapy.

6. **Plasmablastic lymphoma** is a variant of diffuse large B-cell lymphoma that often presents in the **nasopharynx**.

   a. Patients with plasmablastic lymphoma usually also have positive test results for **EBV**.

   b. Plasmablastic lymphoma usually occurs in immunosuppressed patients.

III. Salivary Glands

A. Inflammatory Disorders

1. **Sialoadenitis** may be an acute or chronic inflammatory condition caused by obstruction (eg, stones), infection (eg, mumps), or radiation therapy for head and neck carcinomas.

2. **Sialoadenosis** is hyperplasia of the salivary gland tissue related to several systemic conditions, including alcoholism, AIDS, malnutrition, and diabetes mellitus.

3. **Sjögren syndrome** is a chronic autoimmune destruction of the salivary glands (and lacrimal glands); it is associated with autoantibodies to **Ro/SSA and La/SSB.**

B. Primary Salivary Gland Neoplasia

1. Malignancy is more common in smaller glands: minor (buccal mucosa) > sublingual > submandibular > parotid.

2. Larger glands may contain lymph nodes that may be reactive or neoplastic (eg, lymphoma or metastatic disease such as squamous cell carcinoma and melanoma).

3. Therefore, **fine-needle aspiration (FNA)** biopsies are recommended to determine whether surgical excision is necessary and provide a provisional diagnosis.

4. **Lymphoepithelial cysts** and **mucoceles** may arise from obstruction; notably, lymphoepithelial cyst should prompt suspicion for **HIV** infection.

5. Primary salivary gland neoplasms may be benign or malignant.

   a. **Pleomorphic adenoma** is a common benign tumor.

(*1*) It usually presents as a mass in the parotid gland.

(*2*) It is a mixed tumor composed of benign epithelium and myxoid stroma (Figure 4–3A).

b. **Warthin tumor** is a common benign "tumor" associated with smoking that may actually represent a reactive process leading to cysts lined by metaplastic oncocytes overlying reactive lymphoid follicles (Figure 4–3B).

c. **Oncocytoma** is a benign "tumor."

(*1*) It may represent a hyperplastic metaplasia or a primary neoplasm (Figure 4–3C).

(*2*) Similar to a Warthin tumor, it may be bilateral.

d. **Mucoepidermoid carcinoma** (MEC) is the most common malignant salivary gland tumor, especially in children (Figure 4–3D).

(*1*) Low-grade MEC is composed mostly of mucus-producing glandular tumor cells (muco-).

(*2*) High-grade MEC is composed mostly of squamous cell carcinoma (-epidermoid).

(*3*) MEC is often associated with a marked inflammatory response to the mucin and keratin.

e. **Adenoid cystic carcinoma** is an infiltrative malignant neoplasm.

(*1*) It commonly encases nerves and has high recurrent potential, even after treatment.

(*2*) It is composed of cribiform glands containing hyaline material; nuclei are deceptively bland (Figure 4–3E).

f. **Acinic cell carcinoma** is a rare malignant neoplasm.

(*1*) It arises from the enzyme-secreting acinar cells.

(*2*) Tumor cells have characteristic delicate cytoplasm containing zymogen granules (Figure 4–3F).

g. **Ductal carcinoma** arises from the salivary duct and resembles ductal carcinoma of the breast (see Chapter 12); therefore, the differential diagnosis includes metastatic carcinoma and high grade MEC.

FINE-NEEDLE ASPIRATION BIOPSY

- *FNA is often the first diagnostic step when evaluating salivary gland lesions as well as thyroid, lymph nodes, and breast masses.*
- *A thin 22- to 25-gauge needle is passed into the lesion collecting cells, which are then smeared on a glass slide and stained.*
- *The slides are evaluated by a pathologist and diagnosed with similar sensitivity and specificity to excisional biopsies.*
- *The objective is to exclude cases that do not require surgery and provide a provisional diagnosis to guide treatment.*

IV. Neck

A. Benign Cysts

1. **Branchial cleft cyst** is a developmental remnant, or "inclusion cyst," of a branchial arch.

a. They occur in the anterolateral neck.

b. The location raises a worrisome differential diagnosis:

(*1*) Malignant salivary gland neoplasm

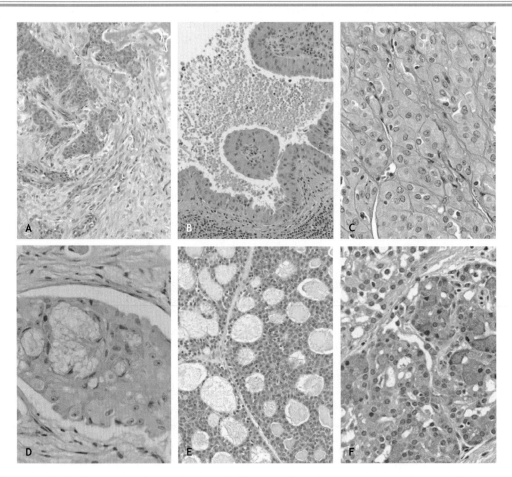

Figure 4–3. Salivary gland neoplasms. A: Pleomorphic adenoma is a mixed tumor (like a fibroadenoma of the breast) composed of both benign epithelial and myxoid stromal elements. **B:** Warthin tumor is associated with smoking, which causes oncocytic metaplasia of the ducts overlying reactive lymphoid follicles. **C:** Oncocytoma is composed of polygonal epithelial cells with numerous mitochondria, which make the tumor cells appear pink and granular. **D:** Mucoepidermoid carcinoma is the most common malignant salivary gland neoplasm, especially in children. Low-grade tumors are composed of malignant *muc*inous glands and high-grade tumors look like squamous cell carcinoma (*epidermoid*). **E:** Adenoid cystic carcinoma is more common in adults. It has characteristic cribriform glands containing hyaline material (arrow). Notice that tumor cells are deceptively bland given the aggressive nature of this malignant neoplasm. **F:** Acinic cell carcinoma (shown here) and salivary duct carcinoma (looks like breast cancer) are rare.

(2) Metastatic disease (eg, carcinoma, melanoma)

(3) Lymphoma

c. In children and young adults, it is likely a benign cyst.

d. In older adults, the lesion is probably malignant.

e. The diagnosis is often made by FNA showing mature squamous cells and a few ciliated columnar epithelial cells.

2. Thyroglossal duct cyst is a remnant of the thyroglossal duct, the migratory track from the mouth to lower neck during development.

a. The cysts occur in the midline of the neck.

b. The diagnosis is often made by FNA showing reactive squamous cells, rare ciliated epithelium, and thyroid epithelium.

B. **Primary Neoplasms**

1. Most malignant neoplasms in the neck are usually **metastatic** carcinoma, melanoma, or lymphoma leading to enlarged cervical or supraclavicular lymph nodes.

2. Submandibular gland neoplasms may occur in the upper neck.

3. Paraganglioma is a neuroendocrine neoplasm of the autonomic nervous system.

a. It may arise from the carotid body in the neck.

b. Similar to pheochromocytoma (see Chapter 11), these tumors may secrete neuroendocrine peptides leading to clinical symptoms (eg, **hypertension**).

V. **Larynx**

A. **Inflammatory and Infectious Disorders**

1. Laryngitis is an acute inflammatory condition of the larynx.

a. It is often caused by **viral** organisms but can also be caused by inhaled irritants, such as tobacco **smoke.**

b. Less common infections of the larynx include diphtheria (*Corynebacterium diphtheriae*) and tuberculosis, which are highly infectious and contagious.

2. Epiglottitis is an acute infectious process of the epiglottis, usually caused by *H influenzae* and β-hemolytic streptococci.

a. There can be significant **swelling** of the epiglottis, leading to varying degrees of airway obstruction.

b. This condition is an **airway emergency,** often necessitating tracheostomy for airway control.

3. Reactive nodules can form on the vocal cords, such as the so-called **singer's nodule.**

a. Singer's nodules are bilateral due to voice overuse.

b. Nodules can be caused by inhaled irritants (tobacco smoke).

B. **Benign Neoplasms**

1. Papillomas are caused by human papillomavirus (HPV) similar to skin warts and lesions on the cervix and anus.

a. Low-risk HPV genotypes (eg, 6 and 11) are associated with relatively benign low-grade dysplasia.

b. High-risk HPV genotypes (eg, 16, 18) are associated with an increased risk of high-grade dysplasia and invasive carcinoma.

c. The histologic features are virtually identical to those seen in the cervix (see Chapter 13).

d. Treatment is excision or laser ablation.

2. **Papillomatosis** means multiple papillomas.
   a. Recurrent papillomatosis is the most common benign neoplasm of the larynx in children and is a cause of airway obstruction.
   b. It is caused by HPV genotypes 6 and 11, often by vertical transmission during delivery.
   c. Treatment is surgery, sometimes requiring multiple surgeries.

C. Malignant Neoplasms
   1. The most common malignancy of the larynx, and upper respiratory tract, is **squamous cell carcinoma.**
   2. Presenting clinical symptoms include hoarseness, pain, dysphagia, and hemoptysis.
   3. In evaluating laryngeal squamous cell carcinoma, the following important **staging** factors should be determined:
      a. Precise location, such as supraglottis, glottis, subglottis
      b. Involvement of **vocal cord,** including fixation
      c. Involvement of the thyroid cartilage
   4. There are a few distinctive variants:
      a. **Verrucous carcinoma** is a well-differentiated carcinoma with wart-like gross and microscopic features.
         (1) It is distinguished by deceptively bland nuclei and broad pushing borders representing expansile invasion, rather than infiltration.
         (2) Superficial biopsies may be falsely diagnosed as low-grade dysplasia or wart.
         (3) Diagnosis requires demonstration of expansile invasion.
         (4) Treatment is surgical resection not radiation.
      b. **Basaloid variant** is a poorly differentiated carcinoma resembling basal cell carcinoma of the skin, but is significantly more aggressive and has a very poor prognosis.
   5. Adenocarcinoma arising from mucous glands and minor salivary gland neoplasms can rarely develop in the larynx.

CLINICAL PROBLEMS

1. Sjögren syndrome is associated with which of the following autoantibodies?
   A. p-ANCA
   B. c-ANCA
   C. anti-Ro/La autoantibodies
   D. anti-EBV IgG and IgM antibodies
   E. None of the above

2. Wegener granulomatosis is associated with which of the following autoantibodies?
   A. p-ANCA
   B. c-ANCA
   C. anti-SSA/SSB autoantibodies

D. anti-EBV IgG and IgM antibodies

E. None of the above

3. A 68-year-old man with an 80 pack-year history of tobacco use but no prior history of malignancy complains of a painless mass in the left parotid gland. What is the most likely diagnosis?

A. Mucoepidermoid carcinoma

B. Warthin tumor

C. Adenoid cystic carcinoma

D. Squamous cell carcinoma

E. Paraganglioma

4. A 72-year-old patient with diabetes complains of severe pain and bloody discharge of the right ear. Which of the following would a Gram stain of material from surgical debridement be expected to show?

A. Gram-positive cocci

B. Gram-negative cocci

C. Gram-positive bacilli

D. Gram-negative bacilli

E. Septate, branching hyphae

5. A 17-year-old girl arrives at her primary care physician's office with a painless mass in the left side of her neck close to the angle of the mandible. Each of the following entities is in the differential diagnosis EXCEPT:

A. Thyroglossal duct cyst

B. Branchial cleft cyst

C. Mucoepidermoid carcinoma

D. Reactive lymphadenitis

E. Hodgkin lymphoma

6. A 90-year-old man complains of a painless, crusting nodule on the superior pinna of his right ear. All of the following are possible diagnoses EXCEPT:

A. Actinic keratosis

B. Basal cell carcinoma

C. Squamous cell carcinoma

D. Relapsing polychondritis

E. All the above are possible

7. A 24-year-old man in your clinic practice underwent a CT scan of his sinuses. The report states there is a mucocele involving the left maxillary sinus. All of the following can be underlying disorders EXCEPT:

A. Allergic sinusitis

B. Cystic fibrosis

C. Sinonasal papilloma causing ostial obstruction

D. Pleomorphic adenoma

   E. All of the above

8. A 33-year-old woman complains of episodic dizziness, palpitations, and headache. On examination, her blood pressure is 162/89 mm Hg. Imaging of her adrenal glands fails to demonstrate a mass. What is the most likely scenario and location of the lesion?

   A. Schwannoma; left cerebellopontine angle

   B. Schwannoma; left carotid body

   C. Meniere disease; left utricle

   D. Paraganglioma; left carotid body

   E. None of the above

9. Nasopharyngeal carcinoma is associated with which of the following?

   A. c-ANCA

   B. p-ANCA

   C. anti-SSA/SSB

   D. anti-EBV IgG and IgM antibodies

   E. None of the above

10. A 52-year-old patient with chronic alcoholism is seen in follow-up after a hospital admission for gastrointestinal bleeding. On physical examination, bilateral parotid gland swelling is noted. Which of the following is the most likely etiology?

   A. Sialoadenosis

   B. Sialoadenitis

   C. Sjögren syndrome

   D. Warthin tumor

   E. Pleomorphic adenoma

ANSWERS

1. The answer is C. Sjögren syndrome is associated with anti-Ro/SSA and anti-La/SSB autoantibodies. c-ANCA is associated with Wegener granulomatosis, while p-ANCA is associated with polyarteritis nodosa.

2. The answer is B. As described above, c-ANCA is associated with Wegener granulomatosis.

3. The answer is B. Warthin tumor is seen in older male smokers. Mucoepidermoid carcinoma is possible here but is usually seen in younger patients. Adenoid cystic carcinoma usually involves the minor salivary glands. Squamous cell carcinoma can metastasize to the parotid, but this would be unlikely without a history of a primary head or neck squamous cell carcinoma. Paraganglioma would not be on the differential.

4. The answer is D. Malignant otitis externa is most commonly associated with *Pseudomonas aeruginosa*, which is a gram-negative bacillus.

5. The answer is A. Thyroglossal duct cysts are midline lesions. All of the other entities are diagnostic possibilities in this scenario.

6. The answer is D. Relapsing polychondritis is a systemic inflammatory disease, which would involve both ears. The presentation would not be that of a solitary nodule but of diffuse inflammatory symptoms (rubor, calor, dolor, tumor).

7. The answer is D. All of the conditions except pleomorphic adenoma would predispose to development of chronic sinusitis. While pleomorphic adenoma is a mass lesion capable of causing obstruction, it usually presents in the parotid gland, not the nasal cavity.

8. The answer is D. While a schwannoma can present with vertigo, the hypertension would be more characteristic of a paraganglioma, which is a neuroendocrine tumor. Paraganglioma is closely related to pheochromocytoma, which presents in the adrenal medulla.

9. The answer is D. Nasopharyngeal carcinoma is EBV-related.

10. The answer is A. Sialoadenosis would be the most common diagnosis in this clinical scenario. Sialoadenitis is an acute inflammatory disorder, usually related to salivary duct obstruction. Sjögren syndrome may cause bilateral salivary gland enlargement but would be less likely in this case. Warthin tumor can be bilateral but would present as discrete parotid masses rather than diffuse enlargement. Pleomorphic adenoma usually presents as a solitary mass involving the parotid gland.

CHAPTER 5
ORAL CAVITY AND DENTITION

Every tooth in a man's head is more valuable than a diamond.
—Miguel de Cervantes, *Don Quixote*, 1605

I. Teeth

A. Dental Caries

1. **Dental caries** (tooth decay) is a microbial disease that results in the destruction of the mineralized tissues of teeth.
2. Specific bacteria, including *Streptococcus mutans, Lactobacillus* **sp.** *and Actinomyces* **sp.,** accumulate within a biofilm known as **dental plaque** on tooth surfaces.
3. Bacteria within dental plaque metabolize sugars and other carbohydrates provided in the diet to produce acids that demineralize teeth and enzymes that digest the organic matrix.
4. The initial lesion of dental caries appears as a white spot on the tooth surface; subsequent destruction of **enamel, cementum,** and **dentin** will produce a cavitated lesion.
5. Dental caries, when left untreated, may progress toward the dental pulp with subsequent inflammation and necrosis of the pulp.
6. Dental caries can be prevented or disease progression can be modified through proper oral hygiene, diet, and fluoride.

B. Pulpitis

1. **Pulpitis** is inflammation of the dental pulp tissue that can be caused by dental caries, trauma, or severe thermal injury.
2. Pulpitis may be acute or chronic, localized or generalized, asymptomatic, or symptomatic (**toothache**).
3. Assessment of history and various clinical tests are used to determine whether pulpitis is reversible or irreversible.
4. **Reversible pulpitis** means that the dental pulp is capable of returning to normal health following removal of the stimulus.
5. **Irreversible pulpitis** means that the dental pulp is injured beyond the ability of the tissue to return to normal health.
6. Pulpal necrosis may follow untreated irreversible pulpitis (as in advanced dental caries with bacterial invasion of the dental pulp), or may suddenly follow a traumatic event to the tooth.

7. In some circumstances, pulpitis may progress to involve the bone around the apex of the affected tooth and may produce an abscess, and even **osteomyelitis**.

C. Gingivitis
   1. **Gingivitis** is inflammation of the adjacent soft tissues.
   2. Most cases are caused by the accumulation of dental plaque.
   3. Gingivitis may be localized or generalized.
   4. Early findings include mild redness of the marginal gingiva.
   5. As gingivitis progresses, gingival tissues become more red, edematous, and will bleed with gentle probing or tooth brushing.
   6. **Chronic hyperplastic gingivitis** results when inflammation produces a significant degree of gingival enlargement.
   7. **Necrotizing ulcerative gingivitis** is a specific form of gingivitis caused by infection with fusiform bacteria and spirochetes usually associated with significant psychological stress.

D. Periodontitis
   1. **Periodontitis** is inflammation of gingival tissues and destruction of the tissues that support the teeth within the jaws, namely the periodontal ligament and alveolar bone.
   2. Shifts in the proportions of pathogenic organisms in dental plaque associated with poor oral hygiene are important in the pathogenesis.
   3. Gingivitis precedes the development of periodontitis, although many cases of gingivitis will not progress to severe periodontitis.
   4. Periodontitis produces increased depth of the gingival sulcus with continued bone loss, resulting in deep periodontal **pockets.**
   5. Progressive bone loss results in tooth loss.
   6. Chronic periodontitis is typically a disease of adults.
   7. **Aggressive periodontitis** may be observed in children and young adults in cases of rapid significant bone loss.

II. Odontogenic Cysts and Neoplasms

A. Odontogenic Cysts
   1. **Radicular cyst** (periapical cyst; apical periodontal cyst) is a lesion that develops in association with the **root** of a tooth that has been devitalized secondary to either pulpal necrosis or endodontic therapy.
      a. Radicular cysts are often asymptomatic.
      b. Radicular cysts are well-defined, unilocular radiolucencies.
      c. Radicular cysts are most often associated with non-vital teeth in the maxilla (Figure 5–1).
   2. **Dentigerous cyst** (follicular cyst) is a developmental odontogenic cyst arising in association with the **crown** of an unerupted tooth.
      a. Dentigerous cysts most commonly affect young adults.
      b. Dentigerous cysts are most commonly observed in association with impacted teeth.
      c. Potential complications of dentigerous cysts include tooth displacement; resorption of adjacent teeth; secondary infection; and, in the case of large mandibular lesions, fracture.

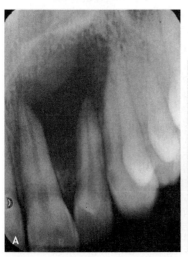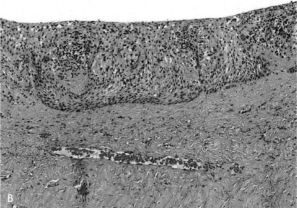

Figure 5–1. Radicular cyst. A: Radiolucent cyst arising after traumatic injury to the incisor root resulting in pulpal necrosis. **B:** Extension of the inflammatory reaction to the periapical bone stimulated proliferation of odontogenic epithelial remnants to form an epithelial lined cyst.

3. **Eruption cyst** is a cyst that develops as a result of dilatation of the follicular space over the crown of an erupting tooth producing a swelling of the gingiva.
4. **Lateral periodontal cyst** is a developmental odontogenic cyst most often discovered as an incidental radiographic finding.
   a. Lateral periodontal cyst occurs most typically in adults.
   b. Lateral periodontal cyst is usually a unilocular, radiolucency found in the mandibular premolar and canine area.
5. **Odontogenic keratocyst** (keratocystic odontogenic tumor) is a developmental odontogenic cyst with characteristic histopathologic features and significant clinical behavior.
   a. The posterior mandible is the most common site (60–80%).
   b. Odontogenic keratocysts appear as unilocular or multilocular radiolucencies (Figure 5–2A).
   c. Odontogenic keratocyst is often asymptomatic, although larger cysts may be associated with pain, swelling, or drainage.
   d. Odontogenic keratocysts show histopathologic features that include a uniformly thick layer of stratified squamous epithelium with a parakeratotic surface and a basal layer of palisaded, columnar epithelium (Figure 5–2B).
   e. Conservative treatment of odontogenic keratocyst may be associated with a significant **recurrence rate.**
   f. Odontogenic keratocysts, usually multiple and asynchronous, may indicate that the patient has the **nevoid basal cell carcinoma syndrome** (Gorlin-Goltz syndrome).

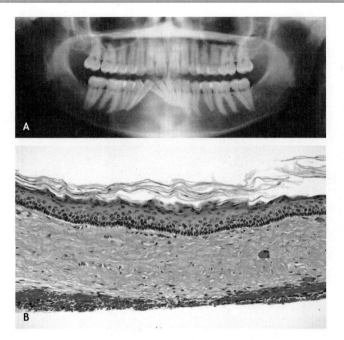

Figure 5–2. Odontogenic keratocyst. A: Radiolucent lesion of the anterior mandible associated with displacement of adjacent teeth. **B:** Characteristic features include a uniformly thick layer of stratified squamous epithelium with parakeratosis. These lesions may recur.

ODONTOGENIC CYSTS

- *The jaws are relatively unusual among the bones because of the relative frequency of cystic lesions.*
- *The process of odontogenesis provides a potential source of epithelial cells that under certain circumstances may proliferate, resulting in the formation of a variety of cystic lesions.*
- *Odontogenic cysts are usually classified on the basis of **location** in the jaw and relationship to the tooth as well as histopathologic findings.*

    B. **Odontogenic Neoplasms**

       1. **Odontoma** is the most common odontogenic tumor, although it should be regarded as a **hamartoma** rather than a true neoplasm.

          a. Odontoma occurs mostly in children and young adults.

          b. It consists of the elements of a tooth including enamel, dentin, cementum, and dental pulp.

          c. **Compound odontoma** consists of tooth elements with an orderly arrangement that form numerous miniature teeth.

       2. **Ameloblastoma** is a benign but locally aggressive neoplasm derived from odontogenic epithelium, resembling ameloblasts.

          a. Ameloblastoma most commonly affects young adults.

          b. It occurs most commonly in the posterior portion of the mandible, although ameloblastoma may arise in any portion of the tooth-bearing regions.

          c. Ameloblastoma is a unilocular or multilocular radiolucent lesion (Figure 5–3).

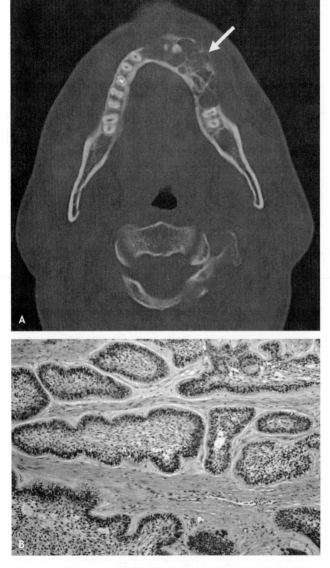

Figure 5–3. Ameloblastoma. A: Radiograph showing locally destructive odonto-genic tumor by CT scan. **B:** Ameloblastoma recapitulates the enamel producing cells characterized by nesting with a peripheral layer of palisaded columnar cells resem-bling ameloblasts.

d. Most cases are within the jaw although some develop within gingival soft tissues (**peripheral ameloblastoma**).

  3. Calcifying epithelial odontogenic tumor (Pindborg tumor) is a benign neoplasm derived from odontogenic epithelium.

     a. It arises most frequently in the posterior mandible and is frequently associated with an unerupted tooth.

     b. Histologic sections show cords of polyhedral odontogenic epithelial cells associated with eosinophilic, hyalinized, amyloid-like extracellular matrix and calcifications.

  4. Odontogenic myxoma is a benign locally aggressive neoplasm derived from dental papilla.

     a. Odontogenic myxoma affects young adults.

     b. It is a radiolucent lesion with well-circumscribed scalloped borders and a loculated pattern.

     c. Cortical expansion and bone reabsorption may be seen.

  5. Malignant odontogenic tumors are very rare but include malignant ameloblastoma, ameloblastic carcinoma, clear cell odontogenic carcinoma, and intraosseous carcinoma.

ODONTOGENIC NEOPLASMS

CLINICAL CORRELATION

- *Odontomas typically arise during the period of normal tooth development.*
- *Failure of a tooth to erupt at the normal time should prompt investigation into the possibility of odontogenic cysts or tumors.*

III. Inflammation

  A. Reactive Lesions

    1. Traumatic fibroma is a reactive fibrous nodule.

     a. Traumatic fibroma is most commonly observed in the buccal mucosa along the bite line, although other sites of occurrence include labial mucosa, lateral tongue, and gingiva.

     b. The lesion consists of a nodular mass composed of relatively acellular densely collagenous connective tissue.

    2. Pyogenic granuloma is a red lobulated exophytic nodule that may show surface ulceration.

     a. It occurs commonly on gingiva, but other oral mucosal locations prone to trauma may also be affected.

     b. It is a reactive hyperplasia of endothelial cells forming lobules of capillaries within inflamed collagenous stroma.

     c. Pyogenic granulomas are common in pregnant women.

    3. Peripheral ossifying fibroma is a nodular proliferation with bone formation occurring *exclusively* in the gingiva.

     a. Grossly, it is a well-defined red nodule (Figure 5–4A).

     b. Microscopically, it is moderately cellular with collagenous stroma and production of osseous matrix (Figure 5–4B).

    4. Peripheral giant cell granuloma is a nodular proliferation of multinucleated giant cells in a vascular stromal matrix.

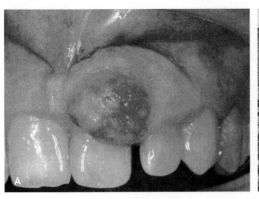
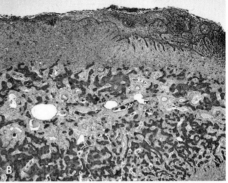

Figure 5–4. Peripheral ossifying fibroma. A: Gross image of a well-defined reactive nodule, which over time produces a bone-like osseous matrix **(B)**.

B. Mucus Escape Reaction (Mucocele)
  1. **Mucus escape reaction** develops following traumatic severance of a minor salivary gland duct with resultant spillage of mucinous salivary secretions into the submucosal connective tissue.
  2. It occurs most commonly in the lower lip (Figure 5–5A), but other sites include the floor of mouth (ranula), ventral tongue, buccal mucosa, and palate.
  3. Histologic sections show basophilic mucin associated with inflammation and granulation tissue (Figure 5–5B).

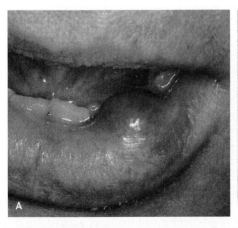
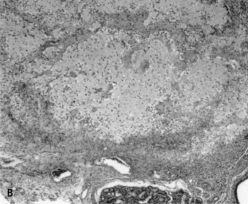

Figure 5–5. Mucocele. A: Gross image of a blue nodule arising in the vermilion of the lower lip. **B:** Traumatic damage to a minor salivary gland duct had released mucin into the submucosal tissue, leading to mucin pools associated with inflammation.

C. Aphthous Stomatitis
   1. **Aphthous stomatitis** is a common oral disorder of uncertain etiology although it probably represents immune dysregulation.
   2. A variety of risk factors have been described including stress, hormonal changes, trauma, dietary allergies, and deficiencies.
   3. Aphthous ulcers (**canker sores**) are typically painful ulcers occurring in oral squamous mucosa (eg, buccal mucosa, ventral tongue) that heal spontaneously within 7–10 days, but may recur.

IV. Infections
   A. **Herpes simplex virus** (HSV) transmission is primarily through direct contact with saliva containing viral particles.
      1. **Herpetic gingivostomatitis** develops in a minority of infections.
         a. Painful vesiculo-ulcerative lesions develop.
         b. There is also fever, headache, and cervical lymphadenopathy.
      2. Recurrent HSV infection most commonly affects the vermilion border of the lips (**herpes labialis**), although intraoral lesions may occur on the attached gingiva and hard palate mucosa.
         a. Recurrent herpes simplex lesions are preceded by a **prodrome** of tingling, itching, or burning.
         b. A cluster of vesicles form that ulcerate and crust.
      3. A diagnosis of primary and recurrent HSV infections can usually be made on the basis of characteristic history and clinical features.
         a. Oral exfoliative cytology may demonstrate typical viral cytopathologic effects (**m**ultinucleation, nuclear **m**olding, and chromatin **m**argination, known as **Tzanck** cells).

   B. **Herpes zoster virus infection** involving the second or third divisions of the trigeminal nerve and may produce oral lesions.
      1. Clusters of vesicles rupture resulting in painful ulcers.
      2. Unilateral zonal distribution is characteristic.
      3. Oral exfoliative cytology preparations show similar viral cytopathic effects as observed in HSV infections.

   C. **Hand-foot-and-mouth** disease is caused by **coxsackievirus.**
      1. Oral lesions are generalized throughout the oral cavity.
      2. These lesions are accompanied by vesicular lesions on the hands and feet.

   D. **Candidiasis** is usually caused by opportunistic infection by *Candida albicans,* which is part of the normal oral flora in 50% of individuals.

   E. **Deep fungal infections** (histoplasmosis, blastomycosis, coccidioidomycosis and cryptococcosis) may cause oral lesions, usually secondary to pulmonary disease with hematogenous spread or oral inoculation by infected sputum.
      1. Deep fungal infections produce chronic ulcerations.
      2. Special histochemical stains (Grocott-Gomori methenamine silver (**GMS**), or periodic acid-Schiff (**PAS**) highlight fungi in sections.

CANDIDIASIS

• *Predisposing factors to the development of candidiasis include broad-spectrum antibiotics, immunocompromise, diabetes, leukemia, xerostomia, and dentures.*
• *Management of candidiasis, especially in recurrent or chronic cases, includes not only appropriate antifungal therapy, but also evaluating the patient for predisposing conditions.*

CLINICAL CORRELATION

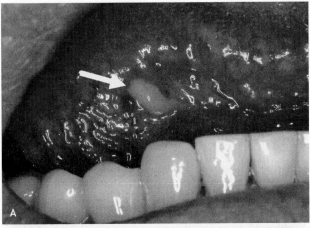

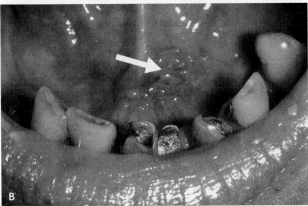

Figure 5–6. Leukoplakia and erythroplakia. A: Ventral-lateral tongue presenting with a white patch (arrow) of leukoplakia that proved to be mild dysplasia. **B:** Velvety red patch (arrow) of erythroplakia in the floor of the mouth demonstrated superficially invasive squamous cell carcinoma.

V. Dysplastic and Malignant Oral Lesions

A. Leukoplakia and Erythroplakia

1. **Leukoplakia** is a **white patch** on the oral mucosa that cannot be characterized clinically as any other specific disease process (Figure 5–6A).
    a. The etiology of leukoplakia is unknown, although many cases are associated with tobacco use.
    b. Leukoplakia typically occurs in middle-aged patients.
    c. Most lesions are on the lower lip vermilion, buccal mucosa, or gingiva.
    d. Most leukoplakia lesions reveal benign **hyperkeratosis.**
    e. About 20% of these lesions are dysplastic; therefore they should be biopsied to exclude carcinoma.

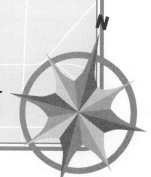

CHAPTER 6
HEART AND CIRCULATION

*The heart of a fool is in his mouth, but
the mouth of a wise man is in his heart.*
—Benjamin Franklin

I. Ischemic Heart Disease

A. Epidemiology

1. **Atherosclerosis** is the leading cause of morbidity and mortality in developed countries around the world.

   a. Major risk factors include:

      (1) **Cigarette smoking**

      (2) **Hypertension**

      (3) **Dyslipidemia**

      (4) **Diabetes mellitus**

      (5) **Family history**

   b. Minor risk factors include:

      (1) Male gender

      (2) Obesity

      (3) Hyperhomocysteinemia

      (4) Increased levels of low-density lipoprotein (LDL)

   c. Some patients with ischemic heart disease will not have any identifiable risk factors.

2. Atherosclerosis of the coronary arteries is the most common cause of ischemic heart disease.

3. **Arteriosclerosis** and atherosclerosis are not synonymous; arteriosclerosis is **nonspecific** "hardening of the arteries."

B. Pathophysiology of Atherosclerosis

1. The leading hypothesis is that atherosclerosis is a reactive mechanism induced by **intimal injury.**

   a. Injurious agents to the intima include oxidized LDL, mechanical, toxic, viral, immunologic, and metabolic products like homocysteine.

   b. **Endothelial injury** leads to influx of inflammatory cells, cytokine elaboration and eventually smooth muscle proliferation.

   c. Intimal collections of **foamy macrophages** are the initial microscopic finding, leading to a grossly visible fatty streak.

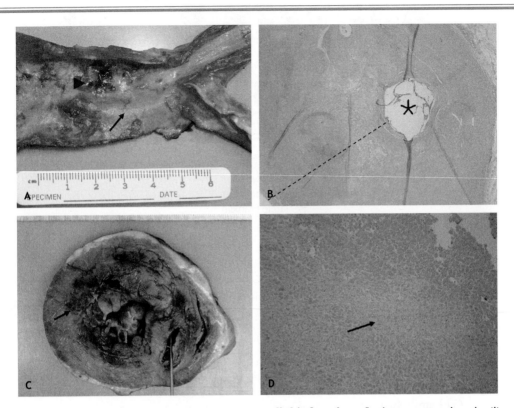

Figure 6–1. Atherosclerosis leading to myocardial infarction. A: Aorta opened at the iliac bifurcation to reveal fatty streaks (arrow) and ulceration (arrowhead). **B:** Atherosclerosis of the coronary vessels leads to progressive stenosis of the lumen (asterisk) by plaque, which may rupture, leading to complete occlusion by a thrombus. **C:** Myocardial infarction (arrow) leads to myocyte death and necrosis **(D)** with sequential development of inflammation (arrow), granulation tissue, and scar.

> d. **Atheroma** (fatty core) arises in the vessel wall.
> e. **Luminal narrowing** occurs when fibrous tissue and smooth muscle cells surround the lipid core forming a stable plaque.
>
> 2. An unstable plaque develops when fissuring and disruption of the fibrous cap exposes the core, leading to thrombosis and stenosis.
> 3. Atherosclerotic plaques occur in multiple vascular locations, including the aorta (Figure 6–1A), coronary, carotid, proximal cerebral, superior mesenteric, and iliac arteries.

C. Acute Coronary Syndrome/Unstable Angina

> 1. The pathologic lesion of unstable angina is atherosclerotic plaque rupture, which leads to thrombosis and incomplete occlusion of an epicardial coronary artery (Figure 6–1B).

2. The presentation of acute coronary syndrome is similar to acute myocardial infarction.

3. Vasospasm may also contribute to acute changes in the luminal diameter, leading to variable ischemia.

4. Atherosclerotic plaque morphology that leads to unstable angina is typically soft, usually an atheroma.

D. **Acute Myocardial Infarction**

1. Symptoms depend on the location and severity of the infarction.
   a. The most common presentation is acute chest pain (angina).
   b. Ischemia may cause **cardiogenic shock**, congestive heart failure (CHF), and pulmonary edema.
   c. If critical conductive areas are ischemic, then an arrhythmia can result, such as ventricular tachycardia or **fibrillation**.
   d. Ischemia of the papillary muscles can lead to acute mitral **valvular insufficiency** and CHF.
   e. It can present as sudden cardiac **death**.
   f. Significantly, it can be clinically *silent*, especially in patients with diabetes mellitus or rare neuropathies.

2. The pathologic lesion associated with acute myocardial infarction is coronary atherosclerotic plaque rupture leading to thrombosis and occlusion sufficient to cause significant cardiac ischemia.

3. There is a well-described timeline of pathologic findings that evolve during an acute myocardial infarction (Figure 6–1 C-D).
   a. Onset: No grossly visible or microscopic features
   b. Hours later: Myocyte "waviness" by light microscopy
   c. One **day** after: Myocyte necrosis and **neutrophilic** infiltrate
   d. One **week** later: Macrophages and **granulation tissue**
   e. One **month** after: White fibrous **scar** forms

4. **Irreversible injury** may occur within **20 minutes** of ischemia.

5. There are several complications of acute myocardial infarction that can occur early or late in the disease course.
   a. **Arrhythmia** can occur at presentation or as a late complication due to conduction system disturbance, or myocardial damage resulting in scarring and electrical impulse reentry.
   b. Altered **contractility** with pump failure due to myocardial ischemia, especially when large amounts of myocardium are ischemic, such as with left main coronary artery disease.
   c. Mitral valve insufficiency due to papillary muscle dysfunction can lead to acute CHF.
   d. Myocardial **rupture** can occur, usually in non-hypertrophic myocardium, 3–7 days after an infarct due to weakening of the infarcted tissue.
   e. Right ventricular infarction can occur when the right coronary or posterior descending artery are involved in a posterior wall infarct, sometimes presenting with hypotension and elevated jugular venous pressure.
   f. Postinfarct **pericarditis** can occur days after an infarct due to inflammation (**Dressler syndrome**).
   g. Mural thrombi can form due to a hypocontractile ventricular wall following an infarct.

h. Ventricular aneurysm may occur if a large area of myocardium has been involved and no longer contracts properly.

i. Progressive **CHF** can occur if enough myocardium has been damaged and the remaining viable myocardium cannot meet demand.

CHEST PAIN

- *The presence of specific physical findings can help in the formation of a useful differential diagnosis and guide therapy.*
- *Inspiratory crackles may indicate pulmonary edema.*
- *A new murmur may be indicative of valvular insufficiency.*
- *An S$_3$ gallop indicates left ventricular dysfunction.*
- *A pleural or pericardial rub can point to pleuritis or pericarditis.*
- *It is important to remember that a normal physical examination does not exclude potentially serious causes of chest pain.*
- *Ischemia can only be ruled out by serial ancillary tests (serum markers, electrocardiogram (ECG), stress test, and angiography).*

    E. Serum Markers of Myocardial Injury

      1. Patient blood is tested in the pathology laboratory for serum markers that rise after myocardial ischemia.

        a. Myoglobin is ubiquitous in cardiac and skeletal muscle; therefore, it is not specific for myocardial damage, but it is an early sensitive marker appearing within 2 hours of injury.

        b. Creatine kinase represents a number of muscle enzymes that are relatively specific for various tissues:

          (1) There are three isoenzymes: CK-BB (brain), CK-MM (skeletal muscle), and **CK-MB** (heart).

          (2) CK-MB represents 10–20% of the total CK in the heart, a much higher concentration than in other muscles, so myocardial injury causes an elevation of CK-MB relative to the total amount of CK in the serum **(CK-MB/CK ratio is predictive).**

          (3) CK-MB begins to rise **4 hours** after infarction, peaks at 2 days, and then begins to fall.

          (4) Treatment-related reperfusion will cause an early peak and fall; extension of the infarction will cause a later or more prolonged peak and fall.

          (5) Serial CK-MB levels are the most helpful way of utilizing the test.

        c. Cardiac troponins are specific structural proteins bound to the thin filament within the cardiac myocyte.

          (1) Troponins are generally not present in the serum.

          (2) Elevated troponin indicates **myocyte damage.**

          (3) Mildly elevated cardiac troponin can be seen in pericarditis, myocarditis, renal failure, sepsis, and pulmonary embolism.

          (4) Troponins rise within **4 hours** of infarction, peak in 24 hours, but **stay elevated** for 5–10 days.

      2. The combination of CK-MB and troponin levels provides good sensitivity and specificity to detect myocardial infarction and provide an idea of when the infarction occurred.

F. Chronic Ischemic Heart Disease

1. The pathologic lesion associated with chronic ischemic disease is a fixed, or gradually progressive, stenotic atherosclerotic plaque of an epicardial coronary artery (Figure 6–1B).

   a. Multiple coronary arteries may be involved, including the left anterior descending (LAD) artery, right coronary artery (RCA), and posterior descending artery (PDA).

   b. Symptoms are a function of degree and extent of disease.

   c. There may be multiple remote myocardial infarctions affecting heart function and conductivity.

2. Exertion-related angina pectoris or symptoms secondary to CHF are usually the presenting manifestations.

3. There can be development of **collateral** coronary circulation to areas of ischemic myocardium.

4. Grossly, the heart can be heavy and enlarged, with features of both ventricular hypertrophy and dilation.

II. Valvular Heart Disease

A. Degenerative Valvular Disease

1. **Calcific aortic stenosis** is the most common valvular disease.

   a. Calcification in an anatomically normal valve is thought to occur by age-related changes.

   b. Calcifications involve the fibrous portion of the cusps leading to small masses preventing complete opening of the valves (Figure 6–2).

   c. Rheumatic heart disease can lead to calcific aortic stenosis, which will present earlier than the "senile" type.

   d. Congenital bicuspid aortic valves are predisposed to calcific aortic stenosis.

   e. Complications of aortic stenosis include left ventricular hypertrophy, arrhythmia, **syncope**, and CHF.

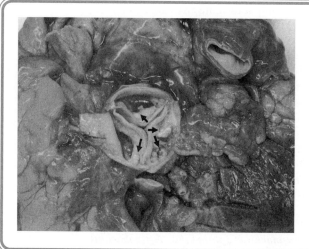

Figure 6–2. Calcified vegetations on tricuspid aortic valve. Senile calcification occurs with age, creating nodules in the outer aspects of the cusps (arrows). Severe calcification may lead to aortic stenosis.

2. **Mitral valve prolapse** or myxomatous degeneration of the mitral valve is common.
    a. Only a small number of patients suffer serious complications.
    b. The most common presentation is an incidental murmur.
    c. The pathologic features include intercordal ballooning of the leaflets (floppy leaflets), elongated tendinous chordae, annular dilation, and deposition of myxoid material in the leaflets.
    d. Myxomatous degeneration of the mitral valve can be a manifestation of a systemic connective tissue disease, such as Marfan syndrome.
    e. Complications of myxomatous degeneration of the mitral valve include arrhythmias, thrombi leading to embolic events, and mitral insufficiency leading to CHF.

B. Rheumatic Heart Disease
    1. **Acute rheumatic fever** is an immunologically mediated systemic inflammatory disease typically occurring 1–6 weeks following group A **streptococcal pharyngitis**.
    2. Acute rheumatic carditis leads to the complications of chronic rheumatic heart disease.
    3. The pathologic lesion is the **Aschoff body**, which is a lesion of lymphocytes and macrophages surrounding bundles of collagen.
    4. Other manifestations of acute rheumatic carditis include myocarditis, pericarditis, and **valve vegetations**.
        a. Acute rheumatic valvulitis leads to thickening, fibrosis, and fusion of the mitral or aortic valve's chordae tendineae.
        b. **Mitral stenosis** is almost always caused by rheumatic disease; long-standing mitral stenosis can lead to atrial fibrillation and pulmonary hypertension.

C. Infective Endocarditis
    1. Infective endocarditis has a 100% mortality rate if untreated.
        a. It is colonization of cardiac valves by microbes.
        b. It can involve normal valves, but usually involves valves damaged by prior disease, such as rheumatic heart disease.
    2. Infective endocarditis can be divided clinically into acute and subacute forms, each with different clinical presentations, causative organisms, and treatment regimens.
    3. Acute infective endocarditis is a fulminant disease.
        a. Complications occur early in the disease course.
        b. The causative organism is usually ***Staphylococcus aureus***.
        c. It may present as an invasive infection with myocardial abscess or valve destruction.
    4. Subacute infective endocarditis has a slower clinical course.
        a. Subacute infective endocarditis can present insidiously, sometimes as just a low-grade **fever**.
        b. The causative organisms are less virulent and include:
            (1) Viridans streptococci
            (2) Streptococcus bovis
            (3) Enterococci
            (4) Haemophilus parainfluenzae, Haemophilus aphrophilus, Actinobacillus, Cardiobacterium, Eikenella, and ***Kingella*** (HACEK)

    c. The **HACEK** organisms used to be very difficult to isolate and were categorized as "culture negative," but they are now recognized as fastidious and slow growing.

    d. The so-called "culture negative" infective endocarditis (fever, valve disease, vegetations on echocardiography, with or without emboli, and negative cultures) is usually caused by *Coxiella burnetii* and *Bartonella* species.

5. The **Duke criteria** provide a clinical framework for making the diagnosis of infective endocarditis.

    a. The major criteria are:

        (1) Continuous bacteremia with an organism that typically causes infective endocarditis

        (2) A new or worsening regurgitant murmur

        (3) **Vegetations** visualized by echocardiography

    b. The minor criteria are:

        (1) Fever

        (2) Blood cultures showing an uncharacteristic organism

        (3) Echocardiographic findings consistent with the diagnosis but not meeting major criteria

        (4) Embolic phenomena, such as septic infarcts

        (5) Immunologic phenomena, such as glomerulonephritis, or a positive rheumatoid factor

    c. To make a diagnosis of infective endocarditis using the Duke criteria, the patient should meet two major criteria, one major and three minor criteria, or all five minor criteria.

6. Pathologic criteria for making the diagnosis of infective endocarditis require demonstrating microorganisms within vegetations, section of cardiac tissue, or in an embolus.

D. Noninfective Endocarditis

1. Marantic endocarditis or nonbacterial thrombotic endocarditis is characterized by small vegetations consisting of platelets, fibrin, and leukocytes on the valve leaflets.

    a. The vegetations are sterile and nondestructive.

    b. This condition is associated with malignancy or sepsis.

    c. Emboli from the vegetations are common, resulting in infarction of involved organs.

    d. A thrombophilic state is thought to be the mechanism; there is usually accompanying venous thrombosis and pulmonary emboli.

    e. **Trousseau syndrome**, a hypercoagulable state with chronic **disseminated intravascular coagulation (DIC)** and migratory thrombophlebitis, is a closely related disorder; it is often seen in mucinous adenocarcinomas.

2. Libman-Sacks endocarditis is associated with systemic lupus erythematosus **(SLE)**.

    a. Mitral or tricuspid valvulitis can lead to development of sterile vegetations consisting of fibrinous material and "**hematoxylin bodies.**"

    b. These vegetations can look like vegetations from nonbacterial thrombotic endocarditis or infective endocarditis.

    c. Unlike the other forms of endocarditis, these vegetations can occur on *both sides of the valve.*

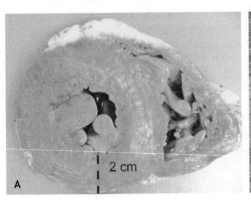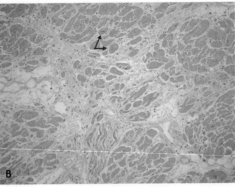

Figure 6–3. Concentric left ventricular hypertrophy. A: Hypertension causes compensatory concentric hypertrophy of the left ventricle. **B:** Plump myocytes have enlarged "box-car" nuclei (arrows).

III. Hypertensive Heart Disease

   A. **Pathophysiology**
   1. Systemic arterial hypertension is a common disease with significant morbidity and mortality.
   2. The disease appears to be **multifactorial** (caused by both environmental factors and genetic predisposition).
   3. It can also be secondary to other pathology, such as **pheochromocytoma** or **renal artery stenosis**.
   4. Hypertension can lead to changes in the heart as it compensates for the extra workload imposed upon it.
      a. Hypertension leads to increased **afterload**, so the heart compensates by increasing muscle mass (Figure 6–3A).
      b. The increased wall thickness leads to decreased compliance of the left ventricle, resulting in increased left ventricular filling pressure, or **preload**.
         (1) There can be compensatory left atrial enlargement, which can lead to **atrial fibrillation.**
         (2) The increased filling pressures can lead to CHF due to diastolic dysfunction.
   5. An anatomic diagnosis of hypertensive heart disease requires:
      a. **Concentric** left ventricular hypertrophy (thicker than 2 cm)
      b. No concurrent cardiovascular pathology that could lead to left ventricular hypertrophy (such as aortic stenosis)
      c. Evidence of clinical hypertension, or pathologic evidence of hypertension in other organs (Figure 6–4)
   6. Microscopic changes include myofiber disarray with myocyte hypertrophy and enlarged **"box-car" nuclei** in a background of increased interstitial fibrosis (Figure 6–3B).

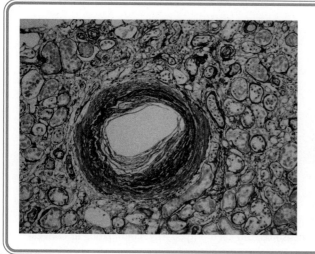

Figure 6–4. Renal artery arteriosclerosis. Malignant hypertension may cause characteristic "onion-skinning," which is a combination of smooth muscle hyperplasia and basement membrane material (stained black).

B. Cor Pulmonale (Right Ventricular Hypertrophy)
  1. Pulmonary diseases, such as chronic obstructive pulmonary disease (**COPD**), interstitial lungs diseases, or thrombotic pulmonary vascular disease, can lead to increased right ventricle afterload.
  2. Increased **afterload** leads to compensatory hypertrophy.
  3. In acute conditions that lead to increased pulmonary arterial pressure, such as massive pulmonary embolism, there is not time for hypertrophy to develop, but marked dilation and dysfunction occur.

IV. Cardiomyopathies

A. Dilated Cardiomyopathy
  1. Dilated cardiomyopathy is defined by progressive four-chamber dilation of the heart with contractile dysfunction.
    a. It is an enlarged "floppy" heart (Figure 6–5A).
    b. Endomyocardial biopsy may reveal the etiology (Figure 6–5B).
    c. Contractile dysfunction leads to reduced pumping action and symptoms of progressive CHF.
  2. The disease is multifactorial, resulting from variable disease processes and genetic predisposition, including:
    a. Toxins (**alcohol**, doxorubicin, cocaine)
    b. Metabolic diseases (**thyroid** disease, **thiamine** deficiency)
    c. **Myocarditis** (viruses, bacteria, parasites)
    d. Neuromuscular diseases (**muscular dystrophies**)
    e. Immunologic (SLE, post-transplant rejection, sarcoidosis)
    f. Hematologic (anemia, leukemic infiltration)
    g. **Genetic factors** with variable inheritance patterns
      (1) Affected genes are usually part of the **cytoskeleton.**
      (2) X-linked cardiomyopathy involves the **dystrophin** protein.

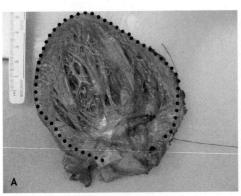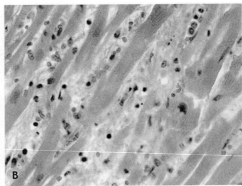

Figure 6–5. Dilated cardiomyopathy. A: Enlarged "floppy" heart with U-shaped left ventricle. **B:** Myocarditis (inflammation of the heart) may cause dilated cardiomyopathy, culminating in congestive heart failure.

3. Severe coronary artery disease with or without myocardial infarction can result in cardiac dilation with ventricular dysfunction, but this is not considered a true cardiomyopathy.
4. The valves should not have any significant pathology, although due to dilation, secondary valvular insufficiency can occur.
5. Several significant complications can develop.
   a. Left ventricular hypocontractility results in diminished forward flow and systemic **hypoperfusion.**
   b. Left ventricular hypocontractility also leads to increased left ventricular filling pressures, pulmonary vascular congestion, **pulmonary edema,** and right heart failure.
   c. **Arrhythmia** is a common complication.
   d. **Mural thromboemboli** can develop.

CONGESTIVE HEART FAILURE

CLINICAL CORRELATION

- *An echocardiogram and chest radiograph are indicated for patients with clinical symptoms of CHF (dyspnea, orthopnea, paroxysmal nocturnal dyspnea, and peripheral edema) and characteristic physical examination findings (elevated jugular venous pressure, inspiratory crackles, cardiac gallop or murmur).*
- *Echocardiography is a **Doppler ultrasound** examination of the heart.*
- *The chest radiograph can help confirm the diagnosis with typical features (enlarged cardiac silhouette, pleural effusions, Kerley B lines, and pulmonary edema).*
- *The left ventricular **ejection fraction** is a useful index in the diagnosis and quantification of CHF (an ejection fraction less than 40% is indicative of dysfunction).*

   B. Hypertrophic Cardiomyopathy
      1. Hypertrophic cardiomyopathy is defined by thickening of the ventricular myocardium without any ventricular dilation.
      2. There is no chamber dilation, so on gross inspection, the heart will look normal in size, but will be increased in mass.

3. There will be markedly increased thickness of the ventricular myocardium, specifically the **septal myocardium**.
    a. The classic gross finding is asymmetric hypertrophy of the septum with impingement on the anterior mitral leaflet.
    b. There is marked disarray of the myocytes, especially in the septum with myocyte hypertrophy and interstitial fibrosis.
4. The main cause of hypertrophic cardiomyopathy is **genetic mutation**.
    a. Several genes that encode components of the cardiac myocyte sarcomere have been identified, including point mutations in β-myosin heavy chain, α-tropomyosin, troponins, and myosin-binding proteins.
    b. Mutations in these genes affect cardiac **contractility**.
5. The complications of hypertrophic cardiomyopathy are different than dilated cardiomyopathy.
    a. There is **hypercontractility** of the ventricle with impaired relaxation, leading to increased filling pressures (diastolic dysfunction) with **pulmonary vascular congestion** and edema.
    b. There can be occasional functional left ventricular outflow obstruction leading to **syncope**.
    c. Both ventricular and atrial arrhythmias can occur, especially **atrial fibrillation** due to left atrial enlargement from the elevated left ventricular filling pressure.
6. Multiple diseases may mimic hypertrophic cardiomyopathy, due to thickening of the ventricular myocardium, for example:
    a. Cardiac **amyloidosis**
    b. Systemic arterial **hypertension**
    c. **Aortic stenosis** with left ventricular hypertrophy
    d. Age-related subaortic septal hypertrophy

C. Restrictive Cardiomyopathy
    1. This condition is similar to hypertrophic cardiomyopathy in that there is preserved systolic function but a decrease in compliance.
    2. Impaired ventricular compliance leads to increased filling pressures or diastolic dysfunction.
    3. The heart is grossly normal.
        a. The ventricles are not dilated or thickened.
        b. The ventricles can show increased subendocardial fibrosis.
    4. The endomyocardial biopsy will show increased interstitial fibrosis and possibly a more specific etiology.
    5. There are several possible causes of restrictive cardiomyopathy.
        a. **Löffler endomyocarditis**: Fibrosis of the endocardium with striking **eosinophilic** infiltration and mural thrombi.
        b. **Amyloidosis**: Deposition of amyloid in the myocardium.
        c. **Radiation**: Myocyte damage leads to myocardial fibrosis.
        d. **Endocardial fibrosis**: Seen in tropical areas, it afflicts younger adults and **children** with a progressive subendocardial fibrosis eventually involving the atrioventricular valves.
        e. **Endocardial fibroelastosis**: An unusual disease of infants, usually in association with other congenital anomalies.
    6. Restrictive cardiomyopathy can be confused with other clinical entities, such as chronic constrictive pericarditis.

V. Congenital Heart Disease

A. Septal Defects

1. **Ventricular septal defects** are the most common congenital defect.
   a. There is a **left-to-right** shunting of blood, with the severity depending on size, location, and concurrent anomalies.
   b. Membranous defects are more common than muscular defects.
   c. Membranous defects tend to be larger and more severe with a greater likelihood of shunting and late complications, such as **Eisenmenger syndrome** (right-to-left reversal of flow due to pulmonary hypertension, culminating in cyanosis).
   d. Many ventricular septal defects occur with other anomalies, such as **tetralogy of Fallot** (Figure 6–6).

2. **Atrial septal defects** (ASD) are the second most common cardiac defect.
   a. They are associated with left-to-right shunting, unless pulmonary hypertension develops (Eisenmenger syndrome).
   b. There are three major types of atrial septal defects.
      (1) **Secundum** defects (90%) are located at the fossae ovalis.
      (2) **Primum** occurs next to the atrioventricular valves.
      (3) **Sinus venosus** defects are located at the superior vena cava entry to the right atrium.

3. **Atrioventricular septal defect** (AVSD) is an uncommon defect.
   a. Embryologically, there is failure of the superior and inferior endocardial cushions to fuse, creating a defect where potentially all four chambers of the heart may communicate.
   b. There are two main types of AVSDs.
      (1) The incomplete type is characterized by an ostium primum ASD and a cleft mitral valve.
      (2) The complete type is characterized by a combined atrial and septal defect that results with all four chambers in communication.

4. **Patent foramen ovale** is not an anomaly but rather a failure of complete closure, which occurs in about 20–30% of normal individuals.

B. Cyanotic Congenital Heart Defects ("T" syndromes)

1. **Tetralogy of Fallot** is the result of the infundibular septum being abnormally positioned anterior and superior.
   a. There are four main features (Figure 6–6B):
      (1) Subpulmonic stenosis
      (2) Ventricular septal defect
      (3) Overriding aorta
      (4) Right ventricular hypertrophy
   b. The degree of subpulmonic stenosis determines the severity of the defect and its clinical presentation.
   c. **"Boot-shaped"** heart is due to right ventricular hypertrophy.
   d. If the subpulmonic stenosis is mild, there will be left-to-right shunting resulting in the so-called "pink tetralogy."

2. **Truncus arteriosus** results from abnormal separation of the aorta and pulmonary artery leading to a shared trunk serving both the right and left ventricles (Figure 6–6C); the consequence is pulmonary overload and cyanosis.

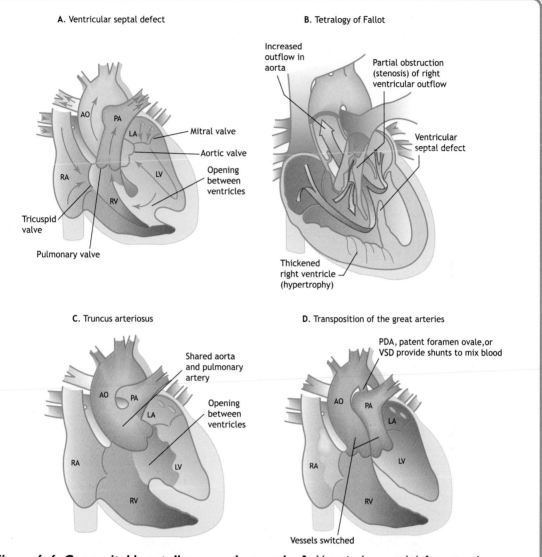

Figure 6–6. Congenital heart disease and cyanosis. A: Ventricular septal defects are the most common heart malformation. They lead to a left-to-right shunting of blood. **B–D:** In contrast, tetralogy of Fallot, truncus arteriosus, and transposition of the great arteries lead to right-to-left shunting, leading to cyanosis. AO, aorta; LA, left atrium; LV, left ventricle; PA, pulmonary artery; RA, right atrium; RV, right ventricle.

3. **Transposition** of the great vessels means the aorta arises from the right ventricle and the pulmonary artery arises from the left ventricle (Figure 6–6D).
   a. There is complete separation of the pulmonary and systemic circulations, a condition that is incompatible with life.
   b. To live, a shunt has to exist for mixing blood, usually in the form of an ASD, ventricular septal defect, or patent ductus arteriosus.

DUCTUS ARTERIOSUS

DEVELOPMENTAL
INSIGHTS

- *The ductus arteriosus is necessary for life in utero.*
- *It shunts blood from the pulmonary artery to the aorta, effectively bypassing the developing lungs.*
- *It closes shortly after birth becoming the ligamentum arteriosum; however, if it remains patent (or persistent) it creates a left-to-right shunt that, if prolonged, may cause pulmonary hypertension.*
- *It is associated with a characteristic cardiac murmur, the so- called **"machinery"** murmur, which is a continuous murmur throughout systole and diastole.*
- *Ironically, a patent ductus arteriosus occurring in conjunction with other anomalies, such as coarctation or transposition, can be lifesaving.*

4. **Tricuspid atresia** is occlusion of the tricuspid valve due to unequal developmental division of the atrioventricular canal.
   a. A concurrent ASD, or patent foramen ovale, allows maintenance of proper circulation via right-to-left shunting.
   b. A ventricular septal defect (VSD) allows blood to flow into the pulmonary artery.
   c. The consequence is a hypoplastic right ventricle.
5. **Total anomalous pulmonary venous connection/return** (TAPVR) occurs when the pulmonary veins fail to connect to the left atrium.
   a. Primitive venous channels from the lungs enter into the systemic venous system, usually the left innominate vein.
   b. A patent foramen ovale or an ASD allows blood to enter the left atrium and systemic circulation.
   c. The consequence is pulmonary circulatory overload with right ventricular hypertrophy and right atrial enlargement.

C. **Coarctation of the Aorta**
1. Coarctation means narrowing or constriction.
2. There are two types: the infantile form and the adult form.
   a. The infantile form arises proximal to the ductus arteriosus and results from hypoplasia of the distal aortic arch.
   b. The coexistence of a patent ductus arteriosus can lead to shunting of unoxygenated blood to the lower half of the body, leading to cyanosis.
   c. The adult form arises at the **ligamentum arteriosum** where there is a ridge of tissue, causing narrowing.
   d. If sufficient constriction occurs, hypertension in the upper extremities and underperfusion of the lower extremities develop, leading to pallor and claudication.
3. Coarctation is more common in males but is associated with **Turner syndrome** in females (X0 karyotype).
4. Coarctation can occur as an isolated defect but often occurs with a bicuspid aortic valve (50% of cases).

VI. Neoplasia of the Heart

A. **Myxomas** are the most common primary tumors of the heart.
1. Most myxomas occur in the left atrium of middle-aged women.
    a. It may cause mitral valve obstruction or regurgitation.
    b. They are grossly soft pale nodules attached to the atrium by a fibrous stalk.
    c. Biopsy reveals a hypocellular tumor composed of **star-like "stellate" cells** in a mucoid background.
2. There is an inheritable form of myxoma that presents as multiple myxomas in children and young adults.

B. **Rhabdomyoma** is a benign primary tumor of the heart.
1. It is seen in children, some with **tuberous sclerosis**.
2. A very distinctive feature of this tumor is the so-called **spider cells** seen on microscopic examination.

C. **Angiosarcoma** is the most common primary malignant tumor of the heart.
1. Angiosarcoma usually arises in the atrium.
2. It is a malignant neoplasm of endothelial cells (see Chapter 15).

D. **Metastatic** tumors are more common than primary heart neoplasia.
1. Metastatic tumors involving the heart include metastatic carcinoma (especially lung and breast), melanoma, and systemic lymphoma.
2. Local extension of primary lung, thymus, and mediastinal germ cell neoplasms may also involve the heart.

VII. Pericardial Diseases

A. Pericardial Effusion
1. It is characterized by a fluid collection in the pericardial space exceeding the normal 25–50 mL.
2. The fluid may be serous, hemorrhagic, or purulent, which may suggest the cause.
3. **Cardiac tamponade** is impaired cardiac filling due to increased fluid pressure in the pericardial space.
    a. **Hemopericardium** is the result of hemorrhage into the pericardial space, resulting in cardiac tamponade.
    b. Hemopericardium can result from myocardial rupture from myocardial infarction, penetrating or blunt trauma, aortic dissection (Figure 6–7), or infectious pericarditis.
4. **Cardiac shadow** is a radiographic feature suggesting chronic pericardial effusion.

B. Acute Pericarditis
1. Acute pericarditis is an inflammatory process involving the epicardial and pericardial spaces.
2. There are several types, which include the following:
    a. Serous pericarditis
    b. Fibrinous pericarditis
    c. Purulent pericarditis
    d. Caseous pericarditis
    e. Hemorrhagic pericarditis

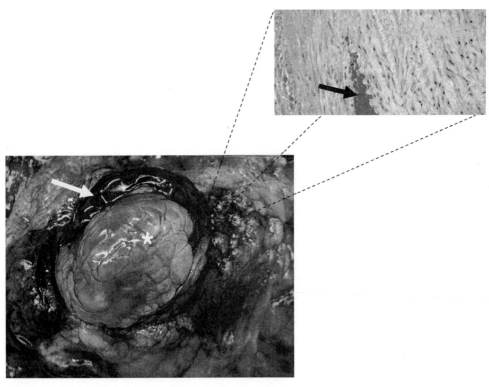

Figure 6–7. Aortic root dissection leading to hemopericardium. Dissection may be caused by hypertension, atherosclerosis, or genetic predisposition (eg, Marfan syndrome). A tear in the wall in the proximal portion of the aorta (type A) may rip into the pericardial sac causing hemopericardium (arrow). The apex of the heart is marked by an asterisk.

   3. Serous and **fibrinous pericarditis** are caused by a heterogenous group of conditions including connective tissue disease, viral infection, post-myocardial infarction, uremia, and trauma.
   4. **Purulent pericarditis** is caused by bacterial organisms.
      a. It is **exudative** rather than serofibrinous, with a larger amount of thick opaque fluid.
      b. The usual organisms responsible are *S. aureus, S. pneumoniae,* group A streptococcus, and the Enterobacteriaceae.
   5. **Caseous pericarditis** is usually caused by *Mycobacterium tuberculosis* or fungi; it causes fibrogranulomatous pericarditis.
   6. **Hemorrhagic pericarditis** is usually the result of malignancy involving the pericardial space; cytologic examination of the fluid can yield a diagnosis if malignant cells are present.
C. **Chronic Constrictive Pericarditis**
   1. Fibrinous and purulent exudates can become organized causing a rind of fibrous tissue enveloping the heart and obliterating the pericardial space.

a. The pericardium becomes adherent to the epicardium.

       b. Concretio cordis is a thick rind of scar tissue encasing the heart resembling a plaster cast.

  2. The pathophysiology of chronic constrictive pericarditis is impaired ventricular filling, with a clinical picture similar to restrictive cardiomyopathy.

PERICARDIAL PATHOLOGY AND AUSCULATORY FINDINGS

CLINICAL CORRELATION

- *Pericardial friction rub may be present in pericarditis.*
- *The friction rub is usually evanescent, with a variable number of ausculatory components throughout the heartbeat.*
- *Cardiac tamponade may sound like a "pericardial knock."*

VIII. Diseases of the Peripheral Vascular System

  A. Systemic Arterial Hypertension

    1. This common disease has a multifactorial etiology, including both genetic and epigenetic causes.

      a. A few rare single gene mutations have been found and a few common genetic polymorphisms (eg, Thr235Met in **angiotensinogen**) are also associated with primary "essential" hypertension.

      b. Environmental factors probably interact with these genetic polymorphisms to lead to elevated blood pressure (increased salt intake, obesity, stress, and smoking).

    2. Essential hypertension is diagnosed only when a secondary cause cannot be identified.

    3. Secondary causes are rare (<5% of cases) but include the following:

      a. Renal artery stenosis caused by **atherosclerosis**

      b. Renal artery stenosis caused by **fibromuscular dysplasia**

      c. Acute and chronic medical renal diseases (see Chapter 10)

      d. Adrenal cortical hyperfunction (eg, Cushing syndrome)

      e. Exogenous hormones and medications (eg, **prednisone**)

      f. Pheochromocytoma

      g. Hyperthyroidism and hypothyroidism

      h. Coarctation of the aorta

      i. Obstructive sleep apnea

      j. Increased intracranial pressure (stroke, hemorrhage, tumor)

    4. Uncontrolled hypertension is the "silent killer."

      a. Hypertension can lead to both ischemic and hemorrhage stroke.

      b. It leads to CHF and arrhythmia.

      c. It causes endothelial damage leading to atherosclerosis.

      d. Vascular damage and elevated blood pressure may cause carotid or aortic dissection (Figure 6–7).

      e. Hypertension leads to renal vascular disease and glomerular injury, culminating in renal dysfunction.

    5. Malignant hypertension is uncommon (<5% of hypertensive patients)

      a. Acute elevations of blood pressure (>200/100 mm Hg) and signs of end-organ damage and hyperplastic "onion-skinning" arteriosclerosis (Figure 6–4) may be present.

      b. If left untreated, malignant hypertension is fatal.

B. Atherosclerosis and Arteriosclerosis
1. There are three distinct forms of arteriosclerosis, each differing in their pathophysiology and clinical presentation.
   a. **Atherosclerosis** is composed of lipid plaques.
   b. **Arteriosclerosis** is not specific but is a term sometimes used to describe vascular wall hyalinization or hyperplasia.
   c. **Mönckeberg** calcific sclerosis is characterized by calcium deposits in the vascular wall that do not lead to stenosis; it is usually seen in the elderly and in certain anatomic sites such as the uterus, breast, and scrotum.
2. Atherosclerosis is composed of lipid, foamy macrophages, smooth muscle cells, and fibrosis (eg, coronary artery disease).
   a. The American Heart Association classification includes:
      (1) Type I (intimal injury; isolated foam cells)
      (2) **Type II** (fatty streak; intracellular lipid)
      (3) Type III (intermediate lesion)
      (4) **Type IV** (atheroma)
      (5) Type V (fibroatheroma; lipid core with fibrous layer)
      (6) **Type VI** (unstable lesion with thrombus formation)
   b. Atherosclerotic plaques develop in large and medium-sized arteries, including the aorta (Figure 6–1A), carotid, iliac, mesenteric, renal, and coronary vessels (Figure 6–1B).
      (1) Plaque rupture leads to thrombosis or embolism.
      (2) Plaque formation can cause vessel wall weakening with aneurysm formation and rupture (Figure 6–8).
      (3) Plaque and thrombosis may slowly progress to gradual stenosis of the vessel (Figure 6–1B).
3. Arteriolosclerosis is seen often in diabetes and hypertension.
   a. Small arteries and arterioles are affected.
   b. There is narrowing of the lumen, resulting in ischemia.
   c. There are two types, hyaline and hyperplastic.
      (1) The **hyaline** type is characterized by exudation of plasma into the vessel wall causing narrowing and ischemia.
      (2) The **hyperplastic** type is characterized by "onion- skinning" of the vessel wall smooth muscle (Figure 6–4).
   d. Both hyaline and hyperplastic arteriolosclerosis are most commonly encountered in examination of kidney biopsies, which are performed in the evaluation of renal disease (Chapter 10).

DEEP VENOUS THROMBOSIS

CLINICAL CORRELATION

- *Deep venous thrombosis (DVT) is quite common, especially in hospitalized patients.*
- *Risk factors are described by **Virchow triad**: alteration in the vessel endothelial lining, alteration of local blood flow, and alteration of blood clotting factors.*
- *Most cases of thrombosis occur in the deep leg veins.*
- *Migratory superficial thrombophlebitis (**Trousseau syndrome**) is seen in patients with underlying adenocarcinoma.*
- ***Phlegmasia cerulea dolens** describes thrombosis of the femoral veins that leads to venous stasis and **painful blue leg**.*
- ***Phlegmasia alba dolens** describes thrombosis of the femoral veins with femoral artery vasospasm that leads to **painful white leg**.*

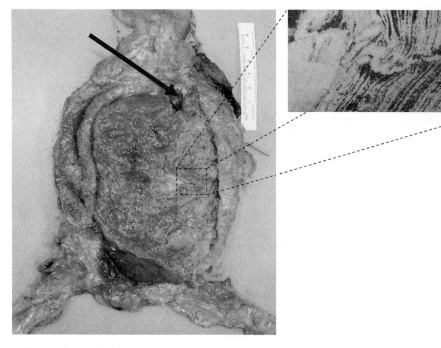

Figure 6–8. Abdominal aortic aneurysm. Atherosclerosis and hypertension may cause destruction and dilation of the aortic wall, especially in the descending aorta near the iliac bifurcation. Turbulence and endothelial damage cause thrombus formation (inset, lines of Zahn forming thrombus). Progressive dilation may culminate in aortic rupture (arrow).

C. **Aneurysm and Dissection**
    1. An aneurysm is a localized abnormal dilation of the vascular wall.
        a. Aneurysms caused by atherosclerosis commonly involve the **abdominal aorta**, leading to dilation, thrombosis, and rupture (Figure 6–8).
        b. Aneurysms caused by cystic medial degeneration of the arterial media (eg, Marfan syndrome) commonly involve the **thoracic aorta.**
        c. Aneurysms can be **hereditary**, such as berry aneurysms of the **cerebral** vasculature associated with autosomal dominant polycystic kidney disease.
        d. Infectious causes include **mycotic aneurysms** and **syphilitic** (luetic) aneurysms.
            (1) Mycotic aneurysms can be seen with endocarditis or sepsis with bacterial seeding of the vessel wall.
            (2) Syphilitic involvement of the **vasa vasorum** can lead to vessel wall weakening and formation of an aneurysm, usually with tertiary syphilis.
        e. A false aneurysm or pseudoaneurysm is a breach of the vessel wall with an extravascular hematoma.
    2. Complications include the following:
        a. **Rupture** leading to massive hemorrhage
        b. **Infection** leading to bacteremia

c. **Thrombosis** leading to distal embolism

d. **Obstruction** of surrounding vessels and organs

e. Contrary to older terminology, development of dissection is usually not associated with an aneurysm.

3. **Dissection** is a hematoma tearing into the wall (Figure 6–7).

a. Predisposing factors include **hypertension** (usually in older men) and connective tissue disorders (eg, **Marfan** syndrome with mutations in the **fibrillin** gene).

b. **Trauma** can also lead to formation of a dissection.

c. The most common lesion associated with a dissection is **cystic medial degeneration** (disruption or fragmentation of the normal elastic component of the arterial wall).

d. **Aortic dissection** is classified by the segment involved.

   (1) **Type A** or **proximal** dissection involves the aortic arch.

   (2) **Type B** or **distal** involves the descending aorta.

e. Complications may be fatal, with hemorrhage into the pericardial space (Figure 6–7), thorax, or abdomen.

D. **Vasculitis**

1. Vasculitis is classified according to blood vessel size: small, medium, or large.

2. **Small-vessel vasculitides** include Wegener granulomatosis, Churg-Strauss syndrome, microscopic polyangiitis, and Henoch-Schönlein purpura.

a. **Wegener granulomatosis** involves the upper respiratory tract, lungs, and kidneys.

   (1) It is associated with **c-ANCA** (antineutrophil cytoplasmic antibody-cytoplasmic pattern).

   (2) It is characterized by necrotizing vasculitis and granulomatous inflammation (Figure 6–9).

   (3) Diagnosis is best made by paranasal sinus biopsy.

   (4) Renal involvement is characterized by a necrotizing segmental glomerulonephritis, which is not specific.

b. **Churg-Strauss syndrome** is a multisystem vasculitis mainly involving the **respiratory** tract.

   (1) It presents with allergic rhinitis, severe **asthma,** fever, and elevated blood **eosinophil** count.

   (2) Involvement of other organs (eg, central nervous system (CNS) is associated with a poor prognosis.

   (3) Biopsy shows a necrotizing eosinophilic inflammatory process and granulomas.

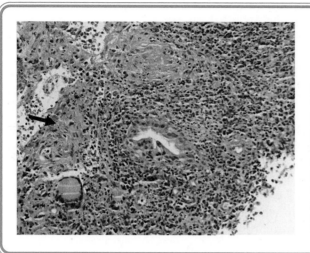

Figure 6–9. Vasculitis. Vasculitis is characterized by inflammation of small (arrow), medium, or large blood vessels. The size of the vessel, site of involvement (nasal biopsy in this case), and serologic studies (c-ANCA) may narrow the differential diagnosis (eg, Wegener granulomatosis).

(4) The diagnosis depends on the triad of asthma, eosinophilia, and biopsy-proven vasculitis.

c. **Microscopic polyangiitis** is a multisystem vasculitis with **pulmonary, renal**, and peripheral **nerve** involvement.
   (1) It is a nongranulomatous necrotizing vasculitis.
   (2) It is associated with a positive **p-ANCA.**

d. **Henoch-Schönlein purpura** occurs mainly in **children.**
   (1) It involves the **skin, gastrointestinal tract,** and **kidneys.**
   (2) The skin biopsy shows a **leukocytoclastic vasculitis** with fibrinoid necrosis, involving superficial dermal vessels and an **IgA** deposition by immunofluorescence.
   (3) Renal biopsy will typically reveal a proliferative glomerulonephritis, which can appear similar to **IgA nephropathy** (see Chapter 10).

LEUKOCYTOCLASTIC VASCULITIS

- *Skin involvement presents as "**palpable purpura**."*
- *The purpuric lesions typically affect the lower extremities.*
- *On biopsy, the superficial dermal vessels will show fibrinoid change, infiltration by neutrophils, and perivascular debris.*
- *Leukocytoclastic vasculitis can be seen in systemic vasculitic syndromes, or isolated to the skin.*
- *When isolated to the skin, it is often secondary to medications, viral infections, or neoplasia.*

   3. Medium-vessel vasculitides include polyarteritis nodosa and Kawasaki disease.

a. **Polyarteritis nodosa** is a necrotizing vasculitis that involves the arteries of **skin, gastrointestinal tract,** and **kidney.**
   (1) Pulmonary involvement is rare.
   (2) The disease is related to chronic **hepatitis B** infection, but can also be associated with hepatitis C and HIV.
   (3) Patients can have a positive **antinuclear antibody (ANA) test** and low levels of complement, suggesting an immune-complex pathophysiology.
   (4) Diagnosis is made by biopsy, or angiography.

b. **Kawasaki disease** is also called **mucocutaneous syndrome**.

  (1) It typically occurs in children.

  (2) The medium-sized vasculitis is usually self-limited, but **coronary aneurysms** can occur (20% of patients).

  (3) It also involves the gastrointestinal tract (muco) and skin (cutaneous).

BUERGER DISEASE

- *Thromboangiitis obliterans is a distinct vasculitis occurring in young **male smokers**.*
- *Patients have an increased prevalence of HLA-A9 and HLA-B5.*
- *Medium-sized arteries of the upper and lower extremities, especially the **tibial** and **radial** arteries, are involved.*
- *Biopsy shows segmental and transmural acute and chronic inflammation with thrombosis.*

  4. **Large-vessel vasculitides** include giant-cell arteritis and Takayasu arteritis.

  a. **Giant-cell arteritis** is a common vasculitis involving patients over age 50 (1/5000 people).

  (1) Clinical presentation is characterized by headache, tenderness over the **temporal** artery, and **visual** symptoms.

  (2) The most common laboratory finding is elevated erythrocyte sedimentation rate (ESR).

  (3) Diagnosis is confirmed by temporal artery biopsy, which shows a transmural chronic inflammatory infiltrate and disruption of the internal elastic lamina.

  b. **Takayasu arteritis** is rare and is most prevalent in young women (age 10–40 years, >80% in women).

  (1) Clinical presentation is characterized by **fever,** night sweats, weight loss, and **ischemia** of involved organs.

  (2) This disease is also called the **"pulseless disease"** due to stenosis of the subclavian artery.

  (3) Diagnosis is usually made by clinical and radiographic findings, because tissue biopsies of the large deep blood vessels (aortic arch, carotids, subclavian, and renal vessels) would result in excessive morbidity.

  (4) Tissue shows granulomatous inflammation of large arteries associated with lumen narrowing or aneurysm.

E. Vascular Malformations and Neoplasia

  1. **Arteriovenous malformations** are a developmental anomaly characterized by abnormal vascular proliferation and connections.

  a. The lesion may be a connection between an artery and vein or proliferation of small capillaries or larger blood vessels.

  b. They may occur anywhere, including skin, brain, and viscera.

  (1) An arteriovenous malformation in the brain may be a source of thrombosis and stroke, requiring "coiling."

  (2) Malformations in the nose, lungs, and gastrointestinal tract may present as bleeding.

  (3) Small benign capillary proliferations in the skin, so- called telangiectasias, increase in number with age, liver disease (**spider telangiectasias**), and may also be a sign of an underlying genetic disorder (Osler-Weber-Rendu).

OSLER-WEBER-RENDU DISEASE

- *Osler-Weber-Rendu disease (also called hereditary hemorrhagic telangiectasia [HHT]) is an autosomal dominant (**endoglin** gene, **ALK1** gene) vascular dysplasia leading to telangiectasias of the skin, mucosa, and viscera.*
- *It may be clinically silent with a mild increase in the frequency of nosebleeds (epistaxis) or gastrointestinal bleeding.*
- *It may be lethal with vascular malformations in the lungs or brain, leading to hemorrhage and death.*
- *The diagnosis is subtle and requires attention to the possibility of HHT in families with frequent nosebleeds and conspicuous cutaneous telangiectasias.*

    c. **Nevus flammeus** (eg, **"port-wine stain"**) is an ordinary birthmark composed of dilated vessels in the dermis; the **Sturge-Weber syndrome** is characterized by port-wine stain in a trigeminal nerve distribution.

2. **Lymphangioma** is a proliferation and dilation of lymphatics.
   a. **Lymphangioma circumscriptum** is a malformation, not a neoplasm, that involves the dermis in infancy; it consists of a well-circumscribed nodule of dilated lymphatic channels.
   b. **Progressive lymphangioma** is a benign slow-growing neoplasm involving the dermis in adults; it consists of an infiltrative appearing tumor composed of dilated lymphatic channels.

3. **Hemangiomas** are benign.
   a. They can be several centimeters in size and are usually red/blue lesions in the dermis, submucosa, or viscera that can be flat or nodular.
   b. Microscopically, they are lobulated, well-circumscribed, and composed of closely packed thin-walled capillaries.
   c. **Hemangioma of infancy** is a proliferation of benign capillaries that may rapidly enlarge during the first year of life, but then **involutes**.
      (1) The distinction from other hemangiomas is significant because of this difference in natural history.
      (2) The distinction may be made by positive immunostaining for **GLUT1** (placental antigen!).
   d. **Cavernous hemangiomas** are a common subtype of hemangioma that are benign, but more commonly involve the viscera and can be locally aggressive leading to clinical symptoms.
      (1) They can involve the central nervous system in a rare entity called **von Hippel-Lindau disease.**
      (2) Clinically, they can mimic malignant neoplasms.
      (3) These lesions are larger with dilated vascular spaces, sometimes with thrombosis and calcification.

4. **Pyogenic granuloma** is a benign lobulated capillary hemangioma that arises in response to **traumatic** injury (eg, after surgery) or hormones (eg, **pregnancy**).
   a. It predominantly occurs in young pregnant women (**granuloma gravidarum**) and regresses after delivery.
   b. The oral cavity and hands are common sites.
   c. Histologic sections show an ulcer with underlying capillary proliferation in a background of acute inflammation.
   d. Excision is the treatment of choice.

5. **Glomus tumor** is a **painful** small (<1cm) benign neoplasm that usually involves the **fingers**.

a. It is derived from the glomus body, a modified **smooth muscle** cell involved in **thermoregulation.**

b. Excision is the treatment of choice.

6. **Kaposi sarcoma** is associated with human herpesvirus 8 (HHV-8).

a. **HHV-8** is a sexually transmitted.

b. It is common in **Mediterranean** countries and **Africa.**

c. The prevalence is low in the United States (except with **HIV**).

d. Kaposi sarcoma has three stages:

(1) Patch

(2) Plaque

(3) Nodular

e. The lesions are grossly red-purple, solitary to multiple, spread proximally, and often become coalescent.

f. On microscopic examination, it is a hypercellular spindle cell proliferation with intervening slit-like spaces containing red blood cells.

g. There are three main classifications of Kaposi sarcoma.

(1) Classic Kaposi sarcoma (described by Kaposi in 1872) is seen in older **Mediterranean** men and usually presents in the lower **extremities.**

(2) **African** Kaposi sarcoma is prevalent in South Africa; it involves **lymph nodes** with very little skin involvement, and follows an **aggressive** clinical course.

(3) **HIV**-associated Kaposi sarcoma is more common than the other two forms and is a leading AIDS-associated tumor.

7. **Bacillary angiomatosis** is also associated with immunosuppression, especially HIV/AIDS.

a. Clinically, it can resemble Kaposi sarcoma but is more nodular, commonly involving the skin, bones, and organs.

b. Bacillary peliosis involves viscera.

c. The causative organism is *Bartonella henselae*, which also causes **cat-scratch** disease in immunocompetent patients.

d. The best way to distinguish bacillary angiomatosis from pyogenic granuloma is a modified **silver stain**, which will demonstrate the causative organism.

8. **Angiosarcoma** can occur anywhere there are **blood vessels.**

a. They most commonly occur in the head and neck of the elderly.

b. Previous **radiation** therapy (eg, post–**breast** cancer treatment) and **lymphedema** (acquired and congenital forms) increase the risk of developing angiosarcoma.

c. **Polyvinyl chlorides**, arsenicals, Thorotrast (radiographic contrast material) increases the risk, especially in the liver.

d. Microscopically, the cells of angiosarcoma can be **spindled** or **epithelioid,** with enlarged, hyperchromatic nuclei; sometimes they will make intracytoplasmic lumens resembling **capillaries.**

(1) Angiosarcoma may be challenging pathologic diagnosis, because low-grade tumors resemble hemangiomas and high-grade tumors resemble carcinoma and melanoma.

(2) Tumor cells stain for endothelial markers **CD31** and CD34.

CLINICAL PROBLEMS

1. An 82-year-old woman has syncope. On her physical examination, she is found to have a systolic murmur. An echocardiogram is performed showing significant left ventricular hypertrophy and an abnormal cardiac valve. Which one of the following is **FALSE?**

   A. This condition is likely associated with a bicuspid aortic valve

   B. Left atrial enlargement will also be found on the echocardiogram

   C. This condition can present with congestive heart failure

   D. Histologic sections of myocardium would show box-car nuclei

   E. All the above

2. The patient complains of 'ripping' chest pain radiating to his back and down his left arm. A chest radiograph shows a widened mediastinum. Which of the following may be associated with this disease?

   A. Mutation in the fibrillin gene

   B. Hypertension

   C. Severe atherosclerosis

   D. Trauma

   E. All the above

3. A 45-year-old man is shoveling snow from his sidewalk when he suddenly collapses and dies. Which one of the following statements is **FALSE?**

   A. The heart may appear grossly normal

   B. Sections of his myocardium show granulation tissue

   C. Left anterior descending coronary artery is occluded

   D. He may have had a history of smoking and hypertension

   E. Left ventricular hypertrophy indicates hypertensive disease

4. A pregnant woman has a bleeding nodule growing on her tongue. Which of the following likely describes the lesion?

   A. Microscopic sections of the lesion would show nests of small basophilic cells with peripheral palisading and cleft artifact

   B. Microscopic sections would show a proliferation of squamous cells with atypia and abnormal keratinization

   C. Microscopic sections would show a proliferation of capillaries with reactive endothelial cells and abundant neutrophils

   D. Microscopic sections would show dense bands of collagen with vertically oriented vessels

   E. Microscopic sections would show acanthosis of the squamous epithelium with parakeratosis and elongation of the rete ridges

5. A patient has nosebleeds, fever, and a cough. A chest radiograph shows bilateral nodular densities in both lung fields. An erythrocyte sedimentation rate is greater than 100 mm/h. An ANCA test is positive. Which one of the following statements is **FALSE**?

   A. Microscopic examination of lung biopsy material could show vessels with necrosis and granulomatous inflammation

   B. This disorder is commonly associated with palpable purpura

   C. The nasal cavity and sinuses may be involved

   D. The patient may have renal involvement

   E. The patient would have a positive c-ANCA

6. Symptoms of congestive heart failure have developed in a 22-year-old man over the last few weeks. He undergoes an evaluation including an echocardiogram, which shows a depressed ejection fraction but no signs of valve disease. Coronary angiography shows no significant obstructive lesions. An endomyocardial biopsy is performed. Which of the following findings would be **MOST LIKELY**?

   A. Marked myocyte hypertrophy with interstitial fibrosis

   B. An inflammatory infiltrate with associated myocyte injury

   C. Deposition of a waxy hyaline substance

   D. Marked fibroelastosis of the endocardium

   E. Marked infiltration by eosinophils

7. A 54-year-old man suddenly dies while eating a meal in a restaurant. Autopsy reveals an area of firm, well-demarcated white discoloration involving the lateral portion of the left ventricle. Several of the coronary arteries show atherosclerotic lesions, none of which are substantially obstructive. There is some degree of left ventricular hypertrophy. Which of the following statements is **FALSE**?

   A. Analysis of the vitreous fluid may be helpful in this scenario

   B. The manner of death is likely due to natural causes

   C. The findings suggest an acute massive myocardial infarction

   D. The presence of a 'nutmeg' pattern of the liver may indicate the presence of congestive cardiac failure

   E. The patient's medical doctor should be contacted for more history

8. A 37-year-old woman has progressive dyspnea, cough, and fever. A chest radiograph shows bilateral infiltrates. She also notes dark brown urine. Which of the following statements is **FALSE**?

   A. Low levels of serum complement may be seen

   B. Blood cultures should be performed

   C. Serum ANCA should be performed

   D. The differential diagnosis includes systemic lupus erythematosus

   E. Polyarteritis nodosa is the most likely diagnosis

9. A 19-year-old man arrives at the hospital following an episode of syncope at school. His physical examination is normal. An electrocardiogram is unremarkable. An

echocardiogram is performed and demonstrates a pedunculated mass within the left atrium. Which of the following statements is **FALSE**?

A. Metastases are more common than primary cardiac tumors

B. Cardiac myxoma usually presents in the right atrium

C. Cardiac rhabdomyoma is associated with tuberous sclerosis

D. Angiosarcoma is the most common malignant primary heart neoplasm

E. Patients with familial atrial myxoma can have associated skin lentigines, adrenocortical nodular dysplasia, and large cell calcifying Sertoli cell tumor of the testis (Carney syndrome)

10. A 32-year-old man arrives at the emergency department with 12 hours of progressively worsening chest pain. The pain is sharp and radiates to his back and left shoulder. His physical examination is unremarkable. Which of the following statements is **FALSE**?

A. Normal myoglobin and troponin I excludes myocardial infarction

B. A normal chest radiograph does not rule out aortic dissection

C. The pain may be musculoskeletal in origin

D. The pain may be gastrointestinal in origin

E. An elevated myoglobin would be indicative of myocardial damage

ANSWERS

1. The answer is A. A bicuspid aortic valve with complicating aortic stenosis typically presents much earlier in life than calcific degenerative aortic stenosis of a tricuspid aortic valve.

2. The answer is E. Aortic dissection is associated with Marfan syndrome (fibrillin gene), hypertension, atherosclerosis, and trauma.

3. The answer is B. Sudden death likely occurs from an acute thrombus occluding a coronary artery leading to acute infarction, arrhythmia, and death. The heart may appear grossly normal. Hours after the infarction, microscopic examination may show "wavy" myocytes, but no inflammation; a day later neutrophils; a week later granulation tissue forms.

4. The answer is C. Pyogenic granuloma is a benign hyperplasia of capillaries that may arise after trauma (eg, surgery) and sometimes de novo in pregnant women.

5. The answer is B. Palpable purpura is associated with leukocytoclastic vasculitis. Wegener granulomatosis is associated with a positive c-ANCA (proteinase-3). It involves the upper respiratory tract, lungs, and kidneys.

6. The answer is B. Given the history and test findings, myocarditis is the most likely answer. Option 'a' described findings of a hypertrophic cardiomyopathy, which would have been easily seen on the echocardiogram. Option 'c' describes amyloidosis, also

easily diagnosed based on clues seen on the echocardiogram. Option 'd' and 'e' describe endocardial fibroelastosis and Löffler endomyocarditis, respectively.

7. The answer is C. The gross appearance of the myocardium is indicative of a prior myocardial infarction. Several late complications can occur after a myocardial infarction, including congestive heart failure and arrhythmia. When unwitnessed death occurs outside of the hospital, the decedent's medical provider should always be contacted for more history.

8. The answer is E. Polyarteritis nodosa typically does not involve the pulmonary vessels.

9. The answer is B. Myxomas of the heart most often occur in the left atrium, arising from the atrial septum near the fossa ovalis. Metastatic tumors are more common. The familial tumor syndromes are a favorite of the boards, including Carney syndrome (compare to Carney triad).

10. The answer is E. While myoglobin is elevated in myocardial damage, it is nonspecific and can be elevated due to any skeletal muscle injury.

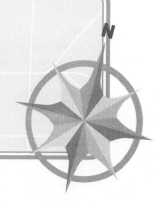

CHAPTER 7
LUNG

. . . the child that tastes of salt when kissed
—ancient European folklore

I. Congenital Anomalies

A. Bronchopulmonary Anomalies

1. **Pulmonary hypoplasia** may arise from the absence of amniotic fluid during lung development (eg, Potter sequence: renal agenesis → oligohydramnios → pulmonary hypoplasia).

2. Most cysts are residual **bronchogenic**, esophageal, or enteric primitive foregut that develop into **cysts** around the **hilum**.

3. **Congenital cystic adenomatoid malformations** are hamartomas in the lungs leading to few (type 1) or multiple (types 2–3) cysts.
   a. Type 1 is most common and more easily treated by surgery.
   b. Type 3 is least common and has a poor prognosis.

4. Pulmonary sequestration is a complete or partial separation of a bronchial segment from the bronchial tree (no airway connection).
   a. **Intralobar sequestrations** are enclosed by lung pleura and prone to recurrent infections.
   b. **Extralobar sequestrations** are not associated with the lungs and may be found anywhere in the thorax.

LUNG BUDS

- The respiratory diverticulum (lung bud) arises from the ventral wall of the foregut during the fourth week of gestation.
- Tracheoesophageal ridges separate this rudimentary pouch from the dorsally located esophagus.
- The lung bud develops caudally into two main bronchi which, in turn, branch as three secondary bronchi on the right and two on the left.
- As the individual bronchioles continue to divide, the alveolar epithelium changes from flattened cuboidal to type I pneumocytes, so gas exchange becomes possible by the seventh month.
- Type II pneumocytes produce surfactant that reduces surface tension, thereby preventing alveolar collapse during expiration.

B. **Cystic Fibrosis**
   1. Cystic fibrosis is the most common lethal genetic disease affecting people of Northern European descent.
      a. The incidence in whites is 1/3200; blacks 1/15,000.
      b. It is an **autosomal recessive gene** and many **Northern European** whites are heterozygous carriers (1/20).
   2. The primary defect results from abnormal function of an epithelial **chloride channel** protein encoded by the *CFTR* gene on 7q31.2.
      a. The effects are widespread, leading to thick mucoid fluids in the respiratory tract, gastrointestinal tract, reproductive tract, pancreatic ducts, and abnormal epidermal salt secretion.
      b. The clinical consequences are obstruction, including bronchiectasis, meconium ileus, infertility, pancreatic insufficiency, and abnormal sweat test (5× increase in NaCl).
   3. Pulmonary changes are the most serious complication.
      a. Thick mucus secretions lead to obstruction of bronchioles giving rise to bronchiectasis and superimposed lung infections (***Pseudomonas aeruginosa, Haemophilus influenzae***, and ***Staphylococcus aureus***).
      b. Recurrent infection is common and abscesses may form.
      c. By age 18, most patients suffer from chronic ***Pseudomonas* infection**.
   4. Cardiopulmonary complications, including chronic obstructive pulmonary disease (**COPD**), and right-sided heart failure (**cor pulmonale**) are the most common causes of death.
   5. Improved control of infections and lung transplantation surgery have improved life expectancy (median age of survival is 37 years).

II. Pulmonary Infections

A. **Pneumonia**
   1. Pneumonia is defined by the clinical pattern and causative organism (Table 7–1).
   2. Symptoms include respiratory distress, productive cough, tachycardia, and fever.
   3. Signs of pulmonary consolidation, such as crackling breath sounds, egophony, and dullness to percussion, are often present.
   4. **Acute community-acquired pneumonia** (CAP) is caused by a diverse array of bacteria.
      a. ***Streptococcus pneumoniae***, also known as pneumococcus, is an encapsulated, α-hemolytic, gram-positive diplococcus, and it is the leading cause of CAP requiring hospital admission.
      b. ***H influenzae*** is a gram-negative coccobacillus with six serotypes (a–f); children are now routinely vaccinated against the most virulent strain, type b.
      c. ***Moraxella catarrhalis*** is a gram-negative diplococcus, and although it remains a leading cause of **otitis media** in children, it may also cause lower respiratory tract infections.
      d. ***S aureus*** (the Greek *staphyle*, meaning "a bunch of grapes," affixed to the Latin *aureus*, meaning "golden") describes the microscopic (clusters of gram-positive cocci) and the gross (creamy yellow colonies) features of the organism.
      e. ***Klebsiella pneumoniae*** is a gram-negative rod that is commonly implicated in cases involving **aspiration of gastric contents**, and it is characterized by parenchymal hemorrhage resulting in thick, bloody, mucoid sputum classically described as "currant jelly sputum."

Table 7–1. The clinical pattern of pneumonia and common causative organisms.

Variant	Clinical Pattern	Common Causative Organisms
Bronchopneumonia	Patchy multifocal consolidation	*Streptococcus pneumoniae, Staphylococcus aureus, Haemophilus influenzae, Escherichia coli, Klebsiella pneumoniae, Enterobacter, Pseudomonas aeruginosa;* anaerobes
Lobar pneumonia	Lobar consolidation	*S pneumoniae*
Atypical pneumonia	Inflammation within alveolar interstitium	*Mycoplasma, Legionella,* viral (adenovirus, influenza, respiratory syncytial virus)

  f. *P aeruginosa* is a gram-negative rod that has a characteristic **sweet, fruity odor**.

  g. *Legionella pneumophila* is a weakly gram-negative, aquatic bacillus with two clinical presentations.

   (1) The genus *Legionella* was named after an outbreak of severe pneumonia among the attendees of an American Legion convention during the US bicentennial celebration in Philadelphia **(legionnaires disease).**

   (2) A milder, non-pneumonic variant is known as **Pontiac fever** following an outbreak in Michigan in 1968.

 B. Atypical ("Walking") Pneumonia

  1. Walking pneumonia is named for its characteristically protracted course with gradual resolution, as well as its lack of alveolar exudate, and its multifactorial etiology (Table 7–2).

  2. *Mycoplasma pneumoniae* is a common cause of walking pneumonia.

   a. Infection by *M pneumoniae* may be distinguished from viral atypical pneumonia by the presence of elevated **serum cold agglutinins** in approximately half of *Mycoplasma* infections.

   b. The **absence of a cell wall** limits the effectiveness of antibiotics such as penicillins, cephalosporins, and vancomycin, but a full recovery from mycoplasmal pneumonia can be expected with a macrolide (azithromycin or erythromycin).

  3. Severe acute respiratory syndrome (SARS) quickly garnered worldwide attention when more than 8000 cases with over 700 deaths were reported in 2002 and 2003.

   a. Although apparently originating in China, local transmission was reported in several areas of Southeast Asia as well as in San Francisco, Vancouver, and Toronto.

   b. The causative agent is the **SARS coronavirus** (SARS-CoV), a positive-sense, single-stranded RNA virus, which produces nonspecific symptoms

Table 7–2. Clinical features of different types of atypical pneumonia.

Condition	Clinical Features
Mycoplasma	Most common atypical pneumonia; young adults; paroxysmal cough; positive cold-agglutinin test
Psittacosis (*Chlamydia*)	Inhalation of dried infectious bird feces
Q fever (*Coxiella burnetii*)	Most common rickettsial pneumonia; infected dust or unpasteurized milk
Rabbit fever (*Tulleremia*)	Rare, but highly infectious; veterinarians, hunters
Respiratory syncytial virus	Higher incidence during winter; infants
Histoplasmosis	Endemic to Midwest river valleys
Coccidioidomycosis ("Valley fever")	Endemic to southwestern United States (especially California's San Joaquin valley)
Blastomycosis	Endemic to central and southeastern United States and Ontario
Cryptococcosis	Pigeon feces, bird nests, and guano; immunocompromised
Pneumocystis (PCP)	AIDS-defining opportunistic infection

including fever above 38 °C, cough, myalgia, and gastrointestinal complaints, followed by profound respiratory distress often requiring mechanical ventilation.

C. Tuberculosis (TB)
1. TB is an infection by ***Mycobacterium tuberculosis***.
2. TB is the leading fatal infectious disease worldwide with approximately
3. **million deaths** annually.
   a. Humans are the only known reservoir for *M tuberculosis*.
   b. It is estimated that 50% of humans may be carriers!
3. The most frequent route of transmission is inhalation of droplets expelled from an infected host.
   a. Once drawn into the airspaces, the bacilli are ingested by pulmonary macrophages and transported to regional lymph nodes.
   b. The inoculum required for infection is relatively small, as few as 10 organisms per droplet may cause infection.
4. *M tuberculosis* is slow-growing and incites a chronic histiocytic "necrotizing granulomatous" response (Figure 7–1).
   a. Patients should submit sputum for smear and culture.

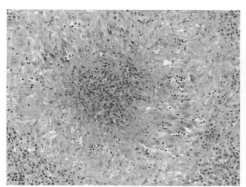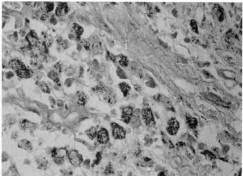

Figure 7–1. Tuberculosis and necrotizing granulomatous disease. Histologic sections of the lung reveal nodules of histiocytes with necrotic centers. Staining sections for acid-fast bacteria (AFB) shows histiocytes filled with "red snappers," elongated AFB, tuberculosis.

    b. The bacilli require at least 4 weeks for visible growth on solid **Lowenstein-Jensen culture media**.

    c. Because the bacilli retain many stains after decoloration with acid-alcohol, they are often referred to as **acid-fast bacilli** (AFB) (Figure 7–1).

5. Infection follows one of several patterns depending on the sites of involvement and the host response.

    a. Pulmonary TB typically presents with a productive cough (occasionally with hemoptysis), fever accompanied by "**drenching night sweats**," anorexia, and weight loss.

    b. Tuberculous spondylitis (**Pott disease**) is an extrapulmonary extension usually to the **thoracic spine**.

    c. Infected lymph nodes may become completely replaced by chronic granulomatous inflammation with **caseous** necrosis, the so-called **tuberculous lymphadenitis** (scrofula).

    d. Less commonly, there may be genitourinary, gastrointestinal, meningitic, and cutaneous (lupus vulgaris) involvement.

6. The **tuberculin skin test** provides surveillance and screening.

    a. A standard amount of purified protein derivative (PPD skin test) is injected intradermally, and the amount of induration between 48 hours and 72 hours at the injection site is a surrogate for immune response and hence previous exposure.

    b. Results must be correlated with the patient's age and individual known risk factors, including immunosuppression.

7. Treatment is a prolonged course of antibiotics; failure to follow this regimen encourages the development of resistant TB strains.

III. Acute Lung Injury

    A. Pulmonary Edema

        1. Fluid extravasation from the pulmonary capillary vasculature into the alveoli and interstitium leads to pulmonary edema.

2. There are several etiologies, but they may be grouped into three primary pathophysiologic mechanisms.

  a. The **alveolar-capillary barrier** may become more porous, allowing extravasation of fluid and cells.

  b. An **imbalance of Starling forces** (increased pulmonary capillary pressure or decreased plasma oncotic pressure) will draw fluid from the vasculature into the tissue.

  c. **Lymphatic obstruction,** often secondary to mass effect of a tumor, will cause upstream lymphatic congestion.

3. Chest radiography is used to distinguish cardiogenic from other forms of pulmonary edema.

  a. Enlargement of the cardiac silhouette, basilar edema, bilateral pleural effusions, and **Kerley lines** are all suggestive of **cardiogenic** pulmonary edema.

  b. Diffuse edema is more characteristic of noncardiogenic etiologies.

4. Serum levels of **brain natriuretic peptide** (BNP) also help differentiate congestive heart failure from pulmonary causes.

  a. BNP is an endogenous hormone secreted by the cardiac ventricles in response to increased filling pressures.

  b. Values between 100 pg/mL and 400 pg/mL are nonspecific indicators of cor pulmonale and embolism.

5. Histology shows a proteinaceous fluid exudate into alveoli.

KERLEY LINES

- *Kerley lines are the radiographic evidence of pulmonary fluid accumulation.*
- *Kerley A lines are typically longer, located within the inner half of the lungs, and course diagonally toward the hila. These represent distention of lymphatic channels.*
- *Kerley B lines are more commonly observed, are located toward the subpleural surfaces, and usually indicate pulmonary edema.*

  B. Acute Respiratory Distress Syndrome (ARDS)

  1. ARDS is a severe form of acute lung injury, which is clinically characterized by dyspnea, profound hypoxemia, decreased lung compliance, and diffuse bilateral infiltrates on a chest radiograph.

  2. There are many causes, including severe infection, trauma, drugs, and collagen vascular diseases.

  3. **Diffuse alveolar damage (DAD)** is the histologic counterpart of ARDS and displays a sequence of histologic phases from early to late.

    a. During the acute exudative phase, there is intra-alveolar edema and hemorrhage.

    b. In the later fibrotic phase, fibroblasts proliferate and replace the damaged alveoli and interstitial tissue with relatively less compliant scar.

  4. Pulmonary function typically does not return to baseline following resolution of DAD.

TRANSFUSION-RELATED ACUTE LUNG INJURY (TRALI)

- *TRALI is currently the leading cause of transfusion mortality.*
- *Donor antibodies to recipient leukocyte antigens activate complement and encourage granulocytes to aggregate within the pulmonary microvasculature.*

- *The diagnosis is based on clinical findings that are similar to ARDS but arise within **6 hours** after transfusion.*
- *TRALI has a 5–10% mortality rate, but with interim ventilatory support, most symptoms resolve within 96 hours.*

IV. Obstructive Pulmonary Diseases

A. Chronic Bronchitis

1. Clinical diagnosis requires a chronic productive cough for **3 months** during at least **2 successive years** in the absence of any other etiology.
2. Subsequent impairment of mucociliary clearance of bacteria and mucus progressively limits alveolar gas exchange.
   a. Compensatory changes in pulmonary blood flow through poorly ventilated lungs results in hypoxemia, hypercapnia, and respiratory acidosis.
   b. Pulmonary artery vasoconstriction and cor pulmonale gives patients the gross appearance of "**blue bloaters**."
   c. Accumulated secretions lead to bacterial infections.

B. Emphysema

1. Like chronic bronchitis, the symptoms of emphysema include both cough and shortness of breath.
2. The destruction of alveolar walls and the relative dilation of the remaining airspaces are grossly evident, leading to bullae (Figure 7–2).

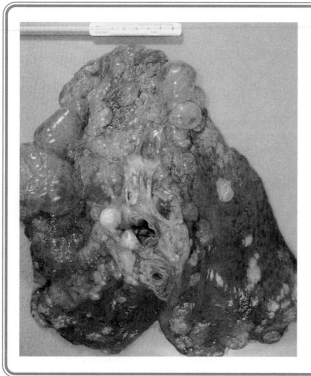

Figure 7–2. Emphysematous bullae in a lung from an elderly man with a long history of smoking and chronic obstructive pulmonary disease. Bullae may rupture leading to pneumothorax.

a. The irreversible loss of individual alveoli has two consequences: the loss of elasticity essential for effective exhalation, and decreased surface area for gas exchange.

b. Compensation requires hyperventilation.

c. Low flow through a relatively well-oxygenated lung leads to muscle wasting in patients giving them the gross appearance of "**pink puffers.**"

d. **Tobacco smoke** is the leading cause of emphysema.

e. A rare cause of emphysema is **α_1-antitrypsin deficiency**; it leads to **panacinar emphysema** (rather than centrilobar) that is also accelerated by smoking tobacco.

THE EFFECTS OF SMOKING

- *Tobacco smoke consists of a complex mix of pulmonary irritants, including acetone, ammonia, arsenic, formaldehyde, nicotine, carbon monoxide, hydrogen cyanide, tar, cadmium, and toluene.*
- *Chronic exposure to these substances encourages the leukocyte-mediated damage of respiratory mucosa and the development of subsequent chronic bronchitis and emphysema.*
- *Tobacco smoke may also exacerbate asthma symptoms.*
- *Squamous cell carcinoma and small cell carcinoma are strongly associated with a history of smoking.*

    C. **Asthma**

      1. Asthma affects **5% of people** and usually presents in **childhood**.

      2. Clinical manifestations include cough, shortness of breath, and **wheezing** reversible with a bronchodilator (eg, albuterol).

        a. The lung fields may appear hyperinflated on chest films as the decreased airway caliber prevents effective expiration.

        b. Common triggers may be **environmental** allergens (extrinsic asthma) or vigorous **exercise** (intrinsic asthma).

        c. Further diagnostic evaluation may include pulmonary function tests (spirometry), peak-flow monitoring, serum eosinophil and IgE levels, and methacholine- or histamine-challenge testing.

      3. Although microscopy is rarely part of the routine asthma workup, several findings are quite characteristic.

        a. There is bronchial smooth muscle hypertrophy.

        b. Eosinophil-derived protein crystalloids (**Charcot-Leyden crystals**), and mucus (**Curschmann spirals**) may be seen.

      4. Asthma is usually effectively managed by bronchodilator, but corticosteroids are used when necessary.

      5. **Status asthmaticus** is an acute, severe attack that does not respond to the usual asthma therapies; it can be life-threatening and requires immediate medical attention.

ATOPY

- *Atopy is an exaggerated tendency to respond to common environmental allergens with increased serum levels of IgE and eosinophils.*
- *Asthma, allergic rhinitis, and eczema (the **atopy triad**) are often clinically associated with each other.*
- *Early exposure to certain infections (hepatitis A virus and mycobacteria), indoor contaminants (pet dander), or particulate air pollution have been correlated with lower incidence of allergic conditions, so genetically determined susceptibility may be modified by subsequent environmental conditions.*

D. Bronchiectasis
   1. Bronchiectasis is an **irreversible bronchial dilation** caused by the destruction of the airway wall and subsequent accumulation of mucus, inflammation, and infection.
   2. Bronchial **obstruction** is the leading cause of bronchiectasis (eg, tumor or cystic fibrosis).
   3. Patients typically have a productive cough, dyspnea, and wheezing.
      a. A chest radiograph may show parallel linear markings (tram tracks) radiating from the hila into the lower lung lobes.
      b. **Hemoptysis** indicates damage to dilated bronchial arteries.
   4. The constellation of bronchiectasis, sinusitis, hearing loss, and decreased fertility is suggestive of **Kartagener syndrome**, an ultrastructural defect in ciliary microtubules lining the upper respiratory tract and eustachian tubes.

V. Diffuse Interstitial Disease

   A. Pulmonary Fibrosis
      1. Idiopathic pulmonary fibrosis is a chronic, progressive fibrosis of the lung interstitium.
         a. As the name implies, the pathogenesis has not yet been determined.
         b. Lung transplantation is sometimes attempted, but the overall prognosis is poor.
         c. Biopsy reveals characteristic differences in "**space and time**" with patchy fibroblastic foci (Figure 7–3), the so-called **usual interstitial pneumonia** (UIP).
      2. Nonspecific interstitial pneumonia (NIP) displays more uniform involvement of alveolar septae.
      3. **Bronchiolitis obliterans organizing pneumonia** (BOOP) is a form of organizing pneumonia marked by fibroblastic proliferations that extend into the lumina of terminal bronchioles.
         a. At least half of all cases are idiopathic (cryptogenic organizing pneumonia).

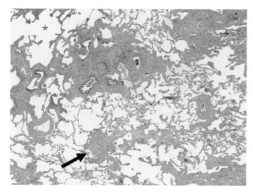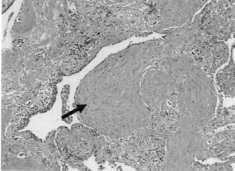

Figure 7–3. Honeycomb lung. Usual interstitial pneumonia with variation in histologic pattern (ruptured dilated alveoli and solid areas of scar tissue and temporal sequence (some solid areas are new myofibroblastic proliferations, arrow other areas are fibrotic).

Table 7–3. Common pneumoconioses.

Condition	Mineral Dust (common sources)
Anthracosis	Carbon dust (urban, smoker)
Asbestosis	Asbestos (old insulation)
Baritosis	Barium dust (mining)
Berylliosis	Beryllium (aviation, electronics)
Coal pneumoconiosis	Coal dust (carbon and silica)
Silicosis	Silica dust (glasswork, masonry)

      b. BOOP has also been associated with multiple conditions including infections, collagen vascular diseases, malignancies, drug toxicity, and radiation therapy.

      c. Unlike UIP and NIP that have no effective treatment, some cases may be controlled by continued corticosteroid therapy.

   4. **Pneumoconioses** result from inhaled mineral dusts (Table 7–3).

      a. Anthracosis, a consequence of urban living, is apparent grossly as irregular patches of black discoloration and microscopically as dark particles engulfed by macrophages.

      b. **Ferruginous bodies** are asbestos fibers coated with endogenous iron and calcium (see inset in Figure 7–6).

      c. Inhalation of asbestos, coal dust, or silicates has been linked to **Caplan syndrome**, the concurrence of rheumatoid arthritis and pneumoconiosis.

      d. Silicosis also confers an increased susceptibility to TB, a combination known as **silicotuberculosis.**

 B. Interstitial Granulomatous Disease

   1. **Hypersensitivity pneumonitis** results from exuberant antibody production to an inhaled substance.

      a. Acute symptoms include dyspnea, fever, and cough within 4–6 hours after heavy exposure; recurrent or chronic exposure may induce permanent fibrosis.

      b. Numerous antigens have been reported (Table 7–4).

      c. Biopsy findings reveal interstitial chronic inflammation and poorly formed noncaseating granulomas.

   2. **Sarcoidosis** is usually a diagnosis of exclusion.

      a. It is most common in young (20- to 50-year-old) **African Americans** (females are affected more than males).

      b. Clinical symptoms include nonproductive cough, dyspnea, chest pain, fever, and unintended weight loss.

      c. Chest radiograph may show bilateral **hilar adenopathy**.

      d. Lung or thoracic lymph node biopsy usually shows noncaseating **"naked" epithelioid granulomas.**

Table 7–4. Antigens associated with hypersensitivity pneumonitis.

Conditions	Environmental antigens
Byssinosis	Airborne cotton, linen, and hemp
Cheese washer lung	Fungi (*Penicillium casei*) in casings
Farmer's lung	Thermophilic actinomycetes in hay
Humidifier lung	Thermophilic bacteria in water heaters
Hot tub lung	*Mycobacterium avium* complex
Malt worker's lung	*Aspergillus clavatus* in moldy barley
Pigeon breeder lung	Avian proteins in feathers and excreta

 e. In most cases, there is an associated elevation of serum **angiotensin-converting enzyme** levels.

 f. The course of disease is variable; while many patients have spontaneous resolution, others with more extensive extrapulmonary disease, particularly cardiac and neurologic, have a poor prognosis.

VI. Vascular Disease

 A. Pulmonary Emboli

  1. Emboli usually arise from the deep veins of the **lower extremities**, and larger emboli may lodge within the pulmonary artery, the so-called **saddle emboli**, fatally compromising cardiopulmonary flow.

  2. Emboli may arise from **thrombi** (eg, **coagulopathy**); or, they may be composed of fat, **bone marrow**, neoplastic cells, pathogens, **amniotic fluid**, or even air.

  3. In patients with cardiac septal defects, an embolus may detour into the left heart as a **paradoxical embolus** to organs and the brain.

  4. Despite the lungs' dual arterial supply, infarction is possible if bronchial supply is diminished (eg, elderly).

   a. Acute infarctions are hemorrhagic, painful, and often present as hemoptysis.

   b. Peripheral wedge infarctions are the most common.

PULMONARY VASCULATURE

- *The lungs, like the liver, are endowed with a dual arterial supply (pulmonary and bronchial arteries).*
- *The pulmonary arteries transport relatively deoxygenated blood to the alveoli for gas exchange.*
- *The bronchial arteries support the pulmonary parenchyma.*
- *All blood drains into pulmonary venous return.*

 B. Pulmonary Hypertension

  1. There are several causes, including cardiac anomalies (septal defects), venous congestion, and veno-occlusive disease.

  2. Primary pulmonary hypertension is idiopathic.

3. Elevated pulmonary pressure leads to vascular proliferation, medial smooth muscle hyperplasia, and eventually cor pulmonale, ventricular arrhythmias, myocardial infarction, and death.

4. Early treatment of the underlying cause may be effective, otherwise the prognosis is poor.

C. **Diffuse Pulmonary Hemorrhage Syndromes**

1. **Goodpasture syndrome** is the combination of pulmonary alveolar hemorrhage and acute glomerulonephritis.

   a. It is most frequently observed in young adult males.

   b. Goodpasture disease more specifically refers to glomerular injury mediated by anti-glomerular basement membrane antibodies.

   c. Patients are treated with aggressive plasma exchange to remove the offending antibody as well as corticosteroid therapy.

2. Idiopathic pulmonary hemosiderosis (IPH) is rare and characterized by variably recurrent episodes of intra-alveolar hemorrhage.

   a. Most cases involve children (1 to 7 years old).

   b. There is no known immunologic association with IPH.

   c. Sputum samples reveal numerous hemosiderin-laden macrophages.

3. **Wegener granulomatosis**, a rare systemic vasculitis of small and medium-sized vessels, may lead to cough and hemoptysis, in addition to the characteristic nasal ulcerations, **"saddle-nose" deformity**.

VII. Neoplasia

A. **Adenocarcinoma**

1. **Adenocarcinoma** is currently the **most common** lung cancer.

   a. It is associated with smoking and patient age.

   b. The distinction between small cell and non–small cell carcinoma is significant, because small cell carcinoma is almost always metastatic at the time of diagnosis and surgery is therefore not indicated (Table 7–5).

2. Adenocarcinoma usually occurs in the **peripheral** pleural aspect of the lung, rather than near the hilum.

3. Presenting symptoms and signs include shortness of breath, weight loss, **hemoptysis**, and a **spiculated** lesion near the pleural surface.

Table 7–5. Characteristic features of primary pulmonary carcinomas.

Malignancy	Characteristic Features
Adenocarcinoma	Peripheral, malignant glands
Bronchioalveolar	Alveolar architecture and is often multifocal
Squamous cell carcinoma	Central, squamous sheets and keratin pearls
Small cell carcinoma	Central, necrosis, mitoses, high N:C ratios
Carcinoid (low grade)	Central (classic), or peripheral (spindled)

4. Bronchioalveolar lavage (cytology), or lung biopsy will show groups of malignant glandular cells with enlarged, irregular nuclei, prominent nucleoli, and delicate cytoplasm.
   a. Well-differentiated tumors are arranged in **glands**.
   b. Poorly differentiated tumors are arranged in sheets and infiltrating single cells.
5. The **bronchioloalveolar subtype** of adenocarcinoma exhibits a characteristic **lepidic** growth pattern lining alveolar spaces.
6. Most primary lung adenocarcinomas immunostain for thyroid transcription factor 1 (TTF-1), which also stains thyroid tumors.
7. Adenocarcinoma is associated with a few paraneoplastic syndromes, including **Trousseau syndrome**, an acquired coagulopathy associated with visceral carcinoma that results in migratory thrombophlebitis; and, secondary hypertrophic pulmonary osteoarthropathy, which involves both digital clubbing and periostosis of tubular bones.
8. Treatment is resection and chemoradiation.
9. Prognosis is related to tumor stage.
   a. **Stage 1** is restricted to lung.
   b. **Stage 2** has positive lymph nodes.
   c. **Stage 3** is invasion of chest wall, or nearby organs/tissues.
   d. **Stage 4** has distant metastases.
10. It has greater metastatic potential than squamous cell carcinoma.

B. Squamous Cell Carcinoma
   1. Squamous cell carcinoma is strongly associated with smoking.
   2. Tumors are usually central (hilar) and present as locally invasive, destructive, obstructive, and cystic masses.
   3. Presenting signs and symptoms include pain, obstruction, and hemoptysis.
   4. Repeated sputum samples, or tissue biopsy, yield keratinizing squamous cells (Figure 7–4), often with inky black nuclei.

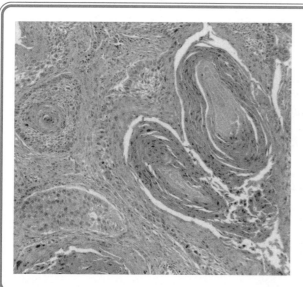

Figure 7–4. Squamous cell carcinoma usually arises centrally, rather than peripherally, and is composed of sheets of squamous cells with intercellular bridges that make keratin (eg, large pearl in this figure). Together with small cell carcinoma (oat cell), squamous cell carcinoma is usually associated with a history of smoking.

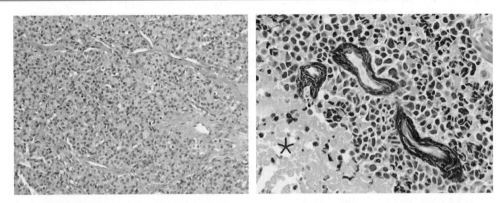

Figure 7–5. Neuroendocrine tumors. Both low-grade (carcinoid on the left) and high-grade (small cell carcinoma on the right with necrosis, asterisk), neuroendocrine carcinoma have metastatic potential. However, small cell carcinoma is almost always metastatic at the time of diagnosis.

     5. Squamous cell carcinoma almost never stains for TTF-1.

     6. Squamous cell carcinoma is strongly associated with multiple paraneoplastic processes.

          a. The most common of these is **hypercalcemia** due to parathyroid hormone-related protein secretion by the tumor.

          b. Tumor may invade the nearby branchial plexus, causing shoulder pain and muscle atrophy, the so-called **Pancoast tumor**.

          c. Involvement of sympathetic nerves at the level of C8-T4 results in **Horner syndrome: ptosis, miosis,** and **anhidrosis**.

   C. Carcinoid Tumor (Low-Grade Neuroendocrine Carcinoma)

     1. Carcinoid tumors are common (5–10% of primary lung neoplasms), slow-growing, low-grade, neuroendocrine tumors with small nuclei, delicate cytoplasm, and rare to absent necrosis or mitotic figures (Figure 7–5), unlike small cell neuroendocrine carcinoma.

          a. They arise from enterochromaffin (Kulchitsky) cells within the gastrointestinal tract, including lungs (foregut derived).

          b. Although low grade, carcinoid tumors can metastasize.

          c. Metastases to the liver may cause carcinoid syndrome (2% of cases), although much less frequently than gastrointestinal carcinoid tumors.

     2. Nearly all low-grade carcinoid tumors arise centrally, near the main bronchial branches.

     3. A subset occurs in the periphery and may have spindle cell morphology (atypical carcinoid).

     4. Approximately 10% of carcinoids secrete excess hormones, especially **serotonin** (5-hydroxytryptamine), which produces flushing, diarrhea, and peripheral edema.

     5. Treatment is surgery and survival is excellent.

D. Small Cell Carcinoma
 1. Small cell (oat cell) carcinoma is a high-grade neuroendocrine carcinoma characterized by rapid **growth**, very high **metastatic** potential, small delicate nuclei, **inconspicuous nucleoli**, very high N:C ratios, high **mitotic** rate, and **necrosis** (Figure 7–5).
 2. Nearly all small cell carcinomas arise centrally and have metastasized at the time of diagnosis (eg, adrenals, liver, brain).
 3. Small cell carcinoma is strongly associated with smoking; typical patients are usually older with a long pack-year history and present with fatigue, weight loss, dyspnea, and hemoptysis.
    a. Intrathoracic spread may cause superior vena cava obstruction, esophageal compression, and palsies of both the phrenic and recurrent laryngeal nerves.
    b. The secretion of peptide hormones induce multiple paraneoplastic syndromes, including the **syndrome of inappropriate secretion of antidiuretic hormone (SIADH)** and the syndrome of ectopic adrenocorticotropic hormone (ACTH).
 4. Nearly all small cell carcinomas of the lung express TTF-1.
 5. Although sensitive to chemoradiation, prognosis is very poor.

E. Metastatic Disease
 1. The lung is a common site for metastases, similar to the liver.
 2. Nearly all types of carcinoma metastasize to the lung in time.
    a. Distinguishing primary lung from metastatic disease is important for both staging and prognosis.
    b. Tumors may be distinguished by histologic features (eg, tall columnar cells with dirty necrosis in metastatic colon cancer), or immunophenotype (eg, estrogen receptor positive metastatic breast cancer).

VIII. Pleura

A. Pleural Effusions
 1. **Transudates** are clear, watery filtrates through intact vessels and possess relatively low specific gravity and few **mesothelial** cells.
    a. These are usually benign.
    b. They usually result from congestive heart failure, portal hypertension, or low albumin.
 2. **Exudates** have a more cloudy appearance, an elevated specific gravity, and greater cellularity.
    a. While infection and malignancy are two of the most common etiologies, autoimmune disease, pancreatitis, trauma, radiation, chemotherapy, and uremia have all been associated with exudates.
    b. Samples should be evaluated by cytology and chemistry to test for tumor cells and measure protein and glucose levels.

B. Pneumothorax
 1. **Primary spontaneous pneumothorax** may occur in otherwise healthy patients who rupture a bleb (eg, Figure 7–2) near the pleural surface.
    a. It presents with acute chest pain and shortness of breath.
    b. Most patients are very tall men 20 to 40 years of age.

2. **Secondary spontaneous pneumothoraces** are associated with numerous forms of parenchymal lung diseases, such as COPD, cystic fibrosis, sarcoidosis, idiopathic pulmonary fibrosis, TB, and malignancy.

3. Both penetrating and nonpenetrating lung injuries may cause **traumatic pneumothoraces**.

4. Regardless of the etiology, the pathophysiology is the same.

   a. The introduction of air (**pneumothorax**), blood (**hemothorax**), or lymph (**chylothorax**), into the pleural cavity collapses the ipsilateral lung and compresses the contralateral lung, compromising gas exchange and producing **hypoxemia**.

   b. Positive pressure also compresses the mediastinum, impairing venous return to the heart and reducing cardiac output.

C. Mesothelioma

1. Mesothelial cells are epithelial (cytokeratin positive) skin-like cells that line the pleura, pericardium, and peritoneal surfaces.

   a. Chronic inflammation may lead to mesothelial hyperplasia.

   b. Mesothelial cells often show reactive nuclear atypia that mimics neoplasia, especially in chronic effusions.

2. **Malignant mesothelioma** of the pleura is a neoplastic proliferation of mesothelial cells that invades surrounding tissue (eg, lung).

   a. Patients may have a history of asbestos exposure (Figure 7–6).

   b. Malignant mesothelioma presents with chronic effusion, pleural rind encasing part of the lung, and shortness of breath.

   c. Prognosis remains poor despite surgery and chemoradiation.

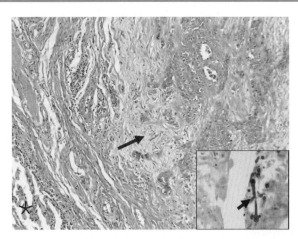

Figure 7–6. Asbestos and mesothelioma. Pleural or peritoneal based mesotheliomas arise from the mesothelial lining and are diagnosed by identifying sheets, glands (arrow), or papillary proliferations invading into surrounding tissues (eg, into lung, asterisk). Asbestos exposure increases the risk of developing mesothelioma and may be diagnosed by identifying ferruginous bodies, a fusiform beaded rod (inset), which is coated with iron.

CLINICAL PROBLEMS

1. A 35-year-old black woman complains of a lingering, nonproductive cough and increasing dyspnea over the past year. A subsequent chest film reveals prominent hilar lymphadenopathy. If her primary care provider suspects sarcoidosis, what additional study would be most appropriate?

   A. PCR mutation analysis of the *CFTR* gene (delta F508)

   B. Serum angiotensin-converting enzyme levels

   C. Sputum culture for acid-fast bacilli

   D. Allergy testing

   E. α_1-Antitrypsin levels

2. Which of the following are **not** associated with cystic fibrosis?

   A. Meconium ileus

   B. Low percentile on growth charts

   C. Inspiratory stridor that decreases with prone positioning

   D. Recurrent cough with thick sputum

   E. Future infertility

3. A 65-year-old man arrives at the emergency department with acute dyspnea. Which of the following assessments could be ordered to distinguish congestive heart failure from a primary pulmonary etiology?

   A. Brain natriuretic peptide

   B. Sputum culture

   C. Chest radiograph

   D. Cardiac muscle biopsy

   E. Bronchoalveolar lavage

4. A patient with Parkinson disease has pneumonia. Chest radiograph shows bilateral consolidation, predominantly in the right lung fields. Culture reveals gram-negative rods. Which organism is most likely?

   A. *Legionella pneumophila*

   B. *Streptococcus pneumoniae*

   C. *Mycobacterium tuberculosis*

   D. *Mycoplasma pneumoniae*

   E. *Klebsiella pneumoniae*

5. A 13-year-old girl with asthma seeks medical attention at her pediatrician's office complaining of shortness of breath. What would sputum cytology tests reveal?

   A. Fungal hyphae

   B. Acid-fast bacilli

C. Keratin pearls

   D. Charcot-Leyden crystals

   E. Atypical squamous epithelial cells

6. A 46-year-old man has recent onset of bloody nose and hemoptysis. Which of the following is the most likely diagnosis?

   A. Tuberculosis

   B. Wegener granulomatosis

   C. Pneumococcal pneumonia

   D. Severe acute respiratory syndrome

   E. Squamous cell carcinoma of the lung

7. A 48-year-old male smoker has multiple centrally located masses on chest radiograph. He also mentions having increasing left shoulder weakness and pain. A review of systems and physical examination is otherwise unremarkable. What is the most likely diagnosis?

   A. Squamous cell carcinoma

   B. Carcinoid tumor

   C. Mesothelioma

   D. Adenocarcinoma

   E. Sarcoidosis

8. A previously healthy 24-year-old man experiences acute onset hemoptysis and renal failure. An assay for which of the following would most likely be positive in this case?

   A. Antinuclear antibody (ANA)

   B. Anti-double stranded DNA antibody

   C. Anti-microsomal antibody

   D. Anti-glomerular basement membrane antibody

   E. Antineutrophil cytoplasmic antibody (c-ANCA)

9. Which immunohistochemical marker would be most useful in distinguishing a primary lung adenocarcinoma from a colonic metastasis?

   A. HMB-45

   B. S100

   C. TTF-1

   D. Pan cytokeratin

   E. CD45

10. An elderly male veteran has recurrent right-sided pleural effusion. Thoracentesis reveals numerous "reactive appearing mesothelial cells." Chest CT scan shows pleural thickening. CT-guided needle core biopsy results show mesothelial-like cells arranged in glands proliferating in the visceral pleura. What is the most likely diagnosis?

   A. Metastatic adenocarcinoma

   B. Malignant mesothelioma

C. Hyperplasia associated with chronic effusion

D. Asbestosis

E. Infection

ANSWERS

1. The answer is B. Sarcoidosis is an idiopathic granulomatous disease with a particular affinity for lymph nodes, especially those around the pulmonary hilum. In more than half of all cases, the granulomata secrete angiotensin-converting enzyme (ACE), so serum ACE levels have been used as surrogate for total disease burden.

2. The answer is C. Decreasing inspiratory stridor with prone positioning is observed in cases of "laryngomalacia," a common condition in which the pliant cartilage of the larynx occludes the airway during inhalation. Absent any knowledge of laryngomalacia, a savvy test-taker arrives at the correct answer by eliminating the known consequences of cystic fibrosis.

3. The answer is A. Brain natriuretic peptide (BNP) is secreted by the ventricles in response to increased tension on cardiac myocytes. An increased level is indicative of congestive heart failure.

4. The answer is E. The findings are consistent with aspiration pneumonia (ie, infection by *Klebsiella pneumoniae*).

5. The answer is D. Charcot-Leyden crystals are a sign of eosinophilic degranulation, and Curschmann spirals are a sign of excess mucus in sputum of asthma patients.

6. The answer is B. A vasculitis could account for the bloody nose and hemoptysis in this case.

7. The answer is A. Squamous cell carcinoma has been extensively linked to a history of smoking. The lesions are typically centrally located within the pulmonary hilum on chest films. Recall they may involve the adjacent brachial plexus, Pancoast tumor, causing shoulder pain and atrophy.

8. The answer is D. The alveolar and glomerular injuries of Goodpasture disease are mediated by anti-glomerular basement membrane antibodies.

9. The answer is C. Thyroid transcription factor 1 (TTF-1) is a marker of lung and thyroid tissue.

10. The answer is C. A diagnosis of pleural malignant mesothelioma requires invasion into surrounding tissues (eg, lung, chest wall). The most likely diagnosis is reactive hyperplasia (pleural rind) from a chronic effusion (likely heart or liver related).

CHAPTER 8
GASTROINTESTINAL TRACT

Meconium happens...
—Amy Heerema-McKenney, MD

I. Esophagus

A. Congenital Anomalies

1. **Esophageal atresia** is the partial failure of tubular development, leaving a non-canalized cord and a proximal blind pouch; it is usually associated with fistula formation.

2. **Tracheoesophageal fistula** occurs when reparative tissue of the incomplete esophagus forms a luminal tract into the airway.

3. There are several types of esophageal atresia.
   a. Type A is isolated atresia with no fistula.
   b. Type B is atresia with proximal fistula.
   c. Type C is atresia with distal fistula (most common).
   d. Type D is atresia with both proximal and distal fistula
   e. Type E is fistula with a completely patent esophagus.

4. All types present with choking, regurgitation, coughing, and cyanosis when feeding.

5. Approximately 10% of patients have multi-system anomalies, including **v**ertebral defect, **a**norectal malformation, **c**ardiac defect, **t**racheo**e**sophageal fistula, **r**enal anomaly, and **l**imb deformities (**VATER** or **VACTERL** syndrome.

B. Structural Pathology

1. **Stenosis** leads to progressive narrowing of the lumen.
   a. It is usually caused by inflammation, caustic injury, and scleroderma.
   b. Histologic sections show extensive submucosal fibrosis with atrophy of the muscular layer.

2. **Mucosal webs** are semicircumferential ridges of mucosal tissue protruding into the lumen of the esophagus.
   a. Upper webs are associated with iron deficiency anemia, koilonychia, and atrophic glossitis (**Plummer-Vinson syndrome**).
   b. Webs may cause dysphagia.
   c. There is also an increased risk of squamous cell carcinoma.

3. **Schatzki rings** are benign mucosal rings in the distal esophagus.

4. **Achalasia** is a disorder of esophageal motility.
   a. A defect of ganglion cells in the esophageal myenteric plexus leads to increased lower esophageal sphincter tone.
   b. The proximal esophagus becomes dilated causing dysphagia.
   c. A classic '**bird's beak**' appearance is seen on barium swallow.
   d. Secondary achalasia may arise from infection by *Trypanosoma cruzi* (**Chagas disease**), which causes destruction of the ganglion cells in the myenteric plexus.
   e. Degenerative diseases of dorsal motor nuclei cause achalasia.
5. Esophageal diverticula are outpouchings of tissue caused by herniation through muscular layers.
   a. Diverticula may consist of mucosal tissue alone (false diverticula) or may include the muscularis propria (true).
   b. **Zenker diverticula** are true diverticula and arise just above the upper esophageal sphincter.
   c. Patients complain of regurgitation of undigested food, typically without dysphagia.
   d. Traction diverticula arise in the mid esophagus.
   e. Epiphrenic diverticula arise immediately above the lower esophageal sphincter.
6. **Hiatal hernia** is a protrusion of the stomach into the thorax between the diaphragmatic crura.
   a. Sliding hernias (95% of cases) involve the proximal stomach.
   b. Paraesophageal hernias involve protrusion of the gastric fundus through the diaphragm, alongside the esophagus.

ESOPHAGEAL BLEEDING

CLINICAL
CORRELATION

- Esophageal **varices** are tortuous, dilated, submucosal veins in the distal esophagus caused by **cirrhosis** and portal hypertension.
- Varices are asymptomatic until rupture, when the condition presents with emergent upper gastrointestinal (GI) bleeding (**hematemesis**).
- **Mallory-Weiss tears** are longitudinal lacerations at the gastroesophageal junction caused by violent coughing or vomiting.
- Boerhaave syndrome refers to a rare transmural rupture of the esophagus (caused by retching), which may lead to massive hemorrhage.

C. Inflammation and Metaplasia
   1. Esophagitis may be caused by infection.
      a. *Candida albicans* is the most common cause of infectious esophagitis, especially in immunocompromised patients.
      b. Cytomegalovirus and herpes simplex virus-1 affect immunocompromised patients, causing "punched-out" ulcers.
   2. Radiation-induced esophagitis consists of mucosal atrophy, submucosal fibrosis, and vascular proliferation.
   3. **Eosinophilic esophagitis** is characterized by large numbers of eosinophils infiltrating the squamous epithelium of the proximal esophagus (allergic condition, rather than reflux).

a. It is most common in young males and is associated with allergies, or it
      may be idiopathic.
   b. Endoscopic examination reveals "felinization," with consecutive mucosal
      rings and furrows.
4. Chemical esophagitis refers to caustic chemical injury.
   a. Alcohol, corrosive acids, alkalis (eg, lye in suicide attempts), tobacco
      smoke, and hot liquids, are caustic, leading to inflammation, ulceration,
      and esophageal stricture.
   b. It may lead to dysphagia.
5. **Reflux esophagitis** is caused by caustic gastric or duodenal juices refluxing
   into the esophagus.
   a. Reflux esophagitis is most frequently associated with gastroesophageal re-
      flux disease (GERD).
   b. **GERD** is caused by reduced lower esophageal sphincter tone (eg, proges-
      terone or some foods) and increased abdominal pressure (eg, pregnancy,
      or weight gain).
   c. The squamous epithelium at the gastroesophageal junction becomes in-
      flamed with an eosinophilic infiltrate and ulceration develops in severe
      cases.
   d. Stimulation of exposed nociceptors by acidic fluid causes burning subster-
      nal pain (heartburn).
6. **Barrett esophagus** is a metaplastic change from the normal squamous epithelium to intestinal-type columnar epithelium with mucin filled goblet cells
   (Figure 8–1).
   a. It arises in patients with long-standing GERD.
   b. Endoscopically, it appears as "tongues" of red, velvety mucosa in the lower
      esophagus.
   c. Intestinal metaplasia may progress to dysplasia, similar to colonic epithe-
      lium, showing low-grade adenomatous change followed by high-grade
      dysplasia and adenocarcinoma.

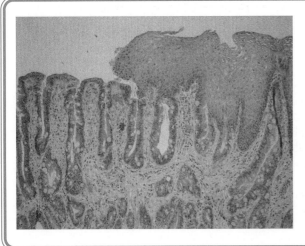

**Figure 8–1. Barrett
esophagus.** Squamocolum-
nar junction with intestinal
metaplasia of glandular mucosa (conspicuous mucin-
filled goblet cells).

d. In turn, patients with Barrett esophagus must undergo periodic endoscopic surveillance, with biopsies of metaplastic mucosa to monitor for developing dysplasia and adenocarcinoma.

D. Neoplasia

1. **Adenocarcinoma** arising from Barrett esophagus accounts for most cases of esophageal cancers in developed nations.
    a. Dysphagia, chest pain, weight loss, and hematemesis are the usual presenting symptoms and signs.
    b. Exophytic lesions may cause progressive narrowing of the esophagus, presenting as dysphagia with solid foods and eventually liquids.
2. **Squamous cell carcinoma** is the most common malignant tumor of the esophagus; it is especially common in northern Iran, China, South Africa, and in parts of France and Italy.
    a. Risk factors include tobacco and alcohol use (accounting for nearly 90% of cases in the United States), gender (male > female), race (black > white), and Plummer-Vinson syndrome.
    b. Most cases occur in the upper two-thirds of the esophagus.
3. **Prognosis** is directly related to stage at presentation.
    a. Stage 1 is local superficial invasion.
    b. Stage 2 is invasion into the wall.
    c. Stage 3 is invasion of adjacent structures.
    d. Stage 4 has distant metastatic disease.
4. **Treatment** for early stage (superficial) tumors is surgical.
    a. Deeply invasive tumors and those with regional lymph node metastases are treated with combined chemotherapy and radiation.
    b. The overall 5-year survival is approximately 30%.
5. Tumors of the esophageal wall include **fibrovascular polyps** (which may be large), smooth muscle neoplasms (**leiomyoma**, leiomyosarcoma), and gastrointestinal stromal tumors (**GIST**).

II. Stomach

A. Hypertrophic Pyloric Stenosis

1. It is caused by smooth muscle hypertrophy resulting in gastric outlet obstruction.
    a. It occurs in 1:5000 births and is more common in males.
    b. Nonbilious vomiting is a presenting symptom in infants.
    c. They may have a palpable "olive-shaped" epigastric mass.
2. Loss of gastric acid from vomiting leads to the classic finding of hypochloremic, hypokalemic metabolic alkalosis.
3. Treatment is surgical splitting of the muscle fibers.

B. Gastritis and Peptic Ulcer Disease

1. **Acute gastritis** is caused by the irritation or breakdown of the gastric mucosa related to nonsteroidal antiinflammatory drugs (NSAIDs), stress, alcohol, smoking, infection, uremia, ischemia, shock, or trauma.
    a. It is a common cause of hematemesis in alcoholics.
    b. It occurs in 25% of patients taking daily aspirin.
    c. Histologically, it is characterized by inflammation that if severe leads to loss of the superficial gastric epithelium (acute erosive gastritis).

Table 8–1. Causes of chronic gastritis.

Type	Cause
Chronic fundal (type A)	Autoimmune gastritis (10%) Autoantibodies are made against parietal cells and intrinsic factor Gland atrophy leads to pernicious anemia
Chronic antral (type B)	*Helicobacter pylori* infection (90%) The most common cause of gastritis Increased risk of peptic ulcers and carcinoma
Hypertrophic (Menetrier disease)	Idiopathic enlargement mucosal folds
Lymphocytic	Infiltration by a large number of lymphocytes; associated with celiac sprue

2. **Chronic gastritis** is characterized by mucosal inflammation with lymphocytes and plasma cells, leading to glandular atrophy and sometimes to intestinal metaplasia (similar to Barrett esophagus); it has multiple causes (Table 8–1).
3. **Stress ulcers** are the full-thickness breakdown of the mucosa.
   a. **Curling ulcers** occur in the proximal duodenum in the setting of severe burns or trauma.
   b. **Cushing ulcers** are associated with intracranial injuries and occur more proximally.

ULCERS IN THE INTENSIVE CARE UNIT

CLINICAL CORRELATION

- *Stress ulcers occur in patients with bacterial sepsis, burns, trauma, or brain injuries with increased intracranial pressure.*
- *Most patients in intensive care units are given strict antacid prophylaxis to prevent gastric erosions or ulcerations.*

4. **Peptic ulcers** are usually solitary and occur most commonly in the stomach and duodenum.
   a. Atypical sites of peptic ulcer disease should implicate other causes such as Zollinger-Ellison syndrome (eg, ulcers in the jejunum, as well as stomach/duodenum).
   b. Peptic ulcers are caused by a combination of impaired defenses and caustic insult from increased gastric acid.
   c. Patients seek medical attention complaining of aching or **burning** epigastric pain, nausea, bloating, or anorexia.
   d. Classically, pain is relieved by food or antacids.
   e. Pain is often **nocturnal** and may radiate to the back or left upper quadrant.
   f. The classic gross appearance is a sharply punched-out, round or oval mucosal defect of variable depth with a clean base.
   g. Hyperemic (red) and edematous mucosa may be present at the periphery, reflecting adjacent chronic gastritis.

h. The most common complication, and often the presenting symptom, is upper GI **bleeding** from erosion into gastric vessels.

i. This bleeding may be recurrent and life-threatening, leading to iron deficiency anemia or massive hemorrhage.

j. Peptic ulcers are associated with the bacillus ***Helicobacter pylori*** in 70% of cases (nearly 100% for duodenal ulcers), which degrades mucosal defenses while increasing acid secretion and inciting a strong immune response.

k. Other causes include long-term NSAID use, reflux of bile acids, Zollinger-Ellison syndrome, and heavy cigarette smoking.

l. Treat with antibiotics, H_2-receptor antagonists, and proton-pump inhibitor therapy ('**triple-therapy**').

m. Without treatment, these ulcers may take many years to heal, and can be complicated by upper GI bleeding and perforation.

C. Gastric Polyps

1. **Fundic gland polyps** are the most common gastric polyp.
   a. They are characterized by cystic dilation of gastric glands.
   b. They are usually caused by proton pump inhibitor therapy.
2. **Hyperplastic polyps** are characterized by tortuous, elongated surface (foveolar) epithelium, with glandular atrophy and mild chronic inflammation.
3. **Adenomatous polyps** are dysplastic growths similar to those in the colon and are precursors for intestinal-type gastric carcinoma.

D. Gastric Adenocarcinoma

1. **Gastric cancer** is the second most common carcinoma worldwide, with high rates in Japan, China, South America, and parts of Europe.
   a. Rates have declined in the United States and United Kingdom.
   b. Mean age at presentation is 55 years.
   c. **Risk factors** include dietary **nitrosoamines** in smoked or cured foods, gender (males > females), chronic gastritis, pernicious anemia, and **achlorhydria.**
   d. There is a slightly increased genetic risk for those with blood group A as well as a family history of gastric cancer or hereditary nonpolyposis colon cancer.
2. Gross pathology reveals exophytic, flat, or ulcerated lesions.
   a. Heaped-up borders and a necrotic base help distinguish carcinoma from a peptic ulcer.
   b. **Linitis plastica** refers to a thickened "leather-bottle" appearance of the stomach caused by diffuse infiltration of the gastric wall by a poorly differentiated signet-ring type of adenocarcinoma.
3. There are two main histologic subtypes of gastric adenocarcinoma.
   a. The **intestinal type** resembles colonic adenocarcinoma and is associated with gastric adenomas and intestinal metaplasia.
   b. The **diffuse type** consists of poorly differentiated mucin- filled cells with a peripheral nucleus (signet-ring cells).
4. Prognosis is usually poor but is related to the stage of disease.
   a. **Stage 1** is tumor limited to gastric wall (survival 70%).
   b. **Stage 2** is tumor penetrating serosa (35%).
   c. **Stage 3** is tumor invading adjacent structures (15%).
   d. **Stage 4** is distant metastases (7%).

5. Due to its insidious course, patients often do not seek medical attention until nodal or distant metastases are present.
    a. Metastases to the ovary are known as a **Krukenburg** tumor.
    b. **Virchow's node** is metastasis to a supraclavicular lymph node.

E. Other Gastric Malignancies
    1. **Gastric lymphoma** is usually a low-grade B-cell lymphoma arising in mucosa-associated lymphoid tissue (MALT type).
        a. It accounts for approximately 5% of gastric malignancies and has a significantly improved prognosis compared with carcinoma.
        b. *H pylori* is associated with up to 90% of cases, and many of these MALT "lymphomas" resolve after treatment.
    2. **GISTs** are the most common mesenchymal tumors of the GI tract.
        a. Most cases arise in the stomach (60% of cases).
        b. They are usually an incidental finding during clinical workup for anemia, abdominal pain, or bowel obstruction.
        c. The tumor is believed to arise from the interstitial cells of Cajal within the muscularis propria.
        d. Histologically, GIST is composed of either elongated spindle cells or epithelioid spindle cells resembling smooth muscle and neural neoplasms.
        e. Most cases (75%) have a mutation in the *c-kit* **gene**, which encodes a tyrosine kinase receptor that may be detected by immunostaining tumor cells for the **CD117** marker.
        f. Notably, some cases are negative for CD117 but have mutations in a related kinase (*PDGFRa*) gene.
        g. Treatment is surgery, but advanced stage tumors may be treated with ki nase inhibitor chemotherapy (eg, imatinib).
        h. Gastric GIST has a better prognosis than more distal tumors.
        i. Prognosis is related to tumor size and mitotic index.

III. Small Intestine

    A. Congenital Anomalies
        1. **Meckel diverticulum** is caused by failure of the embryonic vitelline duct to involute.
            a. It is the most common congenital intestinal anomaly.
            b. It is a "true diverticulum" that includes all three layers of bowel wall (mucosa, submucosa, and muscularis propria).
            c. It follows the **"Rule of 2s."**
                (1) It occurs in 2% of the population.
                (2) It is approximately 2 inches long.
                (3) It is usually within 2 feet of the ileocecal valve.
            d. Meckel diverticula may cause **intussusception,** which occurs when an intestinal segment "telescopes" into adjacent bowel, leading to intestinal obstruction with abdominal pain, vomiting, and eventually infarction (surgical emergency).
            e. It may cause **volvulus,** which is twisting of a segment of bowel around the axis of the mesenteric root or other fulcrum (eg, Meckel diverticulum), leading to compromised venous outflow and infarction.
            f. **Heterotopia** of either gastric or pancreatic tissue is common in Meckel diverticula and may be complicated by peptic ulcer formation that may bleed or perforate, mimicking acute appendicitis.

2. **Duodenal atresia** occurs when the duodenal lumen fails to recanalize during development.
   a. **Bilious emesis** presents in newborns within hours of birth.
   b. 25% of patients with duodenal atresia have **trisomy 21**.
   c. Abdominal radiograph shows classic "**double bubble**" sign.
3. **Omphalocele** is the herniation of abdominal contents (gut, liver, covered by membranous sac) into the **umbilical cord**.
   a. It is caused by abnormal abdominal wall muscle development.
   b. The membranous sac distinguishes it from gastroschisis.
   c. It is associated with cardiovascular anomalies (15–25%).
   d. **Beckwith-Wiedemann syndrome** is characterized by omphalocele, macrosomia, and macroglossia.
   e. Mortality is approximately 40%.
4. **Gastroschisis** involves a failure of abdominal wall closure with extrusion of abdominal contents, which are not covered by a membranous sac and does not involve the umbilical cord.
   a. It is not typically associated with other anomalies.
   b. There is a better prognosis than omphalocele.

B. Small Bowel Herniation
   1. Most come to clinical attention due to pain, a palpable mass, or symptoms of intestinal obstruction.
   2. They are often complicated by incarceration or strangulation.
   3. This may cause mechanical obstruction, compromising venous outflow, leading to infarction (surgical emergency).
   4. Inguinal hernias are the most common type.
      a. **Direct inguinal hernia** is caused by a defect in the transversalis fascia associated with obesity or straining and occurs medial to the inferior epigastric vessels.
      b. **Indirect inguinal hernia** is the most common, is congenital, and herniates through the internal ring of inguinal canal lateral to the inferior epigastric vessels.
   5. **Pantaloon hernia** straddles the inferior epigastric vessels, appearing as both direct and indirect hernias.
   6. **Femoral hernias** are common in females during and after pregnancy; they protrude beneath the inguinal ligament and down the narrow femoral canal, increasing the risk for stangulation.
   7. **Umbilical hernia** is common during pregnancy.
   8. Ventral (incisional) hernia refers to defects in the abdominal wall from a prior surgical procedure.

C. Duodenal Ulcer
   1. The proximal duodenum is the most common site of peptic ulcer formation and is commonly associated with *H pylori* **infection.**
   2. **Gastrinomas** are gastrin-secreting neuroendocrine tumors resulting in markedly elevated serum gastrin levels and may also cause duodenal ulceration.
      a. Gastrinomas are islet cell tumors of the pancreas.
      b. **Zollinger-Ellison syndrome** is caused by gastrin-secreting tumors.
         (1) 90% of patients have duodenal ulcers.
         (2) This diagnosis should be considered if jejunal ulcers are present.

3. **Multiple endocrine neoplasia** type 1 is an autosomal dominant disorder characterized by pituitary adenoma; parathyroid adenomas; and pancreatic islet cell tumors that may be gastrin-secreting and lead to duodenal ulcers.

D. Malabsorption
   1. The small bowel is responsible for absorption of fats, proteins, carbohydrates, vitamins, minerals, and electrolytes.
   2. Patients with malabsorption syndromes have diarrhea or **steatorrhea** (bulky, frothy, greasy stools), abdominal pain, **flatus**, weight loss, and muscle **wasting**.
      a. Malabsorption may be complicated by **deficiencies** in the absorption of fat-soluble vitamins (A, D, E, K), vitamin B_{12}, folate, and iron.
      b. Deficiencies may lead to associated bleeding or anemia.
   3. There are a variety of disorders that may cause malabsorption, including the following:
      a. Lack of villous surface area (eg, **celiac sprue**)
      b. Problems with epithelial transport (eg, **pernicious anemia**)
      c. **Iatrogenic** conditions (eg, post-gastrectomy dumping syndrome).
      d. **Short-gut** syndrome following segmental bowel resections.
   4. **Celiac disease** (gluten-sensitive enteropathy, celiac sprue) is an immune-mediated enteritis causing characteristic villous atrophy of the proximal small intestine with ensuing malabsorption.
      a. The etiology lies in a genetic sensitivity to **glutens** in wheat and related **gliadin** proteins in rye, oats, and barley.
      b. Serum markers include IgA and IgG antibodies to gliadin, tissue transglutaminase, and **endomysial smooth muscle**.
      c. Risk factors include HLA haplotypes DQ2 (95%) and DQ8 (5%).
      d. It is also associated with dermatitis herpetiformis, an IgA-mediated vesicular skin disorder.
      e. Microscopically, there is blunting of intestinal villi with lymphocytic inflammation (enteritis).
      f. Strict adherence to a gluten-free diet treats most patients.
   5. **Tropical sprue** (postinfectious sprue) affects visitors and residents of tropical regions of Africa, Asia, and South America.
      a. It is clinically similar to celiac disease.
      b. Enterotoxigenic *Escherichia coli* has been implicated, and most patients respond to broad-spectrum antibiotics.
   6. **Whipple disease** is caused by infection with *Tropheryma whippleii,* a gram-positive actinomycete.
      a. Malabsorption, arthropathy, or neurologic symptoms may be present due to intestinal, joint, and central nervous system infection.
      b. Duodenal biopsy may show lamina propria distended by numerous foamy macrophages containing periodic acid-Schiff positive lysosomal granules.
   7. **Disaccharidase deficiency** is a congenital or acquired loss of brush border disaccharidase enzymes leading to osmotic diarrhea.
   8. **Lactase deficiency** is common, leading to milk product intolerance.
   9. **Abetalipoproteinemia** is an autosomal recessive deficiency of apolipoprotein B, leading to failed absorption of fatty acids.
      a. Patients can partially metabolize fatty acids in the epithelial cells but cannot form chylomicrons, or low-density lipoproteins, which contain β-lipoproteins.
      b. Triglycerides accumulate in intestinal cell vacuoles.

Table 8–2. Infectious causes of bloody diarrhea.

Pathogen	Presentation	Treatment	'Pearls'
Shigella	Fever Dysentery HUS Invasive	Ciprofloxacin, Ampicillin, TMP-SMZ	Diagnosis is made by stool culture. Epidemics are associated with ingestion of contaminated uncooked food
Salmonella (S typhi)	Invasive May disseminate (typhoid fever)	Quinolones, Cephalosporins	Severe disease associated with S typhi
Campylobacter jejuni	Fever Invasive Bloody	Supportive	Number one cause of food-borne diarrhea in United States
Enterohemorrhagic Escherichia coli (EHEC)	Hemorrhagic colitis, HUS TTP Not invasive	TMP-SMZ, Ciprofloxacin, Supportive	Shiga-like toxin infection associated with ingestion of uncooked meat O157:H7
Yersinia enterocolitica	Fever Cramps Vomiting	Supportive	Infection associated with ingestion of milk, pork, feces
Entamoeba histolytica	Dysentery Disseminates to form hepatic abscesses	Metronidazole	Fecal-oral ingestion of cysts produces "flask-like" ulcers

HUS, hemolytic-uremic syndrome; TMP-SMZ, trimethoprim-sulfamethoxazole; TTP, thrombotic thrombocytopenic purpura.

10. **Pancreatic insufficiency** is a common cause of malabsorption.
    a. Pancreatic enzymes, such as trypsin, chymotrypsin, amylase, and lipase are required for intraluminal digestive functions.
    b. Pancreatic acinar damage in chronic pancreatitis and cystic fibrosis leads to malabsorption of fats and proteins.
11. **Lymphatic obstruction** (lymphangiectasia), by lymphoma or infection, causes severe protein malabsorption.
12. **Infections** may cause malabsorptive diarrhea (Tables 8–2 and 8–3).
E. Crohn Disease
    1. Crohn disease is an inflammatory bowel disease that usually affects the distal **ileum**, but may involve any portion of the GI tract (mouth to anus).
    2. It is most common in the second and third decades of life with a second peak in late middle-age.

Table 8–3. Infectious causes of watery diarrhea.

Pathogen	Presentation	Treatment	'Pearls'
Salmonella	Vomiting Fever Pain (Salmonellosis)	Quinolones and Cephalosporins	Associated with undercooked beef or poultry ingestion. Very common in the United States
Vibrio cholerae	Vomiting 12–48 h dehydration "Rice-water" stool	Aggressive hydration; Quinolones	Cholera toxin in water, raw oysters
Clostridium difficile	Pseudomembranous colitis	Metronidazole	Diagnosis made by identifying C difficile toxin; Associated with broad-spectrum antibiotics
Enterotoxigenic Escherichia coli (ETEC)	Osmotic diarrhea (3–6 days) Fever Cholera-like toxins	TMP-SMZ, Ciprofloxacin	Infant and traveler's diarrhea. Implicated in tropical sprue
Rotavirus	Severe dehydrating nausea and vomiting and low fever (lasts 5–8 days)	Supportive	Most common cause of infantile diarrhea. Seen most often during the winter.
Norwalk virus	Mild diarrhea Nausea and vomiting	Supportive	Fecal-oral transmission Usually seen on cruise ships
Adenovirus	Moderate vomiting	Supportive	Second most common cause of infant diarrhea
Giardia lamblia	Steatorrhea, foul smell, small intestine	Metronidazole	History of camping/hiking
Cryptosporidium	Large-volume fluid loss	Supportive	Seen in immunocompromised persons, especially those with HIV infection

TMP-SMZ, trimethoprim-sulfamethoxazole.

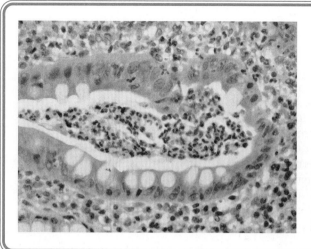

Figure 8–2. Crypt abscess. Active inflammatory bowel disease (Crohn disease and ulcerative colitis) shows neutrophilic infiltration of colonic crypts.

3. Risk factors include Jewish heritage, smoking, and an association with other autoimmune diseases.
4. Crohn disease is characterized by chronic inflammation extending throughout the full thickness of the bowel wall (**transmural enteritis**) to the level of the serosa.
   a. There is acute cryptitis and **crypt abscesses** (Figure 8–2).
   b. There is crypt dropout and **architectural distortion**.
   c. There is chronic inflammation in the bowel wall.
   d. There may be small, poorly formed **granulomas**.
5. Characteristic gross features are caused by the full thickness inflammation, leading to strictures and extension of mesenteric adipose tissue over the serosa, so-called "**creeping fat**."
6. A sharp demarcation between diseased and normal bowel segments creates the characteristic "**skip lesions**" in Crohn disease.
7. Deep narrow fissures may extend deeply through the wall, leading to fistula tract formation with other structures (eg, bowel, bladder, anus, vagina, skin).

SYMPTOMS OF CROHN DISEASE

CLINICAL CORRELATION

- *Symptoms typically begin with intermittent attacks of diarrhea, abdominal pain, and fever, which may remit or progress acutely.*
- *Extraintestinal manifestations include ankylosing spondylitis, erythema nodosum, migratory polyarthritis, primary sclerosing cholangitis (less common than in ulcerative colitis).*
- *Patients with chronic symptoms for many years are at slightly increased risk for carcinoma.*
- *Treatments include systemic corticosteroids, antibiotics, local antiinflammatory medications (aminosalicylates), and immune modulators (azathioprine, anti-tumor necrosis factor).*

   F. Neoplasia
   1. **Brunner gland hyperplasia** is a benign proliferation of submucosal glands in the duodenum that may present as a mass.
   2. **Leiomyomas or lipomas** may develop within the submucosa, as benign neoplasms of smooth muscle and adipose, respectively.

3. Leiomyomas and leiomyosarcoma are rare in the small bowel.
4. **Carcinoid** tumors are well-differentiated neuroendocrine neoplasms that occur throughout the GI tract.
    a. Carcinoid tumors have metastatic potential.
    b. Metastases to the liver may cause **carcinoid syndrome.**
5. Approximately 25% of **GISTs** arise in the small intestine.
6. Neurofibroma is associated with type I neurofibromatosis.
7. **Inflammatory pseudotumor**/inflammatory myofibroblastic tumor is a rare "tumor" of the bowel wall that is composed of mixed inflammatory cells and proliferating fibroblastic and smooth muscle cells.
8. **Lymphoma** may arise in the mucosal lymphoid follicles of the small bowel (Peyer patches) as well as the mesenteric lymph nodes.
9. **Carcinoma** in the small intestine is unusual but occurs in the **periampullary** region of the duodenum with an increased risk in familial adenomatous polyposis.

CARCINOID SYNDROME

- *Carcinoid syndrome occurs because these tumors secrete serotonin and chemicals that cause vasodilation (flushing), diarrhea, and asthma.*
- *Carcinoid syndrome may also cause heart valve damage.*

IV. Colon, Rectum, and Anus

A. Hirschsprung Disease
1. Congenital aganglionic megacolon is caused by migratory arrest of neuroblasts, leading to an absence of ganglion cells in Meissner and Auerbach plexi in the large intestinal wall.
2. This results in ineffective peristalsis, leading to distal intestinal obstruction and proximal dilatation (megacolon).
3. Young children present with chronic constipation, abdominal distention and bilious vomiting.
4. Diagnosis requires **biopsy** of rectal mucosa showing the absence of **ganglion cells.**
5. Treatment requires resection of rectum and affected colon.

B. Vascular Disease
1. **Hemorrhoids** are dilated anal and perianal venous plexuses.
    a. Internal hemorrhoids arise above the anorectal line and are associated with constipation and cause painless bleeding.
    b. External hemorrhoids are painful and may represent prolapsed internal hemorrhoids or perianal hematomas.
    c. Complications include venous thrombosis with severe pain.
    d. Treatment consists of sitz baths, stool softeners, and surgical excision if necessary.
2. **Ischemic bowel** disease encompasses mucosal, mural, and transmural infarction and may be acute or chronic.
    a. Acute occlusion of the superior or inferior **mesenteric** vessels may lead to infarction of large bowel segments.
    b. Arterial thrombosis (less commonly venous) is associated with severe **atherosclerosis; hypercoagulability** disorders; and other vascular disorders, including **vasculitides.**

c. Cardiac vegetations or **atrial fibrillation** increases risk.

    d. Clinical presentation is highly variable, and does not correlate well with the degree of infarction.

    e. Chronic ischemia due to vascular insufficiency leads to mucosal inflammation and colitis.

  3. Arteriovenous malformations (AVM, angiodysplasia) are dilated and tortuous collections of mucosal and submucosa blood vessels.

    a. AVMs are found primarily after age 50, and account for a significant percentage of lower GI bleeding in this age group.

    b. **Hereditary hemorrhagic telangectasia** is a common inherited cause of malformations leading to GI bleeding.

C. Diverticular Disease

  1. Diverticular disease is characterized by outpouchings of the mucosa and submucosa of the bowel wall.

    a. They are very common among older people in developed nations.

    b. Diverticulosis refers to multiple diverticula.

  2. Diverticula are usually asymptomatic.

  3. Diverticulitis presents with colicky lower quadrant pain, tenderness to palpation, fever, and leukocytosis.

  4. Microscopically, most diverticula are "false" and are not surrounded by a muscular layer (distinct from Meckel diverticula).

  5. Complications include rupture, bleeding, abscess, and obstruction.

  6. Diverticulitis is a common cause of **hematochezia** in the elderly.

ACUTE APPENDICITIS

- *The vermiform appendix is a residual tubular extension of the cecal base containing abundant lymphoid tissue, not a diverticulum.*
- *Appendicitis is the most common cause of acute abdomen.*
- *Fever, nausea, and tenderness to palpation are presenting symptoms.*
- *Pain classically begins as periumbilical and then localizes to the right lower quadrant with rebound tenderness.*
- *Inflammation is usually associated with luminal obstruction due to a fecalith or parasite (eg, pinworm).*
- *The inflammation progresses through the wall, creating a fibrinopurulent exudate on the serosa and risk of rupture.*

D. Infection

  1. There are multiple causes of diarrhea (Tables 8–2 and 8–3).

  2. There are multiple parasites that colonize the colon, including the following:

    a. Roundworm (*Ascaris lumbricoides*)

    b. Threadworm (*Strongyloides stercoralis*)

    c. Hookworm (*Necator americanus* and *Ancylostoma duodenale*)

    d. Pinworm (*Enterobius vermicularis*)

    e. Tapeworm (*Diphyllobothrium latum, Taenia* spp.)

    f. Whipworm (*Trichuris trichiura*)

E. Ulcerative Colitis

  1. Ulcerative colitis is the most common form of inflammatory bowel disease affecting the colon (Crohn disease also affects the colon, but unlike ulcerative colitis affects the upper GI tract).

2. Ulcerative colitis is an **immune disease** of uncertain etiology, with a chronic and relapsing course.
3. Rectal bleeding and chronic mucoid diarrhea are present.
4. Relapses, called "flares," vary from infrequent or mild, to catastrophic unremitting episodes, requiring hospitalization.
5. Patients may have a positive **p-ANCA** (see Chapter 6) or anti-*Saccharomyces cerevisiae* antibody (**ASCA**).
6. Extraintestinal manifestations are common, including polyarthritis, erythema nodosum, primary sclerosing cholangitis, and **uveitis**.
7. Ulcerative colitis always involves the rectum, extending retrograde toward the cecum, culminating in **pancolitis**.
8. The mucosa is red, granular, and flattened, with ulceration.
9. Inflammation is confined to the mucosa and submucosa, with no involvement of the bowel wall (unlike Crohn disease).
10. Microscopically, there is acute and chronic colitis with crypt abscesses, distortion of the crypt architecture, and ulceration.
    a. Unlike Crohn disease, there are no fissures, fistulae, skip lesions, or granulomas (Table 8–4).
    b. Infection may mimic ulcerative colitis.
11. Complications include pathologic dilation of the colon, which may be life-threatening (toxic megacolon); perforation, and increased risk of **dysplasia** and adenocarcinoma.
    a. The risk of **adenocarcinoma** is higher than Crohn disease.
    b. Risk is related to the degree and duration of disease (~30% after 30 years with pancolitis.)
12. Patients must have periodic colonoscopic **surveillance** with biopsy to monitor for the development of dysplasia.
    a. Dysplasia may prompt a prophylactic proctocolectomy with creation of an ileal-pouch-anal anastomosis.
    b. 'Pouchitis' occurs in the ileal pouch.

F. Polyps
    1. Benign **hyperplastic polyps** are most common.

Table 8–4. Distinguishing between Crohn disease and ulcerative colitis.

Crohn Disease	Ulcerative Colitis
Ileum/colon, but can be anywhere in gastrointestinal tract	Colon/rectum only
"Skip" lesions, cobblestone mucosa	Rectal involvement, retrograde proximally
Transmural involvement	Mucosal inflammation only
Noncaseating granulomas	Crypt abscesses and ulcers
Strictures, fissures, fistulae	Pseudopolyp formation

a. Microscopically, the crypts have a sawtooth or "star" pattern with cytologically bland intestinal goblet cells.

     b. There is no recognized premalignant risk.

2. Inflammatory polyps are typically large with cystically dilated glands and marked inflammation; **juvenile polyps** occur in children and are similar to inflammatory polyps.

3. Mucosal prolapse syndrome (**solitary rectal ulcer syndrome**) appears as polypoid projections of regenerative and inflamed mucosa.

4. Hamartomatous polyps consist of abnormal polypoid growths of otherwise normal tissue elements.

5. Peutz-Jeghers polyps have a complex branching pattern of connective tissue and smooth muscle.

PEUTZ-JEGHERS SYNDROME

- *An autosomal dominant syndrome characterized by multiple hamartomatous polyps in the GI tract, and pigmentation of mucosa and skin called 'melanin spots.'*
- *There is an increased risk of carcinoma of the pancreas, breast, ovary, uterus, and lung.*

6. Adenomatous polyps are a precancerous lesion; malignant potential increases with size and villous architecture (Figure 8–3).

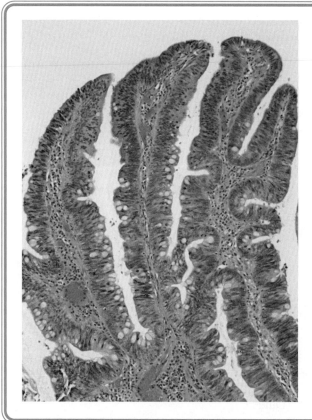

Figure 8–3. Adenomatous polyp. Low-grade dysplasia of colonic epithelium with mucin dropout, elongation, and stratification of nuclei.

7. **Serrated adenomas** have features of both adenomatous and hyperplastic polyps and usually arise in the cecum.

8. **Familial adenomatous polyposis (FAP) syndrome** is an autosomal dominant disease caused by germline mutations in the *APC* gene (adenomatous polyposis coli) on chromosome 5q.

   a. Patients have >100 (usually innumerable) adenomatous polyps throughout the colon and duodenum.

   b. The risk of progression to adenocarcinoma approaches 100%.

   c. Prophylactic colectomy is warranted.

   d. **Gardner syndrome** is a variant that includes desmoid tumors (fibromatosis), epidermoid cysts, and **osteomas** of the jaw.

   e. **Turcot syndrome** describes the combination of FAP and central nervous system tumors, typically medulloblastomas and **glioblastomas.**

9. Hereditary nonpolyposis colorectal cancer (HNPCC) syndrome is also known as **Lynch syndrome.**

   a. It is an autosomal dominant disorder with increased risk of colon cancer, endometrial cancer, and gastric carcinoma.

   b. Mutations occur in **DNA mismatch repair genes,** leading to **microsatellite instability** and widespread genomic errors.

G. Adenocarcinoma

1. Colorectal adenocarcinoma remains one of the most **common** and deadliest cancers in the United States.

2. It typically presents in the sixth and seventh decades of life.

3. Clinical presentation includes **hematochezia** (left-sided tumors), iron deficiency **anemia** (cancer until proven otherwise), obstruction or perforation in advanced cases.

4. Risk factors include adenomatous polyps, familial syndromes or strong family history, and low-fiber/high-fat **diet.**

5. Malignancy develops through the sequential acquisition of mutations in tumor suppressor and oncogenes, leading to adenomatous polyps and ultimately carcinoma (multiple hit hypothesis).

6. Implicated genes include *APC, k-RAS,* and *p53.*

7. Grossly, left-sided tumors are often annular, obstructing ('**applecore,**' 'napkin-ring') lesions, whereas right-sided tumors may become bulky, fungating masses (Figure 8–4).

8. Microscopically, malignant glands range from well-differentiated resembling normal colonic mucosa to poorly differentiated sheets or single infiltrating tumor cells.

9. Metastases occur in local lymph nodes; distant metastases are most common to the liver.

10. Localized colonic tumors are treated with surgery, and patients with nodal or distant metastases receive chemotherapy.

11. Primary adenocarcinomas in the rectum are treated with radiation and chemotherapy prior to surgery.

12. Prognosis is a function of grade, genetic markers, and stage.

   a. **Stage 1** is limited to bowel wall (Dukes A).

   b. **Stage 2** is invasion through the wall (Dukes B).

   c. **Stage 3** has lymph node metastases (Dukes C).

   d. **Stage 4** has distant metastases (eg, liver).

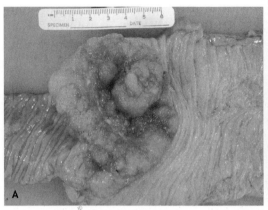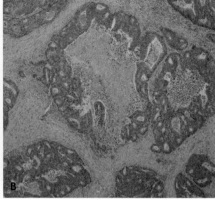

Figure 8–4. Colonic adenocarcinoma. A: Gross photo of fungating lesion in the cecum. **B:** Microscopic photo of colonic adenocarcinoma with complex glandular architecture and central *dirty necrosis*.

H. Anal Dysplasia and Carcinoma
1. Anal squamous dysplasia usually arises from neoplastic transformation by human papillomavirus (**HPV**) similar to dysplasia in the cervix, vagina, vulva, and oropharynx.
   a. Low-grade dysplasia is associated with HPV types 6 and 11.
   b. High-grade dysplasia and carcinoma is associated with HPV types 16 and 18.
   c. Dysplasia may be followed by Papanicolaou smears and biopsy.
2. Low-grade dysplasia presents as a warty condyloma.
3. High-grade dysplasia may progress to invasive carcinoma.
   a. Squamous cell carcinoma is the most common anal tumor.
   b. Adenocarcinoma is usually an extension of rectal cancer.
4. Prognosis depends on grade and stage.
   a. **Stage 1** is smaller than 2 cm.
   b. **Stage 2** is smaller than 5 cm.
   c. **Stage 3** has metastasis to lymph nodes.
   d. **Stage 4** has distant metastases.

CLINICAL PROBLEMS

1. Which of the following would **LEAST LIKELY** account for an ulcer in the distal esophagus?

   A. Herpes simplex virus

   B. Adenocarcinoma of the esophagus

C. Zenker diverticulum

D. Severe reflux esophagitis

E. Lye ingestion

2. All of the following are true regarding Barrett esophagus **EXCEPT:**

A. It develops from long-standing gastroesophageal reflux disease

B. Confers an increased risk of squamous cell carcinoma

C. It is considered a reversible metaplastic condition

D. Requires long-term endoscopic surveillance

E. Histologically characterized by glandular epithelium

3. A male neonate has a distended abdomen and failed to pass meconium. Which of the following is the **LEAST LIKELY** cause of obstruction:

A. Imperforate anus

B. Hirschsprung disease

C. Meckel diverticulum

D. Distal intestinal atresia

E. Intestinal malrotation

4. Forceful nonbilious vomiting presents in an infant who was delivered at full term without complications. Physical examination is notable for a palpable abdominal mass. Which of the following is **MOST LIKELY?**

A. Biliary atresia

B. Phenylketonuria

C. Eosinophilic esophagitis

D. Pyloric stenosis

E. Crohn disease

5. As part of the workup for chronic diarrhea, a 12-year-old girl is found to have a positive anti-endomysial antibody. She undergoes an upper endoscopy with biopsy of the duodenum showing flattened intestinal villi and duodenitis. Which of the following is the **MOST LIKELY** diagnosis?

A. Whipple disease

B. Celiac disease

C. MALT-type B-cell lymphoma

D. Amoebic colitis

E. α_1-Antitrypsin deficiency

6. All of the following are possible complications in patients with long-standing ulcerative colitis, **EXCEPT:**

A. Primary sclerosing cholangitis

B. Stricture of the ileum

C. Adenocarcinoma of the colon

D. Toxic megacolon

E. Uveitis

7. Which one of the following conditions is **NOT** part of the spectrum of pathology associated with Crohn disease?

A. Serosal extension ("creeping") of mesenteric fat

B. Infiltration of the crypts by neutrophils

C. Involvement of the terminal ileum

D. Massive infiltration of the lamina propria by macrophages

E. Presence of occasional noncaseating granulomas

8. Which polyp has the highest risk of progression to carcinoma?

A. Fundic gland polyp

B. Hyperplastic polyp of the colon

C. Hyperplastic polyp of the stomach

D. Adenomatous polyp of the stomach

E. Pseudopolyps in ulcerative colitis

9. Which of the following statements is **NOT** correct regarding Meckel diverticula

A. They may ulcerate due to ectopic acid-producing gastric tissue

B. They are found in 2% of the population

C. They are true diverticula

D. They can act as a fulcrum for intussusception and volvulus

E. They most commonly occur in the proximal jejunum

10. An elderly woman complains of fatigue, anemia, and bright red blood in stool. Which of the following is the **MOST LIKELY** diagnosis?

A. Rectal adenocarcinoma

B. Anal squamous cell carcinoma

C. Endometriosis

D. Small bowel adenocarcinoma

E. Gastric carcinoma

ANSWERS

1. The answer is C. Zenker diverticulum is an outpouching that branches off the upper esophagus. It arises in an area of anatomic weakness called Killian dehiscence.

2. The answer is B. Barrett glandular metaplasia in the lower esophagus is most often a consequence of reflux and increases the risk of developing esophageal adenocarcinoma (not squamous); therefore endoscopic surveillance is recommended.

3. The answer is C. Meckel diverticulum arises in the distal small bowel and is unlikely to present in neonates as obstruction.

4. The answer is D. The provided history is classic for pyloric stenosis.

5. The answer is B. Celiac sprue is a gluten-sensitive enteropathy characterized by diarrhea, duodenal biopsy showing blunting of the intestinal villous mucosa, and serum antibodies to endomysial reticulin.

6. The answer is B. Ulcerative colitis is associated with a few other systemic manifestations, including primary sclerosing cholangitis and uveitis. It may lead to toxic megacolon and over time the risk of carcinoma increases. Unlike Crohn disease, ulcerative colitis does not involve the small bowel.

7. The answer is D. Whipple disease is characterized by massive infiltration of the lamina propria by macrophages (periodic acid-Schiff stain positive).

8. The answer is D. Adenomatous polyps represent low-grade neoplasia, which may progress to high-grade dysplasia and invasive adenocarcinoma. Despite the increased risk of carcinoma in ulcerative colitis, pseudopolyps are hyperplastic and on their own do not increase the risk of cancer.

9. The answer is E. Meckel diverticula occur in the ileum.

10. The answer is A. Approximately 10% of colon cancers occur in the rectum and could be detected by routine annual rectal examination. Bleeding associated with a gastric carcinoma would be digested and appear black. Anal carcinoma is usually human papillomavirus–related and occurs in younger patients; small bowel adenocarcinoma is rare and endometriosis causing rectal bleeding would not be expected in a postmenopausal patient.

CHAPTER 9
LIVER AND BILIARY TRACT

*Hermes, wielder of the caduceus, bound Prometheus to
the mountain where an eagle ate his regenerating liver each day.*
—adapted from Aeschylus

I. Jaundice

A. Mechanism

1. Jaundice describes the yellow discoloration of the skin, sclerae, mucous membranes, and other tissues by excess **bilirubin,** which is the degradation product of **hemoglobin.**
   a. Bilirubin undergoes **glucuronidation** (conjugation) in the liver.
      (1) Conjugated bilirubin (direct) is easily excreted because it is soluble in water.
      (2) Unconjugated bilirubin (indirect) is not.
   b. A rise in either direct or indirect bilirubin raises the blood levels of total bilirubin.
   c. Jaundice is clinically apparent when the serum total bilirubin is above 3 mg/dL.
2. **Unconjugated hyperbilirubinemia** is associated with excess bilirubin production or impaired conjugation.
   a. Hemolysis causes elevated indirect bilirubin.
   b. Impaired conjugation is caused by reduced hepatic uptake resulting from liver disease (eg, hepatitis) or deficiencies.
3. **Conjugated hyperbilirubinemia** is caused by reduced hepatic excretion or impaired bile flow (eg, bile duct obstruction); consequently, the urine contains bilirubin, leading to dark urine.

B. Congenital and Genetic Causes

1. **Neonatal jaundice** occurs during the first week of life.
   a. There is a mild and transient rise in unconjugated bilirubin with a benign clinical course.
   b. It is caused by inadequate production of glucuronyl transferase by the immature liver.
   c. It is treated by UV exposure.

2. **Hemolytic disease** of the newborn is caused by maternal-fetal Rh incompatibility and is more clinically ominous and usually has higher bilirubin levels than benign neonatal jaundice.

3. **Breast milk jaundice** occurs in some breastfed newborns, usually after the first week, and lasts longer than physiologic jaundice.

4. **Gilbert syndrome** is a common cause of slightly increased unconjugated bilirubin, which is usually discovered by family history or an incidental finding in routine laboratory testing.
   a. There is no hepatic impairment or clinical symptoms.
   b. If the patient becomes stressed, it may lead to jaundice.

5. **Crigler-Najjar syndrome** is a severe familial enzyme deficiency with very high unconjugated bilirubin levels.
   a. Type I causes **kernicterus** and is uniformly fatal.
   b. Type II is less severe and responds to phenobarbital treatment, which reduces the unconjugated bilirubin levels.

6. **Dubin-Johnson syndrome** is an autosomal recessive disease with a defective protein carrier in the bile canalicular membrane, which leads to impaired bile excretion, black pigmentation of the liver, and elevated conjugated bilirubin levels.

II. Hepatitis and Cirrhosis

A. Viral Hepatitis

1. Acute viral hepatitis is characterized by jaundice and dramatically elevated liver enzymes (aspartate aminotransaminase [AST] and alanine aminotransaminase [ALT]).

2. Chronic viral hepatitis requires symptoms persisting for longer than 6 months.

3. **Hepatitis A** virus (HAV) is spread through **fecal-oral** transmission.
   a. It usually affects children and adolescents.
   b. Serology demonstrates acute antibodies (IgM anti-HAV).
   c. It is a self-limiting acute disease.

4. **Hepatitis B** virus (HBV) is a DNA virus.
   a. The complete virion is known as the **Dane particle.**
   b. Transmission may be through the **blood** and bodily fluids.
   c. 350 million people are carriers worldwide and there are 185,000 new infections each year in the United States.
   d. **Vertical transmission** (maternal-fetal) is common (90%).
   e. The incubation period averages 6–8 weeks.
   f. HBV infection causes acute hepatitis with resolution (>90%).
   g. It may cause chronic hepatitis, **cirrhosis** (5%), and cancer.
   h. Fulminant hepatitis with extensive necrosis may occur (<1%).
   i. HBV causes characteristic **ground-glass hepatocytes.**
   j. Diagnosis is made by serology.
      (1) **HBsAg** (surface antigen) provides the first evidence of infection and appears in the serum before symptoms.
      (2) **HBcAg** (core antigen) may be the only evidence of infection during the "window period" between the disappearance of HBsAg and the detectability of anti-HBs.
      (3) **HBsAB** (hepatitis B surface antibody) does not rise until the acute infection is over, representing recovery and is detectable for years following **vaccination.**

FULMINANT HEPATITIS

- *There is rapid progression of acute liver failure.*
- *More than 50% of cases are caused by viral hepatitis.*
- *Other causes include acetaminophen, isoniazid, monoamine oxidase inhibitors, halothane, methyldopa, and mushroom toxins (eg, Amanita phalloides).*
- *It is characterized by massive liver necrosis, causing jaundice and mental status changes without signs of chronic liver disease.*

     5. Hepatitis C virus (HCV) is a RNA virus.
       a. Transmission is primarily through the blood.
       b. It was the cause of nearly all transfusion-related hepatitis.
       c. The incubation period is typically 6–12 weeks.
       d. Most patients have only mild symptoms with waxing and waning liver enzyme levels.
       e. Chronic disease develops in most patients with a significantly increased risk of **cirrhosis** and hepatocellular carcinoma (HCC).
       f. Diagnosis is confirmed by detecting HCV by reverse transcription–polymerase chain reaction (RT-PCR), or immunoassay for serum anti-HCV antibody.
       g. Disease is monitored using liver function tests and serial liver needle core **biopsies** to score for **grade** of inflammation and **stage** of fibrosis, culminating in cirrhosis.
       h. Viral hepatitis classically causes **macronodular cirrhosis,** defined as nodules larger than 3 mm, but this pattern may also be seen in Wilson disease and α_1-antitrypsin deficiency.

HEPATITIS C

- *Chronic disease occurs in 85% of patients.*
- *The leading cause is injection drug use.*
- *Cirrhosis will develop in **20%** of patients within 20 years.*

     6. Hepatitis D virus (HDV, delta agent) can only infect hepatocytes in association with infection by HBV.
       a. Viral replication is completely dependent on the HBsAg.
       b. Coinfection of HDV and HBV results in a more severe illness than HBV alone, with up to 5% of patients having fulminant disease (vs 1%).
       c. Superinfection (HDV infection of a hepatitis B carrier) has an even higher rate of chronic progressive disease (80% vs 5%).
     7. Hepatitis E virus (HEV) is an **enterically** transmitted infection that is responsible for water-borne epidemics in equatorial regions.
       a. The disease is usually self-limited.
       b. In pregnant women, it is associated with a high mortality rate (20%).
     8. Epstein-Barr virus causes infectious mononucleosis and may cause a limited hepatitis.
     9. Cytomegalovirus and herpes simplex virus type-1 may cause hepatitis in immunocompromised patients.
     10. Adenovirus is an enteric virus that may affect the liver.
   B. Autoimmune Hepatitis
     1. Autoimmune hepatitis is clinically indistinguishable from chronic viral hepatitis and has a similar risk of cirrhosis.

2. It mostly affects **young women** with HLA-B8 or HLA-DRw3.

3. Histology shows chronic hepatitis with an infiltrate of lymphocytes and **plasma cells**.

4. Serologic diagnosis is based on absent viral serologic markers, elevated titers for antinuclear antibody (**ANA**), anti-smooth muscle antibody (**SMA**), or anti-liver/kidney microsome (**anti-LKM1**).

C. Drug-Induced Liver Damage

1. Some of the most clinically significant drugs leading to liver damage include alcohol (ethanol), acetaminophen, and salicylates.

2. Alcohol (ethanol) abuse is the leading cause of liver disease in the United States.

   a. Alcoholic liver disease is the collective term given to the disorders of steatosis (fatty liver), hepatitis, and cirrhosis.

   b. Hepatic **steatosis** begins as tiny fat droplets (microvesicular steatosis) and progresses to large globules that fill the cytoplasm, displacing the nucleus (macrovesicular).

   (1) Steatosis is reversible.

   (2) Steatosis may progress to hepatitis and cirrhosis.

   c. Alcoholic **hepatitis** may present acutely, especially following excessive alcohol intake.

   d. Biopsy reveals ballooning degeneration of swollen hepatocytes, protein tangles (**Mallory bodies**), cell necrosis (**acidophil bodies**), steatosis, and inflammation (Figure 9–1).

   e. Alcoholic **cirrhosis** is the **irreversible** end-stage form of alcoholic liver disease.

   (1) Alcohol abuse is a leading cause of cirrhosis.

   (2) Classically, alcohol causes **micronodular cirrhosis** (regenerative nodules are less than 3 mm in size).

   (3) Biopsy reveals nodular hepatocyte regeneration surrounded by bridging bands of fibrosis (Figure 9–2).

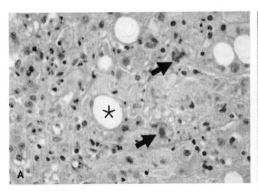
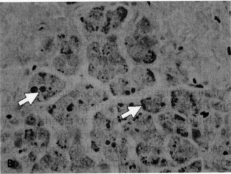

Figure 9–1. Hepatitis. A: Alcoholic hepatitis is common with characteristic Mallory hyaline bodies (arrows) and steatosis (fat deposition, asterisk). **B:** α_1-Antitrypsin deficiency causes liver disease with characteristic periodic acid-Schiff positive/diastase resistant globules of α_1-antitrypsin protein in hepatocytes (arrows).

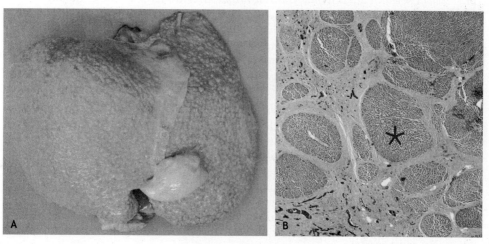

Figure 9–2. Cirrhosis. A: Gross photograph of cirrhotic liver with nodular surface, which histologic sections show to be regenerating nodules (asterisk) of hepatocytes within bridging fibrosis **(B)**.

(4) Patients present with the stigmata of chronic liver disease, or complications of portal hypertension.

(5) There is also an increased risk of HCC.

(6) However, most patients die of hepatic failure, variceal bleeding, or infection.

3. Nonalcoholic steatohepatitis (**NASH**) is clinically and histologically similar to alcoholic liver disease but occurs without heavy alcohol consumption.

    a. NASH is associated with **obesity,** dyslipidemia, and **diabetes.**

    b. NASH may be the cause of **"cryptogenic cirrhosis."**

4. Acetaminophen (N-acetyl-p-aminophenol, APAP) toxicity is covered in Chapter 1.

5. Aspirin treatment of **children** with a viral illness may lead to **Reye syndrome**, which is a rare, potentially fatal, acute mitochondrial disorder involving the liver and brain.

FATTY LIVER OF PREGNANCY

- *Acute fatty liver of pregnancy presents in the third trimester.*
- *Symptoms range from mildly elevated liver function tests to fulminant hepatitis.*
- *The mechanism is thought to be related to defective mitochondrial fatty acid oxidation, leading to steatosis.*

    D. Parasites and Infectious Hepatitis

      1. Bacteria may infect the liver, such as *Staphylococcus aureus, Salmonella typhi,* mycobacteria, and *Treponema pallidum.*

      2. *Echinococcus granulosus* infection, which occurs through ingestion of tapeworm eggs, forms **hydatid cysts;** aspiration or biopsy of these cysts may cause a life-threatening anaphylactic reaction.

      3. *Entamoeba histolytica* causes dysentery and amebic liver **abscess.**

4. *Fasciola hepatica* and *Opisthorchis sinensis* are liver flukes that infest the bile ducts causing biliary fibrosis and increasing the patient's risk of cholangiocarcinoma.
5. *Schistosoma mansoni* and *Schistosoma japonicum* cause **schistosomiasis.**
   a. The larva penetrate the skin, often through the feet.
   b. The larva proliferate in the intestines and portal veins, causing portal vein obstruction, which is the leading cause of **portal hypertension** worldwide.

E. **Metabolic Disorders**
   1. **Hereditary hemochromatosis** is an inherited disorder of iron absorption and accumulation, causing cirrhosis, diabetes, and heart disease (see Chapter 2).
   2. **Wilson disease** is an autosomal recessive disorder of **copper** accumulation that presents in adolescents and young adults.
      a. Copper deposits in the liver, eye, brain, and kidney.
      b. Liver findings range from chronic hepatitis to cirrhosis.
      c. **Kayser-Fleischer rings** are circumferential copper deposits at the periphery of the cornea.
      d. Involvement of the lenticular nucleus of the putamen, a portion of the basal ganglia, causes a movement disorder.
      e. Dementia and psychosis may develop.
      f. Serum studies show decreased levels of the copper-binding protein, **ceruloplasmin.**
   3. **α_1-Antitrypsin (A1AT) deficiency** is a genetic disease that causes pan-lobular pulmonary emphysema and chronic liver disease.
      a. The *A1AT* gene is located on chromosome 14, and there are over 75 allelic variants with co-dominant expression.
      b. The most severe disease is associated with **PiZ homozygotes**.
      c. The PiZ allele is seen in 2–4% of all northern Europeans.
      d. α_1-Antitrypsin deficiency is the most common chronic liver disease in **children.**
      e. Cholestasis is present in infancy, with 75% of patients having an elevated ALT.
      f. Symptoms and liver function tests usually resolve by adolescence, before a second peak in late adulthood.
      g. Late complications include cirrhosis, which develops in 15–20% of those over age 50, as well as an increased risk of HCC.
      h. Liver biopsy reveals red cytoplasmic globules of A1AT highlighted by periodic acid-Schiff (PAS) stain (Figure 9–1).
      i. Diagnosis can be confirmed by low serum A1AT levels.
   4. Congenital storage disorders affect the liver (see Chapter 19).

F. **Hepatic Failure**
   1. Despite the liver's tremendous capacity to regenerate, a loss of more than 85% of parenchyma is enough for the organ to fail.
   2. Liver failure is usually fatal and **transplantation** is required.
   3. Cirrhosis is one of the most common causes of death in the Western world, with most deaths attributable to hepatic failure and complications of portal hypertension.

STIGMATA OF CHRONIC LIVER DISEASE

- *Jaundice and icterus result from hyperbilirubinemia.*
- *Peripheral edema and ascites result from decreased albumin synthesis.*
- *Bleeding is caused by decreased coagulation factor synthesis.*
- *Hematemesis results from varices and portal hypertension.*
- *Palmar erythema, spider angiomas, gynecomastia, and hypogonadism are due to deranged estrogen metabolism and hyperestrogenemia.*
- *Hepatic encephalopathy with asterixis (hand flapping tremor) and altered mental status is due to the inability to excrete ammonia.*
- *Hepatorenal syndrome refers to the complication of acute renal failure associated with hepatic failure, which may be rapidly fatal.*

III. Hepatic Vascular Pathology

A. **Portal Hypertension**
   1. It occurs when resistance to portal blood flow is increased.
   2. In cirrhosis, high portal pressure is caused by sinusoidal and perivenular fibrosis.
   3. High portal pressure leads to 'upstream' **varicosities** (eg, esophagus, rectum) at anastomotic sites between the portal and systemic circulation.
      a. Hemorrhagic esophageal varicosities may be deadly.
      b. Rectal varicosities present as hemorrhoids.
      c. Radiating varicosities of the periumbilical veins are known as **caput medusae**, where they anastomose with epigastric veins.
      d. Pressure in the splenic vein leads to **splenomegaly**.
   4. Posthepatic conditions include hepatic vein obstruction (Budd-Chiari syndrome), and right-sided heart failure.

B. **Budd-Chiari syndrome**
   1. It is associated with **hypercoagulable states** such as polycythemia vera, pregnancy, and tumors, causing **hepatic vein thrombosis**.
   2. It may lead to backflow into the hepatic central vein, causing centrilobular congestion and necrosis with pain and jaundice.

C. **Chronic Congestion**
   1. **Nutmeg liver** is the classic gross presentation of chronic right-sided heart failure leading to chronic centrilobular hepatic congestion and necrosis.
   2. Eventually, this leads to fibrous bridging between central veins (**cardiac sclerosis**), rather than portal tracts (viral cirrhosis).

D. **Peliosis**
   1. Primary sinusoidal dilation causing **blood-filled** collections throughout the liver is peliosis, rather than a hemangioma.
   2. It is associated with anabolic steroids, oral contraceptives, danazol, and *Bartonella henselae* infection.
   3. It may lead to intra-abdominal hemorrhage or hepatic failure.

E. **Veno-occlusive Disease**
   1. It is defined as sinusoidal obstruction because of fibrous obliteration of the central veins.

2. Common risk factors include Jamaican bush tea and high-dose chemotherapy before bone marrow transplantation.
3. Patients have ascites and elevated bilirubin levels.
4. Treatment is supportive.
5. It has a high mortality rate (30%) in patients who have undergone bone marrow transplantation.

IV. Hepatic Neoplasia

A. Hemangioma
  1. Hemangiomas are the most common benign hepatic neoplasm.
  2. They are spongy small nodules, which are usually diagnosed by imaging studies.
  3. They should not be mistaken for metastatic disease or biopsied, which may lead to significant bleeding.

B. Pseudotumor: Focal Nodular Hyperplasia
  1. This is a well-circumscribed mass lesion that usually presents as a spontaneous mass in **young women**.
  2. It is associated with **oral contraceptive** use.
  3. Biopsy reveals a **mixture** of benign hepatocytes and bile ducts, consistent with a hyperplastic lesion rather than a clonal neoplastic proliferation of hepatocytes (eg, HCC).

C. Adenoma
  1. It resembles focal nodular hyperplasia but **lacks bile ducts**, which is consistent with it being a benign low-grade neoplastic proliferation of hepatocytes.
  2. Adenomas also tend to occur in **young women** who take **oral contraceptives** and often regress when the contraceptive is discontinued.
  3. Adenomas are distinguished from HCC by the absence of thickened hepatocyte trabecula, significant cytologic atypia, or invasion of surrounding parenchyma.

D. Hepatocellular Carcinoma
  1. High rates of hepatitis (B and C) in Asia and Africa are associated with the highest rates of HCC.
  2. HCC occurs in 5/100,000 people in North America.
  3. **Cirrhosis** is absent in 50% of cases.
  4. It presents with elevated alpha fetoprotein (**AFP**) (75% of cases).
  5. Biopsy reveals hepatocytes, but no bile ducts, arranged in thickened trabecular plates (>3 cells thick) (Figure 9–3).
      a. **Low-grade** tumors are difficult to discern from adenomas.
      b. **High-grade** tumors are difficult to discern from metastases.
  6. Prognosis depends on the stage of the carcinoma and whether cirrhosis is present.
      a. Stage 1 is a solitary tumor without vascular invasion.
      b. **Stage 2** has vascular invasion or is multifocal.
      c. **Stage 3** is multifocal large tumors (>5 cm in size).
      d. **Stage 4** has distant metastatic disease (usually lungs).
  7. **Fibrolamellar variant** of HCC may have a better prognosis than conventional HCC.
      a. It usually occurs in young adults without a history of prior liver disease.
      b. It is characterized by oncocytic-like hepatocytes (abundant intracellular mitochondria) infiltrating fibrous stroma.

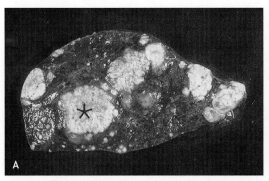
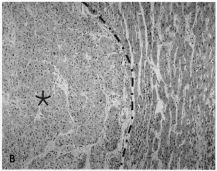

Figure 9–3. Hepatocellular carcinoma versus metastases. A: Gross photograph of liver with multifocal white nodular disease. **B:** Histologic sections show tumor (asterisk), which is sharply demarcated from normal liver (dotted line). Tumor cells vaguely resemble liver, but diagnosis is confirmed by Hepar-1 immunostain and elevated alpha fetoprotein levels.

E. Hepatoblastoma

1. This is the most common liver tumor in children.
2. If left untreated, it is fatal within a few years of diagnosis.
3. Biopsy may reveal tumor cells resembling fetal liver development, malignant appearing HCC, or primitive mesenchyme (eg, cartilage).

METASTATIC DISEASE

- *Most malignant neoplasms identified in the liver are metastases.*
- *Common sites of primary disease include, **colon**, lung, **breast**, **pancreatic** adenocarcinoma, **neuroendocrine carcinoma** (carcinoid or pancreatic islet tumors), and ovary.*
- *Biopsy reveals a **mixed pattern** of normal liver and malignant tumor population, rather than a clonal population of malignant hepatocytes.*
- ***Immunohistochemical staining**, clinical history, and imaging studies are usually sufficient to determine the most likely primary source.*

V. Gallbladder and Bile Duct

A. Congenital Anomalies

1. **Biliary atresia** is the absence or destruction of extrahepatic bile ducts, resulting in complete obstruction to bile flow.
   a. It is a common cause of death from liver disease in children.
   b. It is also a major cause of neonatal cholestasis.
2. **Choledochal cysts** are congenital saccular dilatations of the common bile duct that may cause obstructive symptoms and carry a high risk of stone formation, pancreatitis, and bile duct carcinoma.

B. Intrahepatic Biliary Tract

1. **Primary biliary cirrhosis** is progressive cholestatic liver disease with an autoimmune etiology.

a. It causes **granulomatous** destruction of medium-sized bile ducts with dense lymphoplasmacytic portal infiltrate.

b. **Chronic cholestasis** and **fibrosis** lead to **cirrhosis**.

c. It affects primarily middle-aged women, often with a history of another **autoimmune disease**.

d. Pruritus, malaise, and jaundice are presenting symptoms.

e. Approximately 90% have a positive **anti-mitochondrial** antibody (AMA) by immunofluorescence assay.

f. Direct bilirubin and cholesterol levels are elevated.

g. Hypercholesterolemia leads to characteristic cutaneous **xanthoma** formation.

h. Liver **transplantation** is often required.

2. **Secondary biliary cirrhosis** is caused by extrahepatic bile duct obstruction, leading to intrahepatic biliary inflammation and injury.

a. It is often associated with ascending cholangitis and bacterial infection.

b. Biopsy shows neutrophils, distinguishing it from primary biliary cirrhosis.

3. **Primary sclerosing cholangitis** is a chronic inflammatory disorder of the extrahepatic and intrahepatic biliary tree.

a. Biopsy shows a distinctive "**onion-skin**" bile duct fibrosis.

b. Imaging shows "**string of beads**" highlighting segmental bile ducts stenoses.

c. Approximately 70% of patients also have inflammatory bowel disease, particularly **ulcerative colitis**.

d. There is a markedly increased risk of **cholangiocarcinoma**.

4. **Biliary tree anomalies** are common incidental findings and often associated with polycystic kidney disease.

a. Meyenburg complex (**bile duct hamartoma**) consists of a subcapsular nodular proliferation of benign dilated bile ducts.

b. **Polycystic liver disease** manifests as multiple fluid-containing cysts replacing functional hepatic parenchyma; it may be associated with polycystic kidney disease.

c. **Caroli disease** is a congenital, nonobstructive, segmental dilation of intrahepatic bile ducts.

C. **Extrahepatic Bile Duct**

1. **Choledocholithiasis** refers to the presence of stones within the biliary tree, especially the common bile duct.

a. The stones originate in the gallbladder.

b. Complications include bile duct obstruction, gallstone pancreatitis, hepatic abscess, and cholangitis.

2. **Cholangitis** occurs with bacterial infection of bile ducts, usually by enteric **gram-negative** aerobes.

a. Obstruction from stones is the most common risk factor.

b. Involvement of the intrahepatic biliary tree is called **ascending cholangitis**.

ASCENDING CHOLANGITIS

- *Ascending cholangitis classically presents with **Charcot triad** of fever, jaundice, and right upper quadrant pain.*
- ***Reynold pentad** adds hypotension and altered mental status.*

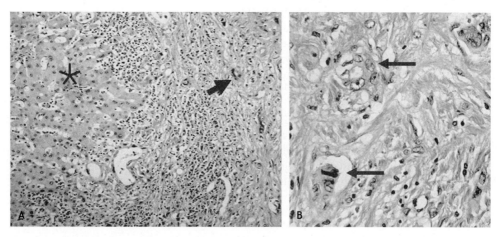

Figure 9–4. Cholangiocarcinoma. A: Klatskin tumor in the hilum of the liver infiltrating into and around normal hepatocytes (asterisk). **B:** The carcinoma is arranged in small scattered glands (arrows) within desmoplastic (scar-like) stroma similar to ductal carcinoma of the breast.

D. Gallbladder
1. **Cholelithiasis** (gallstones) accounts for nearly 95% of all biliary tract disease.
    a. Most cases are asymptomatic (75%), but others cause "colicky" abdominal pain.
    b. **Cholesterol** gallstones are the most common, and are associated with **estrogenic changes** (eg, pregnancy or oral contraceptives) that increase HMG-CoA reductase activity enhancing cholesterol uptake and biosynthesis.
    c. Obese, multiparous, middle-aged women are most at risk.
2. Cholesterolosis refers to the "**strawberry gallbladder**" appearance of tiny scattered gold specks overlying the red gallbladder mucosa; the lamina propria is filled with foamy macrophages.
3. **Cholecystitis** is the most common indication for abdominal surgery and is almost always caused by **gallstones.**
    a. **Acute cholecystitis** presents with severe right upper quadrant pain, leukocytosis, fever, and mild jaundice.
    b. **Chronic cholecystitis** presents with colicky pain after fatty meals, sometimes radiating to the right shoulder.
4. **Rokitansky-Aschoff sinuses** are out pouchings of mucosal epithelium into the muscular wall (gallbladder diverticuli).
5. **Porcelain gallbladder** is extensive dystrophic calcification and wall thickening, which may harbor malignancy.
6. **Gallbladder adenocarcinoma** is very rare, but frequently spreads directly into the liver and is metastatic at the time of diagnosis.

E. Cholangiocarcinoma
1. This malignancy of the biliary tree may present in the liver, hilum (**Klatskin tumor**), or anywhere in the bile duct.

2. The incidence is 0.5/100,000 in North America.
3. Most cases lack clear risk factors, but there is a slightly increased risk associated with primary sclerosing cholangitis, contrast media for imaging studies (eg, Thorotrast), and the liver fluke *O sinensis*.
4. Biopsy reveals infiltrating glands with only moderately atypical nuclei, resembling reactive bile ductules (Figure 9–4); however, malignancy is supported by destructive invasion and a background of desmoplastic (silvery scar-like) stroma.
5. Klatskin tumors in the hilum are usually not operable.
6. Prognosis depends on the stage of disease.
   a. **Stage 1** is confined to the bile duct.
   b. **Stage 2** is invading surrounding structures.
   c. **Stage 3** is invading blood vessels or gastrointestinal tract.
   d. **Stage 4** has distant metastases.

CLINICAL PROBLEMS

1. A 29-year-old woman who takes birth control pills complains of right upper quadrant pain. A mass is found in her liver. Which of the following is most likely?

   A. Metastatic pancreatic ductal adenocarcinoma

   B. Focal nodular hyperplasia of the liver

   C. Hepatocellular carcinoma

   D. Metastatic pancreatic endocrine neoplasm (islet cell tumor)

   E. None of the above

2. Which of the following descriptions of a liver biopsy would be most consistent with a diagnosis of chronic hepatitis C?

   A. Moderate steatosis; mixed lymphocytic and neutrophilic inflammation; Mallory bodies; sinusoidal fibrosis

   B. Mild steatosis; lymphocytic inflammation of portal areas; piecemeal necrosis; bridging fibrosis

   C. Hepatocellular ballooning; globules that are periodic acid-Schiff positive/diastase resistant present within hepatocytes

   D. Bridging fibrosis; mild lymphocytic inflammation; marked hemosiderin deposition within hepatocytes on iron stain

   E. Marked thickening and distortion of hepatocellular plates; marked nuclear atypia of hepatocytes; increased hepatocyte mitoses

3. In a patient with α_1-antitrypsin disease, a liver biopsy would **MOST LIKELY** show:

   A. Enlarged swollen hepatocytes with clear cytoplasm

   B. Periodic acid-Schiff (PAS)-positive deposits within hepatocytes

   C. PAS-positive deposits within the cytoplasm of macrophages

D. Iron stain-positive deposits within the cytoplasm of hepatocytes

E. None of the above

4. Which of the following statements regarding primary sclerosing cholangitis is **CORRECT?**

A. It is frequently associated with autoimmune gastritis

B. Elevated serum anti-mitochondrial antibody (AMA)

C. It is sometimes associated with Crohn disease

D. It is more common in females than males

E. Granulomatous destruction of medium-sized bile ducts

5. Impaired hepatic blood flow in veno-occlusive disease is due to:

A. Thrombosis of the major hepatic veins

B. Sinusoidal fibrosis

C. Nodular regeneration of the parenchyma

D. Fibrous obliteration of terminal hepatic veins

E. Fibrous obliteration of large bile ducts

6. Which of the following statements **BEST DESCRIBES** genetic hemochromatosis?

A. Iron deficiency anemia develops from a mutation in the *HFE* gene.

B. It is an autosomal dominant disorder that can lead to iron overload in the liver and other organs.

C. Patients homozygous for a mutant HFE allele absorb excessive quantities of iron from the diet.

D. Women typically manifest the disease earlier than men, who are protected by higher androgen levels.

E. The disease results in iron deposition primarily within macrophages of the liver, heart, and pancreas.

7. On reviewing a liver biopsy specimen, the following features are identified: steatosis, Mallory bodies, and acute inflammation. Which of the following is the **MOST LIKELY** diagnosis?

A. Glycogen storage disease

B. Acetaminophen overdose

C. Herpetic hepatitis

D. Primary biliary cirrhosis

E. Alcohol-related liver disease

8. A patient with an elevated serum alpha fetoprotein undergoes resection of a liver mass. The mass has the following features: crowded cells growing in thick (4 or more cells) cords/plates, occasional mitoses, an absence of normal bile ducts, and necrosis. Which is the **MOST LIKELY** diagnosis?

A. Hepatocellular adenoma

B. Cholangiocarcinoma

C. Focal nodular hyperplasia

D. Hepatocellular carcinoma

E. Metastatic adenocarcinoma of the colon

9. All the following are associated with hepatitis C, **EXCEPT:**

A. Chronic hepatitis does not develop in most patients.

B. It is the number one cause of liver transplantation.

C. Injection drug use is the number one risk factor.

D. Cirrhosis develops in 20% of patients.

E. It is predisposing factor to hepatocellular carcinoma.

10. A 40-year-old obese woman complains of right upper quadrant pain after eating, which radiates into her back. What is the most likely diagnosis?

A. Duodenal ulcer

B. Hepatoma

C. Cholecystitis

D. Pancreatitis

E. Metastatic adenocarcinoma to the liver

ANSWERS

1. The answer is B. Focal nodular hyperplasia is usually seen in young women and is associated with contraceptive use. It is distinguished from hepatoma by the presence of bile ducts characteristic of a hyperplastic mixed population of cell-types, rather than a clonal proliferation.

2. The answer is B. Chronic active hepatitis is graded according to portal lymphocytic inflammation and hepatocyte necrosis and staged according to degree of periportal fibrosis; bridging fibrosis indicates cirrhosis.

3. The answer is B. α_1-Antitrypsin accumulation in hepatocytes is highlighted by periodic acid-Schiff stain with diastase. Patients also usually have pan-lobular emphysema associated with tobacco smoking.

4. The answer is C. Primary sclerosis cholangitis is associated with inflammatory bowel disease (Crohn disease).

5. The answer is D. Veno-occlusive disease is caused by fibrous obliteration of distal hepatic veins (sometimes seen after high-dose chemotherapy for bone marrow transplant).

6. The answer is C. Hemochromatosis is an autosomal recessive disease; heterozygotes are carriers. If the patient has two copies of the mutant allele, they abnormally reabsorb iron in the gastrointestinal tract, leading to accumulation in the liver, heart, pancreas, and skin.

7. The answer is E. Ethanol is a toxin and causes hepatocyte damage and fatty metaplasia (steatosis). Damage leads to intracytoplasmic Mallory bodies, neutrophil recruitment, and may eventually cause cirrhosis.

8. The answer is D. Hepatocellular carcinoma usually arises in patients with a history of chronic hepatitis and cirrhosis. Alpha fetaprotein levels are significantly elevated. Notably, some cases occur in patients with no history of liver disease (eg, fibrolamellar hepatocellular carcinoma) with a better prognosis.

9. The answer is A. Unlike hepatitis B, most cases of hepatitis C persist as chronic active hepatitis (85% of patients). They also have an increased risk of cirrhosis and need for transplantation.

10. The answer is C. Premenopausal, multiparous, middle-aged women, who are obese, are at particular risk for gallbladder stones and inflammation (cholecystitis).

*Certaine pisse-pot lectures . . . used by all those
who pretend knowledge of diseases, by the urine.*
—1637 by Thomas Brian

I. Congenital and Cystic Diseases

A. Congenital and Cystic Dysplasia

1. **Renal agenesis** (or absence) of both kidneys is incompatible with life; unilateral agenesis is often accompanied by compensatory hypertrophy of the remaining kidney.
2. **Renal hypoplasia** describes a kidney with reduced nephron number.
   a. Most commonly, hypoplasia is the consequence of fewer renal lobes forming during development (Figure 10–1).
   b. Hypoplasia with diffuse nephron absence is called oligomeganephronia.
   c. In both forms, the remaining nephrons are large due to compensatory hypertrophy.
3. **Horseshoe kidney** is a single, horseshoe-shaped organ with fused lower poles (or less commonly, upper poles) that occurs in 0.1–0.2% of the population.
4. **Cystic dysplasia** is characterized by solid and cystic zones of immature collecting ducts, disorganized mesenchymal tissue, and often **cartilage.**
   a. Cystic dysplasia is usually unilateral and is not hereditary.
   b. Grossly, the cysts distort the shape of the kidney, presenting as a renal mass or poor renal function.
   c. Despite the name, there is no premalignant potential.

B. Polycystic Kidney Disease

1. **Autosomal dominant** polycystic kidney disease (ADPKD) results in the gradual development of innumerable **bilateral** renal cysts that usually present in adults and eventually cause renal failure.
   a. ADPKD kidneys are markedly enlarged (4 kg, rather than 0.3 kg), consisting of variably sized cysts containing clear fluid (Figure 10–1).
   b. Cysts may arise from any nephron segment.
   c. ADPKD may also be accompanied by liver cysts (polycystic liver disease) and **intracranial berry aneurysms**.
   d. ADPKD is a genetically heterogeneous disease, but some pathogenic mutations have been identified:

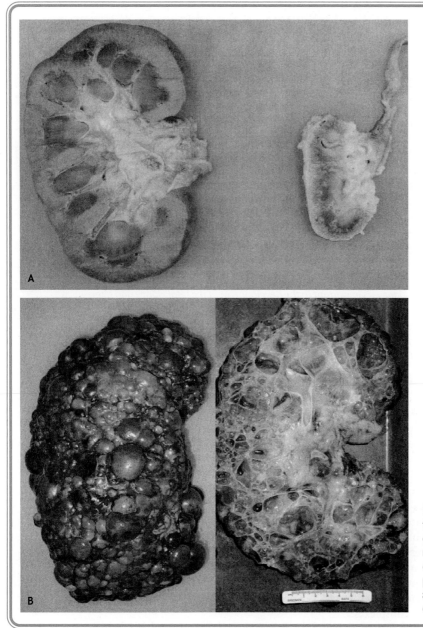

Figure 10–1. Congenital and cystic disease of the kidney. A: Normal adult kidney (left) compared with a hypoplastic kidney and adult autosomal dominant polycystic kidney disease **(B).**

    (1) The **PKD1** gene (chromosome 16p13.3) (85–90% of cases)
    (2) The **PKD2** gene (chromosome 4q21–23)
  2. Autosomal recessive polycystic kidney disease (ARPKD) most commonly is apparent at birth; bilateral kidneys have numerous minute cysts, preferentially in **collecting tubules.**

a. The affected gene has been identified as **PKHD1** (chromosome 6p21), encoding **fibrocystin.**

b. Congenital hepatic fibrosis may also affect these patients.

C. **Cystic Diseases of the Renal Medulla**

1. **Medullary sponge kidney** is a poorly characterized condition presenting in adulthood with multiple collecting duct cysts, which lead to an increased risk of complications, including infection, nephrolithiasis, and hemorrhage.

2. **Nephronophthisis-medullary cystic disease complex** presents most commonly in childhood, and cysts are typically concentrated at the cortico-medullary junction.

D. **Other Cysts**

1. **Acquired cystic renal disease** occurs in patients with end-stage renal disease, including those receiving long-term **dialysis.**

2. Simple cysts may develop in the renal cortex with age.

   a. Cysts may cause hemorrhage or pain.

   b. Cysts must be discriminated from renal cell carcinoma.

OLIGOHYDRAMNIOS

CLINICAL CORRELATION

- *Proper function of the developing kidneys is important to the development of the fetal kidney and fetal lung.*

- *Fluid excreted by the kidneys contributes to amniotic fluid; therefore, lack of adequate kidney function is one of the causes of oligohydramnios contributing to a series of anomalies, including the Potter sequence (see Chapter 19).*

II. Glomerular Diseases

A. **Patterns of Acute Injury**

1. The glomerulus has a limited pattern response to injury.

   a. **Endocapillary proliferation** is **mesangial** and **endothelial.**

   b. **Extracapillary proliferation** is proliferation of cells in the Bowman space, leading to formation of a **crescent,** often occurring with glomerular basement membrane (**GBM**) breaks.

   c. **Exudation** is influx of white blood cells (leukocytes, usually neutrophils), and cytokines secreted by these cells may contribute to glomerular injury.

2. **Hematuria** is often described by patients as tea or cola-colored urine (rather than bright red blood).

   a. Hematuria results from breaks in the GBM, which permit red blood cells into the Bowman space, into tubules, and finally into the urine.

   b. Urinalysis shows **red blood cell casts.**

3. Many glomerular diseases are associated with deposition of antibody or antigen-antibody complexes.

   a. The site of deposition and pattern of damage is determined by factors such as the size and charge of the proteins, and whether the antigen is a component of the glomerulus.

   b. **In-situ immune complex** deposition occurs when the antibody and antigen combine at the site of renal injury.

      (1) The antigen may be 'intrinsic' to the kidney.

         (a) Type IV collagen is an intrinsic antigen in **Goodpasture** anti-GBM disease.

(*b*) Proteins expressed by podocytes may also be the intrinsic antigens in membranous glomerulopathy.

(*2*) The antigen may be "extrinsic" to the kidney.

(*a*) The antigens may be captured by the glomerulus (eg, from microorganisms or drugs).

(*b*) The antigens may be endogeneous from the patient's own cells (eg, nucleic acids from lupus or a tumor).

c. **Circulating immune complexes** are deposited in the glomeruli after the antibody and antigen *combine* in the bloodstream.

ACUTE NEPHRITIC SYNDROME

CLINICAL CORRELATION

- *Acute nephritic syndrome is characterized by elevated serum creatinine and blood urea nitrogen (BUN) levels, hematuria, oliguria, edema, hypertension, and mild proteinuria.*
- *Glomerular lesions leading to acute nephritic syndrome include postinfectious glomerulonephritis, IgA nephropathy, lupus nephritis, and Alport syndrome.*
- *Crescentic glomerulonephritis may cause nephritic syndrome or rapidly progressive glomerulonephritis (RPGN).*

B. **Primary Acute Glomerulonephritis**

1. **Postinfectious glomerulonephritis** is related to antibodies directed at an infecting microorganism.

a. **Strep throat** is the most common inciting infection in temperate climates, but other infections, including chronic infections such as endocarditis, may be causative.

b. Light microscopic findings are diffuse and include global proliferation within glomeruli (Figure 10–2), neutrophil exudation, and red cell casts within tubules.

c. Immune complexes accumulate as "humps" on the epithelial side ("subepithelial") of the GBM, which may be detected by **electron microscopy (EM)** or **immunofluorescence microscopy (IFM);** IFM shows that these humps consist of IgG and C3 (Tables 10–1 and 10–2).

d. Although postinfectious glomerulonephritis is typically a self-limited disease, it may require antibiotic treatment of the underlying infection.

2. **IgA nephropathy (Berger disease)** is an immune deposit disease in which the principal antibody is **IgA** deposited in the mesangium.

a. It is the most common form of primary glomerular disease.

b. Light microscopic finding is mesangial cell proliferation.

c. IFM shows IgA in the mesangium (Figure 10–3).

d. EM shows densities in the same distribution.

e. IgA nephropathy may be associated with the systemic syndrome **Henoch-Schönlein purpura (HSP).**

(*1*) In addition to glomerulonephritis, HSP may include purpuric rash, abdominal pain, and joint pain.

(*2*) HSP is most common in children (ages 3–8), and renal involvement may be more severe in adults.

(*3*) The symptoms can be attributed to a common pathologic lesion in affected sites, that of necrotizing (leukocytoclastic) vasculitis with IgA deposition.

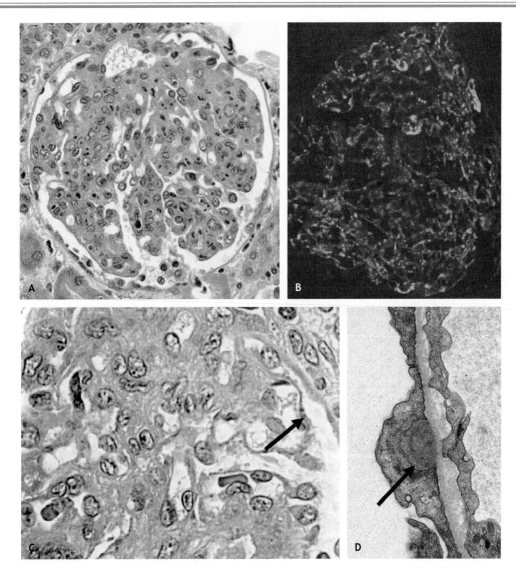

Figure 10–2. Proliferative glomerulonephritis (postinfectious). A: Light microscopy showing glomerulus with increased cellularity, including numerous neutrophils (period acid-Schiff stain, 400 ✕). **B:** Immunofluorescence microscopy for IgG showing scattered immune complex deposits along glomerular capillary walls (400 ✕). **C:** Glomerular basement membrane (GBM) has "hump-like" subepithelial deposits (arrow, between podocyte and GBM), highlighted by electron microscopic image **(D)** showing podocyte surrounding deposit (magnification 10,000 ✕).

Table 10–1. Glomerular Pathology Definitions.

Term	Definition
Subepithelial	Between the podocyte and GBM (on the epithelial side of GBM)
Subendothelial	Between the endothelium and GBM (on the endothelial side of GBM)
Crescent	Extracapillary proliferation of cells, in Bowman space, often associated with necrosis of the glomerular tuft and GBM
Segmental	Involves part of a glomerulus
Global	Involves the entire glomerulus
Focal	Involves only some of the glomeruli
Diffuse	Involves all of the glomeruli

GBM, glomerular basement membrane.

RAPIDLY PROGRESSIVE GLOMERULONEPHRITIS

* *RPGN is a clinical term describing patients with an acute nephritic syndrome and rapid progression to renal failure.*
* *The pathologic correlate is glomerulonephritis with crescents.*
* *Crescents are associated with breaks in the GBM and necrosis of the glomerular tuft.*

   3. Anti-GBM disease is one of the three causes of crescentic glomerulonephritis, usually presenting as RPGN.
      a. Autoantibodies to an intrinsic protein of the GBM cause destruction of the capillary wall.
      b. Type IV collagen is the most common autoantibody target.
      c. Light microscopy shows extracapillary proliferation (crescents) within the Bowman capsule (Figure 10–4A-B).
      d. The characteristic IFM finding is a linear ribbon-like distribution of the IgG antibody along the capillary wall, matching the distribution of antigen (Table 10–2).
      e. Cross reaction of the antibody with pulmonary capillary basement membranes results in lung hemorrhage, and the **pulmonary-renal syndrome (Goodpasture syndrome).**
   4. Pauci-immune crescentic glomerulonephritis is a small vessel vasculitis affecting glomeruli, and other capillaries, and is also known as ANCA-associated glomerulonephritis.
      a. ANCAs are anti-neutrophil cytoplasmic antibodies.
         (1) p-ANCAs are most commonly directed at myeloperoxidase.
         (2) c-ANCAs usually react with proteinase 3.

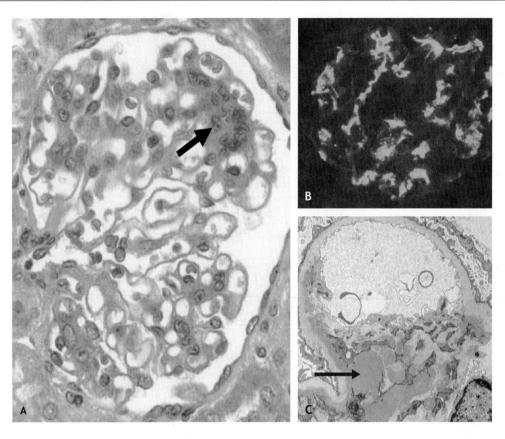

Figure 10–3. IgA nephropathy. A: Light microscopy showing mesangial hypercellularity (arrow) (400 ×). **B:** Immunofluorescence microscopy for IgA with mesangial localization of immune complexes. **C:** Electron microscopy also shows predominantly mesangial localization of deposits (arrow; magnification 6000 ×).

    b. Tissue damage is predominantly due to neutrophil degranulation, and there are no immune complexes deposited in glomeruli by IFM or EM, hence the synonym pauci-immune glomerulonephritis (Figure 10–4C-D).

    c. There are several clinical syndromes associated with ANCAs, but findings are identical on renal biopsy, and clinical correlation is required (for example, see "Wegener granulomatosis" in Chapter 6).

ALPORT SYNDROME (HEREDITARY NEPHRITIS)

- *Alport syndrome results from a defect in an important component of the GBM, the collagen IV α5 chain, (which normally complexes with the Goodpasture antigen, α3 chain).*
- *Since the gene for collagen IV α5 chain is on the **X-chromosome, males** are most often affected.*
- *Patients have hematuria and proteinuria.*
- *Light microscopy shows glomerular scarring (sclerosis).*

CLINICAL
CORRELATION

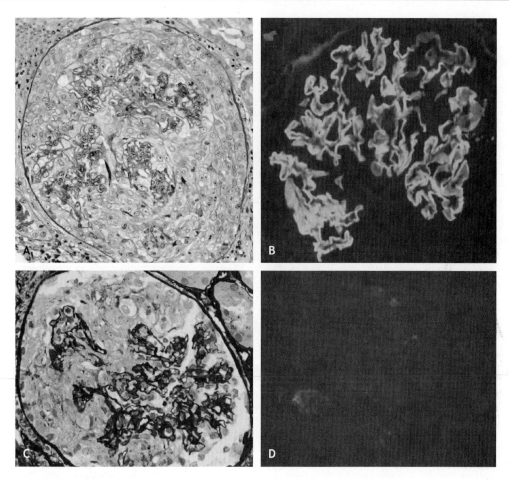

Figure 10–4. Crescentic glomerulonephritis. A: Anti-glomerular basement membrane (GBM) disease, light microscopy showing a crescent filling Bowman space (periodic acid-Schiff stains GBM magenta, 400 ×). **B:** Anti-GBM disease, immunofluorescence microscopy (IFM) showing IgG in an ultrathin linear staining pattern along GBM; no granularity (400 ×). **C:** ANCA-associated glomerulonephritis (pauci-immune glomerulonephritis) showing a crescent almost filling Bowman space (Jones silver stains GBM black, 400 ×). **D:** IFM showing near absence of staining for immune deposits (IgG, 400 ×).

- *EM shows thinning of the GBM, but no immune deposits by IFM.*
- *Nonrenal findings include sensorineural **deafness.***
    5. **Nephrotic syndrome** is a clinical syndrome characterized by heavy proteinuria (>3.5 g/day), edema, hypoalbuminemia, and hyperlipidemia; the serum creatinine is often normal.
        a. **Membranous glomerulonephritis** is a relatively common slowly progressive disease with immune complex deposits accumulating along the subepithelial surface of the GBM (Figure 10–5).

Table 10–2. Key Features of Glomerular Diseases.

Renal Diagnosis	Clinical Presentation	Light Microscopy	Immunofluorescence Microscopy (IF)	Electron Microscopy (EM)
Postinfectious glomerulonephritis	Nephritic	Diffuse global hypercellularity; neutrophils; casts	Coarse granular IgG, C3, widely scattered	Subepithelial humps
IgA	Nephritic	Mesangial expansion and hypercellularity	Mesangial IgA +/− C3	Mesangial deposits
Anti-GBM	Nephritic (RPGN)	Crescents, fibrin, necrosis	Linear IgG +/− C3	No visible deposits
ANCA-associated	Nephritic (RPGN)	Crescents, fibrin, necrosis	Negative	Negative
Alport syndrome	Hematuria or nephritic	Glomerular scarring	Negative	GBM splitting, thinning
Lupus nephritis	Often nephritic	Hypercellularity, wire loop deposits, +/− crescents	"Full house" granular staining	Subendothelial, subepithelial, and mesangial deposits
Membranous	Nephrotic	Thick GBMs; no hypercellularity	Fine granular IgG and C3 capillary loops	Subepithelial deposits
Minimal change disease	Nephrotic	Normal	Negative	Podocyte effacement
Focal segmental glomerulosclerosis	Nephrotic	Segmental scars	Negative or nonspecific IgM, C3	Scars +/− effacement
Diabetic glomerulosclerosis	Often nephrotic	Mesangial nodules (K-W), thick GBMs	Negative	Thick GBMs, mesangial matrix
Amyloid	Often nephrotic	Congo red material in mesangium and vessels	Stains for constituent protein	9–11 nm randomly oriented fibrils
Membrano-proliferative glomerulonephritis	Often nephrotic/ nephritic	'Tram track' double contour GBM, mesangial cellularity	IgG, C3 coarse granular mesangial and capillary loop	Subendothelial deposits

+/−, with or without; GBM, glomerular basement membrane; RPGN, rapidly progressive glomerulonephritis; K-W, Kimmelstiel–Wilson.

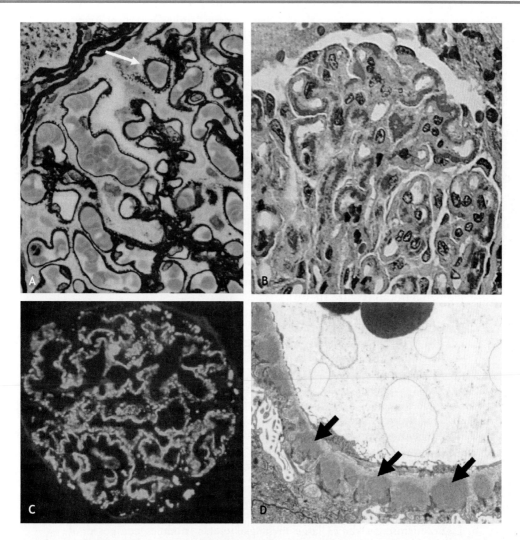

Figure 10–5. Membranous glomerulonephritis. Light microscopy of silver stained (**A**) glomeruli showing small spikes on the outside (epithelial side) of capillary loops (arrow), (**B**) trichrome stained glomeruli showing subepithelial deposits ($630 \times$). **C:** Immunofluorescence microscopy showing IgG staining in a granular fashion along capillary loops. **D:** Electron microscopy showing dark electron dense deposits on the epithelial side of the GBM. New basement membrane forms between the deposits (arrows), resulting in spikes (magnification $12,000 \times$).

(1) Light microscopy shows thickening of the basement membrane between the deposits, resulting in characteristic **"spikes"** on silver stains.

(2) IFM staining shows **bright granular deposits of IgG** along the capillary walls.

(3) EM shows the subepithelial deposits.

(4) Secondary forms of the disease are seen in association with chronic infections, *lupus, drugs,* and some tumors.

b. **Minimal change disease** (lipoid nephrosis) is a common disease in children where the charge barrier of the glomerular capillary wall is lost, resulting in nephrotic syndrome.

(1) Light microscopy is completely normal, hence the name.

(2) There are no deposits by IFM.

(3) The diagnosis is made by EM, which shows loss of the epithelial foot processes, leading to a single continuous epithelial layer, the so-called foot process effacement or fusion (Figure 10–6A).

(4) Minimal change disease is sensitive to corticosteroid therapy; patients often undergo therapy without biopsy.

c. **Focal segmental glomerulosclerosis (FSGS)** is a pattern of injury characterized by collapse and scarring of only portions (segmental) of some glomeruli (focal) (Figure 10–6B).

(1) It begins by involving only a small number of glomeruli, progressively becoming more extensive.

(2) FSGS occurs as a variety of apparently unrelated causes, including hereditary, drug, viral **(HIV)**, or as the end-stage of an underling immune complex disease.

(3) **Black** people are at higher risk for FSGS.

(4) Light microscopy shows scarring, which is usually **irreversible.**

(5) IFM is often negative.

(6) EM shows podocyte foot process effacement.

C. Glomerulonephropathies and Systemic Disease

1. **Diabetic nephropathy** leads to end-stage renal disease in up to 40% of patients with diabetes mellitus.

   a. Proteinuria arises 10–20 years after onset of diabetes, sometimes nephrotic, and often progresses to renal failure.

   b. Light microscopy shows large mesangial matrix nodules composed of proteinaceous eosinophilic material (Figure 10–7) called **Kimmelstiel-Wilson nodules.**

   c. Findings are a consequence of metabolic abnormalities, not immunologic injury; thus, IFM is negative.

   d. EM shows matrix nodules (composed of basement membrane material) and markedly thickened GBM (Figure 10–7).

2. **Amyloidosis** is characterized by "waxy" eosinophilic deposits of amyloid in glomeruli, blood vessels, and other organs throughout the body (including the heart and liver) (Figure 10–8).

   a. Amyloid characteristically stains with **Congo red,** and shows **apple-green birefringence** in polarized light.

   b. Amyloid is composed of fibrils that are approximately 9–11 nm in diameter, formed from abnormally folded proteins forming β-pleated sheets;

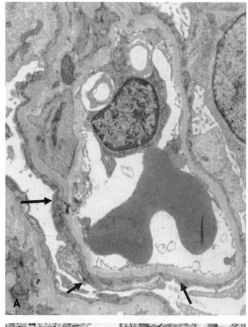

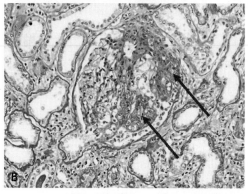

Figure 10–6. Minimal change disease and focal segmental glomerulosclerosis (FSGS). **A:** Minimal change disease is characterized by confluent podocyte cytoplasm without foot processes (arrows, foot processes are effaced; magnification 6000 ×). Histologic sections and immunofluorescence microscopy appear normal (not shown). **B:** FSGS is characterized by partial scarring of the glomerulus (arrows, periodic acid-Schiff stain, magnification 400 ×).

some of the proteins giving rise to amyloid are listed below, and can be detected by IFM.

(1) **Light chains (AL amyloid)** is seen in multiple myeloma.

(2) **Serum amyloid A (AA amyloid)** is derived from an acute phase reactant and is seen in inflammatory diseases.

(3) **β-amyloid protein (Aβ amyloid)** is the protein present in cerebral plaques of Alzheimer disease.

(4) **Transthyretin (TTR)** has a mutant form that is deposited causing familial amyloid polyneuropathy.

3. Systemic lupus erythematosus (SLE) frequently leads to glomerulonephritis, including crescentic glomerulonephritis.

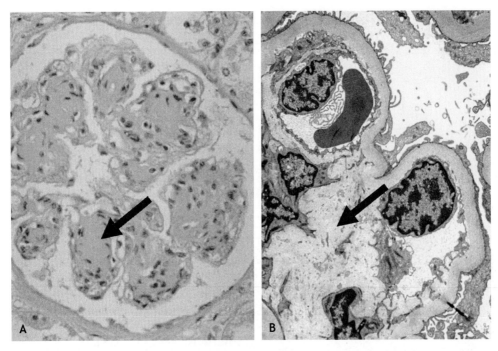

Figure 10–7. Diabetic nodular glomerulosclerosis. A: Light microscopy shows mesangial nodules (Kimmelstiel-Wilson nodules) without increased cellularity (400×). **B:** Electron microscopy shows thickened glomerular basement membrane and excess mesangial matrix (arrow; magnification 7500×).

a. Lupus nephritis is classified according to severity:
  (1) **Class I** (nearly normal) through **class IV** (severe)
  (2) **Class V** (looks like membranous glomerulonephritis)
b. Light microscopy shows bulky subendothelial deposits in glomeruli, causing the so-called wire loops.
c. IFM staining often shows a '**full house**' pattern (positive staining for complement (C3, C1q), immunoglobulin (IgG, IgM, IgA), and EM shows large immune deposits in many locations.
4. **Membranoproliferative glomerulonephritis (MPGN)** gets its name from a distinctive combination of mesangial and endothelial proliferation, along with thickening and duplication of the capillary basement membrane resulting in '**tram tracks.**'
  a. MPGN may occur as a primary immune complex mediated glomerular disease, but most often it is seen secondary to **hepatitis C.**
  b. IFM and EM document the deposition of immunoglobulin and complement (IgG, C3).
  c. MPGN often presents as a mixed nephritic/nephrotic syndrome.
D. Chronic Glomerulonephritis
1. Chronic glomerulonephritis descriptively encompasses segmental and global glomerulosclerosis, tubular atrophy, and cortical thinning.

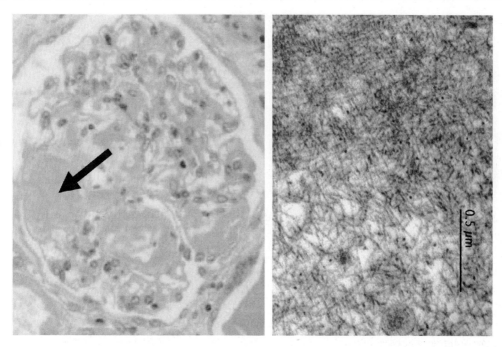

Figure 10–8. Amyloidosis. Light microscopy shows an accumulation of waxy material in the mesangial area (arrow) (400×). Electron microscopy shows randomly oriented 10 nm filaments (magnification 40,000×; scale is 0.5 mcm).

2. Chronic changes are essentially the final common pathway of renal injury and may result from many of the primary diseases described.

III. Tubulointerstitial Diseases

A. Acute Tubular Necrosis (ATN)

1. It presents as acute kidney injury.

2. ATN is caused by loss of tubular epithelial cells.

    a. Renal ischemia is a common cause of ATN because tubular epithelial cells have high metabolic requirements.

    b. Toxic injury may result from drugs (gentamycin), contrast dyes, myoglobin (following rhabdomyolysis), and radiation.

    c. Urinary obstruction may cause ATN (postrenal).

    d. ATN accounts for ~50% of acute renal injury and is often reversible with supportive care (Figure 10–9A).

ACUTE TUBULAR NECROSIS

* *The initiation phase lasts ~1.5 days after renal insult and presents as slightly decreased urinary output and increased BUN.*

* *The maintenance phase is characterized by oliguria (decreased urinary output), high BUN, hyperkalemia, and metabolic acidosis.*

CLINICAL CORRELATION

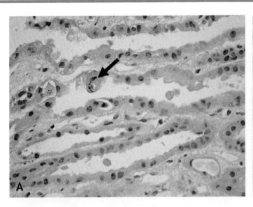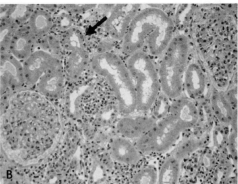

Figure 10–9. Acute tubular necrosis and tubulointerstitial disease. A: Acute tubular necrosis is characterized by dilated tubules lined by injured and proliferating epithelial cells (arrow, 400 ×). **B:** Tubulointerstitial nephritis is characterized by lymphocytes and fibrosis in the interstitium (between tubules), and in cases of renal transplant rejection there are also lymphocytes infiltrating tubule epithelium (arrow, 100 ×).

- *Patients in the recovery phase experience high urinary output (polyuria), hypokalemia, and normalizing BUN.*
- ***Fanconi syndrome*** *is a disorder of renal tubular transport (usually lack of bicarbonate resorption, renal tubular acidosis type II), often due to toxic injury; there is glycosuria, aminoaciduria, and renal tubular acidosis.*

    B. **Tubulointerstitial Nephritis**
        1. Acute drug-induced interstitial nephritis is thought to be an idiosyncratic immune reaction (**hypersensitivity type**) and may be associated with fever, eosinophilia, and rash.
            a. Renal biopsy shows interstitial edema, interstitial inflammation (especially eosinophils), tubular inflammation (tubulitis), tubular injury, and sometimes granulomas.
            b. A number of drugs have been implicated, including sulfonamides, penicillins, thiazide diuretics, nonsteroidal antiinflammatory drugs, allopurinol, and **herbal remedies.**
        2. **Analgesic nephropathy** is a toxic injury characterized by tubulointerstitial nephritis with **papillary necrosis.**
            a. It evolves over months to years of long-term exposure.
            b. Many of the implicated combination analgesics (aspirin + phenacetin) have been taken off the US market.

NONSTEROIDAL ANTIINFLAMMATORY DRUGS (NSAIDs)

CLINICAL CORRELATION

- *NSAIDs can cause renal damage by a number of mechanisms.*
- *NSAIDs may cause renal ischemia due to inhibition of vasodilatory prostaglandin synthesis, particularly in people with other conditions of high renin-angiotensin activity.*
- *NSAIDs may cause acute kidney injury due to hypersensitivity tubulointerstitial nephritis.*
- *NSAIDs are associated with minimal change disease.*
- *NSAIDs are rarely associated with membranous glomerulopathy.*

C. **Pyelonephritis/Reflux Nephropathy**
   1. **Pyelonephritis** is infection of the kidney.
      a. Pyelonephritis most commonly occurs due to an ascending urinary tract infection, presenting with fever and back pain.
         (1) Organisms are most commonly gram-negative intestinal flora **(Escherichia coli, Proteus, Klebsiella, Enterobacter,** also *Streptococcus faecalis*), which colonize the urethra.
         (2) **Instrumentation,** or the short **female urethra,** allows bacterial entry into the bladder where organisms multiply.
         (3) **Vesicoureteral reflux** (VUR) permits bacterial entry into the renal pelvis; predisposition to VUR is most commonly congenital, but can also be acquired or neurogenic.
      b. **Hematogenous pyelonephritis** occurs with seeding of the kidney by organisms traveling through the bloodstream.
      c. **Acute pyelonephritis** is characterized by patchy neutrophilic inflammation involving the interstitium and tubules.
         (1) **White blood cell casts** form in tubules and are excreted into urine.
         (2) There may be necrosis and abscess formation.
      d. **Chronic pyelonephritis** is characterized by destruction of one or more of the renal papillae and dense scarring of the cortex.
         (1) **Reflux** pyelonephritis leads to grossly apparent indented scars at the renal poles.
         (2) **Obstructive** pyelonephritis causes diffuse atrophy.
         (3) 10–20% of end-stage kidney disease can be attributed to chronic pyelonephritis, particularly reflux nephropathy; patients with congenital VUR are especially susceptible.
D. **Cast/Crystal Nephropathies**
   1. **Hyperuricemia** may lead to the precipitation of urate in distal renal tubules/collecting ducts as uric acid crystals or as monosodium urate, leading to tubular obstruction.
      a. Monosodium urate forms needle-shaped crystals (as in gouty tophi) with associated multinucleated giant cells.
      b. Hyperuricemia may also cause renal stones (nephrolithiasis).
   2. **Hypercalcemia** may cause calcium stones in renal tubules, obstructing tubules and causing cellular injury; macroscopic renal pelvic stones may also form.

MULTIPLE MYELOMA

- *Multiple myeloma injures the kidney in several ways, including hypercalcemia, hyperuricemia, and amyloidosis.*
- *Excess free light chains secreted by the plasma cells of multiple myeloma are called **Bence Jones** protein; these light chains appear in the urine in 70% of myeloma patients.*
- *Bence Jones protein may cause toxic injury to renal tubular cells.*
- *Excess light chains may also precipitate as casts (especially in acidic pH) to obstruct renal tubules, and incite an inflammatory reaction, called '**myeloma cast nephropathy.**'*

   E. **Renal Transplant Pathology**
      1. **Rejection** of kidney allografts (transplants) occurs as the recipient's immune system recognizes the kidney as foreign (Figure 10–9B).

a. Rejection is characterized by predominantly T-cell infiltrates in the interstitium and tubules (**tubulitis**).

b. Severe rejection occurs when T-cells attack the vascular endothelium of arteries, causing arteritis (**endothelialitis**).

2. Antibodies are an important cause of hyperacute (immediate) allograft rejection and have a role in humoral rejection at later times post-transplantation.

3. Renal transplant patients are susceptible to infections (eg, BK polyoma virus) because of immunosuppression.

4. High doses of calcineurin inhibitor drugs (cyclosporine, tacrolimus) can also be toxic to the transplanted kidney.

IV. Vascular Diseases

A. Renal Artery Stenosis

1. Constriction of one renal artery may cause hypertension.

   a. **Atherosclerosis** is the most common cause of stenosis.

   b. **Fibromuscular dysplasia** is a family of vascular lesions, many of which are typically seen in **young women;** lesions can result from hyperplasia of the intima, media, or adventitia.

2. The involved kidney shows features of long-term ischemia; it is shrunken with diffuse uniform atrophy.

B. Hypertensive Nephrosclerosis

1. It is the narrowing and sclerosis of small arteries and arterioles due to essential hypertension.

2. The renal changes are called "benign nephrosclerosis," or "arterionephrosclerosis."

   a. The vessels are narrowed by **intimal hyperplasia** and hyalinization (deposits of dense, pink acellular material) and by hypertrophy of the artery's media.

   b. Unlike the uniform atrophy associated with renal artery stenosis, these ischemic lesions are focal, resulting in a coarsely granular renal surface.

C. Malignant Hypertension

1. This rapid disease results in acute vascular lesions and parenchymal injury referred to as "malignant nephrosclerosis."

2. The acute vascular lesions include **fibrinoid necrosis** of renal arteries and arterioles, with a characteristic concentric layered intimal thickening, the so-called **onion skin** lesions.

D. Atherosclerotic Disease

1. Bilateral atherosclerosis of the renal arteries leads to chronic ischemia and renal insufficiency.

2. Atheromatous plaques that are disrupted may fragment; resulting emboli can then occlude intrarenal arteries causing infarction and renal insufficiency, often acutely ("atheroembolic" disease).

E. Vasculitis

1. Almost any form of systemic vasculitis may involve the kidney.

2. Vasculitis usually results in local infarction.

3. Glomeruli are composed of capillaries and the renal injury caused by small vessel vasculitides includes acute glomerular damage.

4. The most common forms are **ANCA-associated,** and they manifest as crescentic glomerulonephritis.

5. Medium vessel vasculitides, such as polyarteritis nodosa, may cause segmental renal infarction affecting renal function.

F. **Thrombotic Microangiopathy**

    1. Thrombotic microangiopathy results from endothelial injury; insults may include infection, antiphospholipid antibodies, complications of pregnancy, and radiation.

    2. Thrombotic microangiopathy is characterized by platelet-fibrin thrombi in capillaries and arteries, resulting in **microangiopathic hemolytic anemia,** as red cells are fragmented passing through damaged capillaries; thus, **schistocytes** can be seen on blood smears.

        a. **Hemolytic uremic syndrome (HUS)** is one of the classic clinical presentations of thrombotic microangiopathy, which as the name implies, is characterized by hemolysis and oliguria with renal failure.

            (1) In **children,** the usual cause is verotoxin produced by *E coli* (O157:H7), or Shiga toxin from *Shigella.*

            (2) **Familial HUS** results from a defect in **factor H,** which normally protects cells from uncontrolled complement activation, since it breaks down C3 convertase.

            (3) Although most patients recover, chronic renal insufficiency develops in some patients later in life.

        b. **Thrombotic thrombocytopenic purpura (TTP)** has the same renal findings, but a different constellation of clinical symptoms.

            (1) Patients develop neurologic symptoms, renal failure, fever, hemolytic anemia, thrombocytopenia, and rash.

            (2) TTP is preferentially seen in patients with defects in the **ADAMTS-13** protease, which cleaves von Willebrand factor multimers, affecting platelet aggregation.

V. Obstruction

A. **Hydronephrosis**

    1. Hydronephrosis is renal pelvis dilation and cortical atrophy, resulting from chronic obstruction of urine outflow.

        a. **Congenital anomalies** are an important cause of hydronephrosis, especially posterior urethral values, ureteropelvic junction (**UPJ**) obstruction, or ureteral stricture.

        b. Transient obstruction from calculi, sloughed papillae, blood clots, and inflammation of lower tract may cause hydronephrosis.

        c. **Benign prostatic hypertrophy** is an important cause of obstruction in older males.

        d. Malignant tumors of the urinary tract may cause obstruction.

        e. Functional obstruction from neurogenic bladder, or pregnancy may also cause hydronephrosis.

B. **Nephrolithiasis (Urolithiasis, Renal Stones/Calculi)**

    1. Kidney stones result from a number of physiologic and metabolic causes but are usually associated with supersaturation of minerals in the renal calyces/pelvis, and are dependent upon **urine pH.**

    2. Stones cause hematuria, obstruction, and severe pain radiating into the groin (**renal colic**).

3. **Calcium oxalate** stones are most common (70%).
   a. Most occur in hypercalcemic states such as bone disease, hyperparathyroidism, or sarcoidosis.
   b. Calcium oxalate stones may also form with high uric acid levels, because uric acid crystals serve as a nucleus.
   c. A minority of calcium stones occur in the setting of hyperoxaluria due to the metabolic disorder **oxalosis,** or increased intestinal absorption.

4. **Struvite** stones are composed of magnesium ammonium phosphate.
   a. Struvite stones are associated with urinary tract infections, especially *Proteus.*
   b. These stones may form 'staghorn' calculi occupying the renal pelvis and branching into calyces, causing severe obstruction and renal cortical atrophy (Figure 10–10).

5. **Uric acid** stones are commonly associated with gout and systemic diseases with abundant cell death (eg, leukemia); however, many patients with uric acid stones do not have hyperuricemia.

6. **Cysteine** stones are primarily associated with lack of tubular resorption of amino acids, a genetic condition.

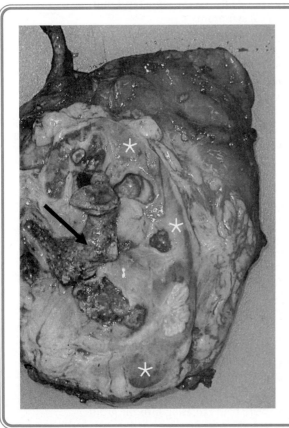

Figure 10–10. Staghorn calculus and renal obstruction. Bivalved kidney with calculus filling the dilated pelvis (arrow), which is most likely a struvite stone. The renal cortex is thinned (asterisk). Note the abundant perinephric fat and the ureter in the upper left of the photograph.

VI. Lower Urinary Tract

A. Urinary Bladder

1. A bladder **diverticulum** is a outpouching of the bladder through a weakness in the muscularis propria (bladder wall).
2. Inflammation of the bladder is called **cystitis** (see Pyelonephritis section for common bacterial organisms).
   a. Nonbacterial organisms causing cystitis include *Candida*, other fungi, and tuberculosis.
   b. Sterile cystitis is often due to **cytotoxic drugs** (chemotherapy), or radiation.
   c. **Interstitial cystitis** is a cause of painful sterile cystitis.
      (1) It is characterized by denudation of the urothelium and fibrosis of the bladder wall with **mast cell** infiltrates and **neural hypertrophy.**
      (2) It occurs mainly in **women** and the cause is unknown.

B. Ureters and Urethra

1. The ureters and urethra are affected by the same inflammatory and neoplastic conditions as the renal pelvis and bladder.
2. Obstruction is a common presenting feature.

VII. Urinary Tract Neoplasia

A. Primary Renal Neoplasms

1. **Renal cell carcinoma** is an adenocarcinoma derived from renal tubular epithelium.
   a. It affects predominantly older men.
   b. Smoking is a significant risk factor.
   c. The classic presentation is hematuria with flank pain and a mass; however, most patients are virtually asymptomatic.
   d. There are several different types of renal cell carcinoma.
      (1) **Clear cell carcinoma** is the most common (Figure 10–11A).
      (2) **Papillary carcinoma** is the second most common type of renal cell carcinoma and may be associated with mutations in the **MET tyrosine kinase receptor.**
   e. Familial renal cell carcinoma is rare, but it occurs in the **von Hippel-Lindau disease (VHL)** along with central nervous system **hemangioblastomas.**
   f. The majority of renal cell carcinomas are sporadic, but most have a defect in the *VHL* **gene** (3p12-26).
   g. Metastatic renal cell carcinoma is poorly responsive to conventional chemotherapy; new agents are undergoing trials.
2. **Oncocytomas** are **benign** renal neoplasms, which can be large.
   a. Oncocytomas are often distinctly "mahogany" brown.
   b. The cells have abundant granular red cytoplasm and small round nuclei (Figure 10–11B).
3. **Wilms tumor (nephroblastoma)** is the most common pediatric renal tumor and is one of the "small round blue cell" tumors of childhood discussed in detail in Chapter 19.

B. Angiomyolipoma

1. Angiomyolipomas are a rare mesenchymal tumor composed of vessels (angio-), smooth muscle (myo-), and fat (lipoma).

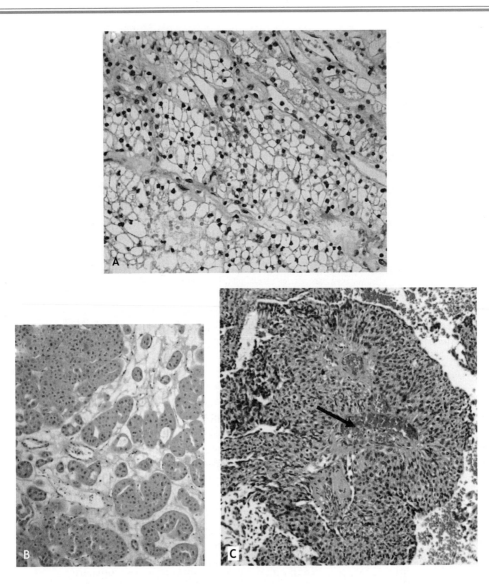

Figure 10–11. Urinary tract neoplasia. A: Renal cell carcinoma, clear cell type, is a primary kidney malignancy with high metastatic potential, which may occur years after primary diagnosis and treatment. It is a highly vascular neoplasm often arranged in sheets of tumor cells with abundant clear cytoplasm and small round nuclei (200 ×). **B:** In contrast, renal oncocytoma is a benign primary kidney neoplasm with no metastatic potential. It resembles oncocytomas of the salivary gland (see Chapter 4) and Hürthle cell neoplasms of the thyroid (see Chapter 11) (50 ×). **C:** Urothelial carcinoma (transitional cell carcinoma) arises from the anywhere along the lower urinary tract, from the renal pelvis, ureter, bladder, and urethra. They are often papillary with long fingers of tumor cells arranged around fibrovascular cores (arrow, 100 ×). They are malignant with metastatic potential and represent the most common malignancy of the urinary bladder.

2. They usually occur in the renal hilum but may involve the kidney.

3. They may be multifocal in patients with **tuberous sclerosis.**

    a. Tuberous sclerosis complex is due to germline defects in one of two interacting tumor suppressor genes, **hamartin (*TSC1*)** or **tuberin (*TSC2*).**

    b. Other lesions in TSC include tubers (central nervous system hamartomas that cause seizures and/or mental retardation), skin angiofibromas, and rhabdomyomas in the heart.

C. Urothelial Carcinoma (Transitional Cell Carcinoma)

    1. Urothelial carcinoma may arise anywhere along the genitourinary tract with urothelial lining, from renal pelvis to urethra.

    2. Urothelial carcinoma most commonly occurs in older **men.**

    3. Other risk factors include **smoking, arylamine dyes,** NSAIDs, cyclophosphamide, and *Schistosoma* infection (endemic in Egypt).

    4. Patients often have painless hematuria.

    5. Urine cytology and cystoscopic tissue biopsy are diagnostic.

    6. Lesions are usually grossly visible and multifocal.

    7. Preinvasive lesions include the following:

        a. Papillary carcinoma is characterized by tree-like branches of fibrovascular cores lined by urothelial carcinoma that may be low grade (small regular nuclei, slow growing), or high grade (pleomorphic nuclei and mitotically active).

        b. Carcinoma in situ is a flat lesion that may be grossly invisible, requiring multiple biopsies for definitive diagnosis.

D. Adenocarcinoma

    1. It may arise from the **urachal** remnant.

    2. However, it most commonly arises together with poorly differentiated urothelial carcinoma.

CLINICAL PROBLEMS

1. A 35-year-old marathon runner comes to the emergency department complaining of muscle pain and dark urine. Urinalysis is negative for red blood cells, and a chemistry panel shows a serum creatinine of 5.7 mg/dL. What is the **MOST** likely finding on renal biopsy?

    A. IgA nephropathy

    B. Minimal change disease

    C. Interstitial nephritis

    D. Acute tubular necrosis

    E. Amyloidosis

2. A 70-year-old man seeks medical attention for hematuria. Select the **LEAST** likely diagnosis.

    A. Urothelial carcinoma

    B. Benign prostatic hypertrophy

C. Renal stones

D. Renal cell carcinoma

E. IgA nephropathy

3. A 35-year-old woman seeks medical attention 2 weeks after her honeymoon. During the trip, she had burning on urination, frequency, and urgency, which she self-treated by drinking cranberry juice. She now complains of fever and left flank pain. What is the **MOST** likely diagnosis?

A. Renal colic

B. Ectopic pregnancy

C. Pyelonephritis

D. Polycystic ovarian disease

E. Renal tuberculosis

4. A 70-year-old previously healthy woman has severe edema, including periorbital edema, and fatigue. She explains that after bone density screening, she got a call to come back for more studies because 'round holes in her bones' were found. Cardiac studies are normal, but urinalysis shows that 8 grams of protein are being excreted per day. Select the pair that describes the **MOST** likely combination of diagnostic test and results:

A. Skin biopsy—mycosis fungoides

B. Kidney biopsy—systemic lupus erythematosus

C. Bone marrow biopsy—acute leukemia

D. Bone marrow biopsy—metastatic carcinoma

E. Bone marrow biopsy—multiple myeloma

5. Which of the following is **NOT** associated with minimal change disease?

A. Heavy proteinuria

B. Negative immunofluorescence microscopy

C. Normal electron microscopy

D. Normal light microscopy

E. Hyperlipidemia

6. What is the syndrome most often associated with the following findings on renal biopsy: crescentic glomerulonephritis, negative electron microscopy, and bright linear GBM staining?

A. Wegener granulomatosis

B. Systemic lupus erythematosus

C. Henoch-Schönlein purpura

D. Thrombotic thrombocytopenic purpura

E. Goodpasture syndrome

7. Crescentic glomerulonephritis is most associated with:

A. p-ANCA

B. HIV

C. Cytomegalovirus

    D. Cryoglobulin

    E. Nephritic factor

8. A child has malaise, and laboratory studies demonstrate a hematocrit of 30%, elevated serum creatinine, and schistocytes on blood smear. Which of the following is the **MOST** likely prodromal syndrome?

    A. Severe headache and stiff neck

    B. Upper respiratory tract infection

    C. Strep throat

    D. Bloody diarrhea

    E. Overwhelming fatigue

9. A 60-year-old man has had type II diabetes mellitus for the last 10 years. His hemoglobin A_{1c} has averaged 7.9% for the last 5 years. Lately, his urine dipstick has revealed proteinuria. Pick the **MOST** likely description of findings on this patient's renal biopsy.

    A. Mesangial nodules and thick glomerular basement membranes

    B. Crescents and vasculitis

    C. Granular subepithelial immune complex deposits

    D. Double contoured glomerular basement membranes "tram tracks"

    E. Interstitial inflammation with eosinophils

10. A 20-year-old black woman has joint aches, a malar rash, and a pericardial rub. Her serum creatinine is 2.3 mg/dL. Which of the following is **LEAST** likely to be seen on her renal biopsy?

    A. Proliferative glomerulonephritis

    B. Crescents

    C. Randomly oriented filaments on electron microscopy

    D. "Full house" immune complex deposits

    E. Subepithelial, subendothelial, and mesangial deposits

11. A teenager is in a motorcycle accident. At the emergency department, he undergoes a CT scan to rule out internal hemorrhage. The CT scan shows that the left kidney is about half the size of the right kidney, but both kidneys have normal shape. What is the best description of his condition?

    A. Autosomal dominant polycystic kidney disease

    B. Autosomal recessive polycystic kidney disease

    C. Unilateral renal agenesis

    D. Unilateral cystic dysplasia

    E. Unilateral renal hypoplasia

12. The location of the deposits in membranous glomerulonephritis suggests:

    A. An antibody directed against an intrinsic antigen on podocytes

    B. An antibody directed against tubular basement membranes

C. A large negatively charged preformed antibody-antigen complex

D. An antibody directed against glomerular basement membrane

E. An antibody to neutrophil granules

13. A biopsy specimen that was obtained from a patient who had undergone renal transplantation shows neutrophils in tubules in the medulla (white blood cell casts). Pick the **MOST** likely diagnosis.

A. Rejection of the transplant

B. Transplant vasculopathy

C. Urinary tract infection

D. Recurrent diabetic nephropathy

E. Toxicity of immunosuppressive drugs

14. A young child is brought to his physician's office, and his mom says that his "eyes look puffy." Laboratory findings show hypoalbuminemia, hyperlipidemia, and proteinuria, but no red blood cells. Serum creatinine is normal. Select the **LEAST** likely diagnosis.

A. Membranous glomerulonephritis

B. Focal segmental glomerulosclerosis (FSGS)

C. Alport syndrome

D. Minimal change disease

E. None of the above

15. A 40-year-old man and his wife come for genetic counseling. The husband has a history of "a couple renal tumors." His surgical history includes a left nephrectomy and surgery on the right kidney to remove two small masses. He reports that his father died at a young age of metastatic carcinoma. Select the **MOST LIKELY** genetic mutation for which this patient should be tested, after appropriate counseling.

A. *FAP*

B. *VHL*

C. *BRCA1*

D. *p53*

E. *MLH1*

16. A 75-year-old man was writhing in pain all night; this morning he passed a stone in his urine. While the man is being examined by his physician, his wife asks the nurse for a refill of his gout medicine. What type of renal stone was passed?

A. Struvite

B. Calcium phosphate

C. Cysteine

D. Uric acid

E. Magnesium ammonium phosphate

17. A 5-year-old boy arrives at the emergency department after crashing on his new bike. He was wearing his helmet and landed in some soft leaves, but he complains of a "really bad bellyache." The CT scan shows a large left renal mass. What is the **MOST** likely diagnosis?

    A. Wilms tumor

    B. Clear cell renal cell carcinoma

    C. Urothelial carcinoma

    D. Papillary renal cell carcinoma

    E. Multiple myeloma

18. A colleague wants to refer a patient with renal insufficiency. The patient has a history of heavy use of nonsteroidal antiinflammatory drugs. What is the **LEAST** likely renal problem in this patient?

    A. Renal papillary necrosis

    B. Tubulointerstitial nephritis

    C. IgA nephropathy

    D. Minimal change disease

    E. Membranous glomerulopathy

19. A middle age woman with acute kidney injury undergoes renal biopsy. The results show interstitial nephritis. According to the thorough history and physical examination, she is otherwise completely healthy and takes no medications. Which elements of her clinical history should be reconfirmed?

    A. Smoking history

    B. Surgical history

    C. Health of the patient's mother

    D. Use of herbal and over-the-counter medications

    E. Exercise program

20. A 20-year-old woman who is 26 weeks pregnant has significantly elevated proteinuria (5 g/day), edema, hyperlipidemia, and hypertension. Which of the following statements is **FALSE:**

    A. This nephrotic syndrome is likely to resolve after pregnancy

    B. She has preeclampsia

    C. Renal biopsy may show glomerular endotheliosis

    D. History of renal disease increases a woman's risk of toxemia

    E. None of the above

ANSWERS

1. The answer is D. Based on the history of exercise, dark urine without red blood cells, and high serum creatinine, acute tubular necrosis (ATN) due to rhabdomyolysis is the best answer, with myoglobulin breakdown products causing pigmentation. IgA presents with hematuria, and serum creatinine may or may not be elevated. Minimal change disease and amyloid most commonly present with nephrotic syndrome and relatively normal creatinine. Interstitial nephritis is associated with white blood cells (especially eosinophils) in the urine and is often associated with drugs or infection.

2. The answer is B. The primary differential diagnostic considerations in hematuria include stones, tumors, and glomerulonephritis. Benign prostatic hypertrophy should not result in hematuria, whereas renal cell and urothelial carcinoma commonly do.

3. The answer is C. Based on the history of apparent urinary tract infection (burning, frequency, urgency) untreated by antibiotics, she likely has an ascending urinary tract infection, in other words, pyelonephritis. Renal colic, ectopic pregnancy and polycystic ovarian disease are lower on the differential, given this patient's history.

4. The answer is E. Multiple myeloma is a plasma cell disease of older patients; neoplastic plasma cells secrete large amounts of abnormal light chains, and this is often spilled in the urine (Bence Jones protein). Certain light chains may accumulate as amyloid fibrils (AL type), a cause of nephrotic syndrome. Multiple myeloma usually causes multiple bony lesions. Mycosis fungoides is a T-cell lymphoma of the skin.

5. The answer is C. In minimal change disease, there is diffuse podocyte injury, resulting in foot process effacement (sometimes called foot process fusion). Light and immunofluorescence microscopy are normal. Minimal change disease presents as nephrotic syndrome, with heavy proteinuria, edema, hyperlipidemia, and normal serum creatinine.

6. The answer is E. Anti-glomerular basement membrane (GBM) disease is the described glomerulonephritis. The anti-GBMs often cross react with pulmonary alveolar capillary basement membranes, causing pulmonary hemorrhage and Goodpasture syndrome. Wegener granulomatosis is another pulmonary-renal syndrome causing crescentic glomerulonephritis and pulmonary hemorrhage, but immunofluorescence microscopy (IFM) studies are negative. Henoch-Schönlein purpura is associated with IgA nephropathy, and systemic lupus erythematosus is associated with widespread granular immune complex deposits on IFM and electron microscopy.

7. The answer is A. ANCAs (anti-neutrophil cytoplasmic antibodies) are associated with pauci-immune crescentic glomerulonephritis. HIV is associated with focal segmental glomerulosclerosis; cryoglobulin and C3 nephritic factor may be associated with different types of membranoproliferative glomerulonephritis. Cytomegalovirus infection causes tubulointerstitial nephritis and is seen in immunocompromised patients.

8. The answer is D. The spectrum of clinical data describes the hemolytic uremic syndrome (HUS, a thrombotic microangiopathy). HUS occurs after an *Escherichia coli* vertoxin or *Shiga* toxin diarrheal illness in children.

9. The answer is A. Diabetic glomerulosclerosis is characterized by Kimmelstiel-Wilson nodules and thickened glomerular basement membrane (GBM). Crescents and vas-

culitis describe ANCA-associated vasculitis; granular subepithelial immune complex deposits are characteristic of membranous glomerulonephritis. 'Tram track' GBMs are classic for membranoproliferative glomerulonephritis (MPGN). Interstitial inflammation is seen in tubulointerstitial nephritis.

10. The answer is C. Randomly oriented filaments (9–11 nm) describe amyloid. All of the other choices are commonly seen in nephritis associated with systemic lupus erythematosus.

11. The answer is E. This is the description of renal hypoplasia. There is no evidence of cystic change; and polycystic kidney disease would affect bilateral kidneys. Agenesis means absence of a kidney (most often bilateral and nonviable); and a cystic dysplastic kidney would not have a normal shape.

12. The answer is A. Membranous glomerulonephritis is characterized by subepithelial deposits, which are located between the podocyte and the glomerular basement membrane.

13. The answer is C. White blood cell casts in tubules characterizes urinary tract infection (pyelonephritis), or reflux, which can certainly happen in transplant patients. Rejection causes a T-cell infiltrates in tubules and vessels.

14. The answer is C. Minimal change, focal segmental glomerulosclerosis, and membranous glomerulonephritis are all causes of the nephrotic syndrome, which fit the clinical data. Alport syndrome causes hematuria.

15. The answer is B. *VHL* is von Hippel-Lindau, which is involved in cases of familial renal cell carcinoma. Patients have multiple bilateral tumors. *FAP* and *MLH1* are involved in colon cancer syndrome (familial adenomatosis polyposis) and hereditary non-polyposis colorectal cancer (HNPCC), respectively. p53 is an important tumor suppressor protein, which mutations resulting Li-Fraumeni syndrome. *BRCA1* is a tumor suppressor with mutations resulting in familial breast and ovarian cancer.

16. The answer is D. Gout is associated with hyperuricemia and uric acid stones. Hyperuricemia may also be associated with calcium oxalate stones, but that was not one of the choices. Magnesium ammonium phosphate is the composition of "struvite" stones.

17. The answer is A. Wilms tumor is the most common pediatric kidney tumor. The other tumors affect adults, with incidence increasing with age.

18. The answer is C. IgA nephropathy has no known association with nonsteroidal antiinflammatory drugs (NSAIDs). Each of the other forms of kidney disease can be associated with NSAIDs, although minimal change disease and membranous glomerulopathy are quite rare associations.

19. The answer is D. Herbal medications and over-the-counter drugs (such as nonsteroidal antiinflammatory drugs) are notorious causes of interstitial nephritis and may not be considered drugs by patients.

20. The answer is E. Preeclampsia presents with proteinuria, edema, and hypertension similar to other nephrotic syndromes but resolves shortly after delivery of the placenta. A history of renal disease may increase a woman's risk of preeclampsia, but in most of these patients, there is no prior history and renal biopsy would be essentially normal with the exception of "glomerular endotheliosis."

CHAPTER 11
ENDOCRINE AND NUTRITION

*There is something fascinating about science. One gets such wholesale
returns of conjecture out of such a trifling investment of fact.*
—Mark Twain

I. Pituitary

A. Pituitary Adenoma

1. Adenoma is the most common neoplasm of the pituitary and has a variable presentation based on either mass effect or hormones.
2. They are classified as either **microadenomas** (<1 cm) or **macroadenomas** (>1 cm).
3. Pituitary adenomas may compress the optic chiasm or invade the cavernous sinus, compromising cranial nerves III, IV, and VI.
   a. They are usually confined to the sella turcica.
   b. Sudden hemorrhage into an adenoma is termed "**pituitary apoplexy**" marked by headache, diplopia, and hypopituitarism.
4. **Prolactinoma** is the most common pituitary adenoma.
   a. Elevated prolactin may suppress follicle-stimulating hormone (FSH) and luteinizing hormone (LH) secretion and lead to **amenorrhea, galactorrhea,** and **erectile dysfunction.**
   b. Macroadenomas may also cause excess prolactin secretion by compressing the pituitary stalk, impeding access to **dopamine.**
   c. Other causes of hyperprolactinemia include physiologic stimuli (stress, pain), systemic disorders (spinal cord lesions, hypothyroidism, chronic renal failure, cirrhosis), and medications (**antipsychotics,** metoclopramide, antihypertensives, oral contraceptives, opioids).
5. The effects of pituitary adenomas that secrete **excess growth hormone** (somatotropin) vary with patient age.
   a. Prior to epiphyseal closure results in **gigantism.**
   b. After epiphyseal closure results in **acromegaly.**
6. Although growth hormone deficiency is often idiopathic in children, it is caused by a pituitary macroadenoma in adults.
7. Corticotropin-secreting adenomas induce the overproduction of corticosteroids and manifest as Cushing disease.
   a. **Cushing disease** is due an adrenocorticotropic hormone (**ACTH**)-**producing tumor** within the pituitary that stimulates the adrenal to secrete cortisol.

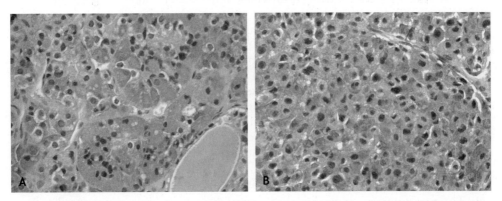

Figure 11–1. Pituitary adenoma. A: Normal pituitary (mixed pattern). **B:** Basophilic adenoma.

 b. Cushing disease (pituitary) is more common than **Cushing syndrome** (adrenal), accounting for 70% of cases.

 c. There may be ectopic production of ACTH from other tumors.

8. Pituitary adenoma is also a component of **multiple endocrine neoplasia (MEN) type I.**

9. Histologic sections show a clonal proliferation of polygonal cells with uniform nuclei, "salt and pepper" chromatin, and variably staining granular cytoplasm (Figure 11–1).

SHEEHAN SYNDROME

• *Sheehan syndrome is hypopituitarism due to ischemic necrosis of an enlarged pituitary during pregnancy.*

• *The absence of function leads to the inability to breastfeed.*

• *The diagnosis may be confirmed by the thyrotropin-releasing hormone (TRH) stimulation test, whereas an injection of TRH fails to raise thyroid-stimulating hormone.*

 B. Growth Disorders

  1. **Constitutional short stature** is characterized by a delay in normal growth velocity; the pubertal growth spurt is delayed, and the patient's adult height will be low-normal.

  2. **Genetic short stature** is characterized by hereditary factors that lead to short stature.

   a. **Dwarfism** is characterized by either hypothalamic or pituitary dysfunction leading to abnormal growth hormone.

   b. **Laron dwarfism** is characterized by the absence of growth hormone receptors.

 C. Diabetes Insipidus

  1. Because the posterior pituitary regulates antidiuretic hormone (**ADH**) secretion, its damage leads to reduced ADH secretion and polyuria (diabetes insipidus).

a. ADH acts on the collecting duct system of the kidney leading to uptake of water and concentrated urine.

b. Lack of ADH leads to volumes of inappropriately **dilute urine.**

2. Affected patients with an intact thirst mechanism and access to water will complain of thirst, polyuria, and polydipsia.

3. Marked **hyponatremia** will develop in patients without access to water or impaired consciousness due to renal losses of free water.

4. There is also a **nephrogenic form** of diabetes insipidus where the kidney is resistant or unresponsive to the action of ADH.

5. Factors leading to central, or pituitary-related, diabetes insipidus include cranial trauma, tumors of the pituitary, surgery, radiation, and inflammatory conditions.

D. **Syndrome of Inappropriate ADH (SIADH) Secretion**

1. There are numerous pathophysiologic states where the posterior pituitary will secrete too much ADH, including the following:

a. Pain

b. Nausea

c. Medication effects

d. Neoplasms

e. Pituitary injury

2. **Ectopic production** of ADH can occur in certain neuroendocrine neoplasms, particularly **small cell carcinoma (oat cell)** of the lung.

3. Despite low serum osmolarity and hyponatremia, the blood volume will be normal and peripheral edema does not develop.

II. **Thyroid**

A. **Congenital Anomalies**

1. Thyroid tissue may be left behind anywhere along the developmental descent path from the floor of the mouth to the lower neck.

2. These lesions may be clinically mistaken as neoplasia.

THYROGLOSSAL DUCT CYST

DEVELOPMENTAL INSIGHTS

• *The connecting thyroglossal duct usually closes between the seventh and tenth weeks of gestation, but segments may remain patent.*

• *Patent ducts may enlarge later in life forming mid-line cysts.*

B. **Disorders of Thyroid Hyperfunction**

1. Symptoms of hyperthyroidism include **heat intolerance,** palpitations, **tremor, fatigue,** muscle weakness, and weight loss.

2. **Graves disease** is the most common cause of hyperthyroidism, affecting 2% of young women.

a. Autoantibodies bind and stimulate thyroid-stimulating hormone (TSH)-receptors.

b. This causes **diffuse enlargement** of the gland sometimes reaching a mass of 80 g (normal 20–30 g).

c. The ophthalmopathy of Graves disease manifests as bilateral **exophthalmos** and results from edema and deposition of mucopolysaccharides within periorbital tissues.

d. **Pretibial myxedema** is secondary to hyaluronic acid deposition and lymphocytic infiltrates within the dermis.

    e. Other changes associated with Graves disease include generalized lymphoid hyperplasia and cardiomegaly.

3. While most patients with **multinodular goiters** are euthyroid, hyperfunctional nodules develop in a small percentage

    a. In this condition, the thyroid gland may achieve truly massive proportions of over **2000 g.**

    b. The pattern of growth can be asymmetric, cause impingement of surrounding structures, and be mistaken for neoplasia.

    c. On gross examination, the cut surface reveals irregular nodules, fibrosis, calcification, and cystic changes.

4. **Hyperfunctioning adenoma,** or "toxic" adenoma, is another cause of hyperthyroidism and thyrotoxicosis.

    a. Most solitary adenomas are benign and nonfunctional.

    b. Somatic "gain of function" mutations in the TSH receptor signaling pathway results in autonomic production of hormone.

    c. The hyperfunctional nodule will "light-up" on a thyroid scan while the rest of the gland is negative.

    d. Treatment is excision of the hyperfunctioning nodule.

5. **Factitious thyrotoxicosis** is thyrotoxicosis without hyperthyroidism and may be caused by prescription medication, or as a "natural" over-the-counter supplement.

6. A **pituitary adenoma** that secretes TSH can result in secondary hyperthyroidism and thyrotoxicosis with both elevated TSH and elevated free thyroxine (T_4) (Table 11-1).

7. **Subacute lymphocytic thyroiditis** differs from Hashimoto thyroiditis, in that it causes **thyroid hyperfunction** and enlargement.

    a. It is also called **painless thyroiditis** because it is usually clinically silent except for thyroid hyperfunction.

    b. It is more frequent in adult women.

    c. It may also arise as postpartum thyroiditis with an increased risk of recurrence with subsequent pregnancies.

    d. Microscopically, there is **lymphocytic infiltration** of the gland with germinal center formation, but unlike Hashimoto thyroiditis, there is no fibrosis or oncocytic metaplasia.

Table 11-1. Thyroid-stimulating hormone (TSH) and free thyroxine (T_4).

Condition	TSH	T_4
Primary hyperthyroidism	↓	↑
Secondary hyperthyroidism	↑	↑
Primary hypothyroidism	↑	↓

THYROTOXICOSIS

- Thyrotoxicosis is a general term for the hypermetabolic state associated with elevated levels of circulating thyroid hormone.
- Aside from increased production, thyrotoxicosis may be due to release of stored hormone, or ingestion of exogenous thyroid hormone.
- Distinguishing among these potential etiologies is important to ensure appropriate therapy.

C. **Disorders of Thyroid Hypofunction**
  1. **Hashimoto thyroiditis** is an autoimmune disease.
     a. It is the most common cause of hypothyroidism where sufficient dietary iodine is available.
     b. Young women are affected 10 times more often than men.
     c. The thyroid can be diffusely enlarged.
     d. Microscopic sections of the thyroid show Hürthle cell metaplasia of follicular cells and extensive infiltration by lymphocytes with well-developed germinal centers.
     e. Thyroid follicles become atrophic with gradual loss of follicular epithelium and colloid.
     f. There is an increased risk of papillary thyroid carcinoma.
     g. Circulating antithyroid antibodies called **antimicrosomal** and **anti-TSH receptor antibodies** are an important target for clinical assays for autoimmune thyroiditis.
  2. **Iodine deficiency** is a common cause of hypothyroidism where dietary iodine is in short supply.
     a. Iodine deficiency leads to development of a **goiter** due to compensatory hyperplasia.
     b. Iodine will reverse the goiter and hypothyroidism.
  3. **Refetoff syndrome** is a disorder of peripheral resistance to circulating thyroid hormone.
     a. A point mutation in the thyroid hormone receptor gene leads to generalized resistance to thyroid hormone and a reduction in basal metabolic rate and **growth retardation.**
     b. The usual tip-off for this entity is clinical hypothyroidism with an elevated TSH and elevated free T_4.
  4. Subacute or **granulomatous thyroiditis (de Quervain thyroiditis)** is less common than Hashimoto thyroiditis but also presents predominantly in women between ages of 30 and 50 years old.
     a. It is thought to be a postviral inflammatory process, following a viral upper respiratory infection, with a seasonal component associated with **coxsackievirus** and **adenovirus.**
     b. There may be antigenic cross-reactivity between viral antigens and thyroid antigens.
     c. The gland is enlarged, firm, and very tender to palpation.
     d. Sections reveal granulomas and abundant inflammation.
     e. Thyroid function is initially increased with release of thyroid hormone due to gland destruction, but over time, function diminishes as waves of inflammation and injury lead to progressive fibrosis.
     f. With recovery, function returns and inflammation resolves in virtually all cases, generally over months.

5. Riedel thyroiditis is very rare and characterized by progressive and extensive fibrosis of the thyroid gland.
  a. Fibrosis may extend from the thyroid gland to involve contiguous structures of the neck leading to recurrent laryngeal nerve paralysis and tracheal compromise.
  b. It is easily mistaken for a malignant process.
  c. The gland is hard, fixed, and often described as **"woody."**
  d. Riedel thyroiditis can be associated with other fibrotic processes occurring in the mediastinum and retroperitoneum.
  e. Circulating anti-thyroid antibodies, as with the other entities described above, can be detected.
6. Palpation thyroiditis can occur after vigorous palpation of the thyroid gland due to mechanical disruption of the thyroid follicles.

D. Neoplasia
  1. Follicular adenoma is a solitary encapsulated nodule separate from the adjacent thyroid parenchyma.
    a. The lesion is composed of a repetitive small microfollicular pattern with minimal colloid (Figure 11–2B).
    b. Tumor cells are cytologically bland and lack features of papillary carcinoma.
    c. The tumor does not invade through its fibrous capsule and no angiolymphatic invasion is present.
    d. Sometimes adenomas develop oncocytic features (or Hürthle **cell** change), the so-called Hürthle cell adenoma.
    e. The differential diagnosis for follicular adenoma includes a hyperplastic nodule in cases of multinodular goiter or other hyperthyroid conditions such as Graves disease.
  2. Follicular carcinoma is distinguished from adenoma by the presence of invasion through the fibrous capsule with angiolymphatic invasion.
    a. It is more common in older women and usually presents as a solitary nodule.
    b. Iodine deficiency appears to be a major risk factor.
    c. Unlike adenoma, follicular carcinoma has metastatic potential, often to bones, sometimes years after diagnosis.
    d. Both follicular adenomas and follicular carcinomas have a high incidence of mutations in the *RAS* **oncogene.**
  3. Papillary thyroid carcinoma is the most common thyroid malignancy, which can present at any age and is more common in women.
    a. Prior exposure to ionizing radiation and Hashimoto thyroiditis appear to be risk factors.
    b. Papillary thyroid carcinomas are often multifocal; therefore, diagnosis in one lobe prompts a complete thyroidectomy.
    c. Histologic sections show branching papillary structures with a fibrovascular core lined by squamoid-like epithelium with enlarged clear nuclei ("little orphan Annie nuclei"), and occasional intranuclear cytoplasmic inclusions (Figure 11–2C-D).
    d. There are several variants of papillary thyroid carcinoma, including the follicular variant (instead of papillary architecture, there is a follicular architecture), tall cell variant, and the diffuse sclerosing variant.

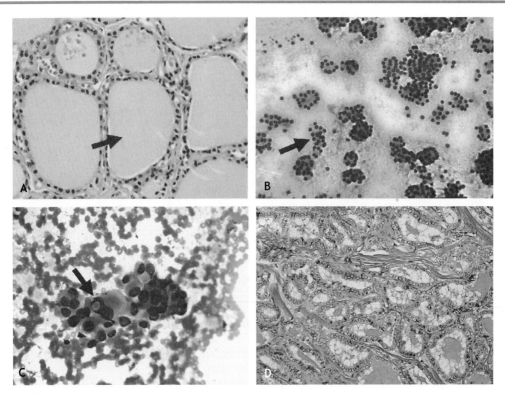

Figure 11–2. Thyroid. Thyroid nodules are common and most are benign; therefore, fine-needle aspiration sampling is used to exclude tumors requiring further surgery. **A:** Normal thyroid tissue has abundant colloid (arrow) and monomorphic bland nuclei. **B:** In contrast, a follicular adenoma/carcinoma would show a repetitive microfollicular pattern (arrow) with minimal colloid. **C:** Papillary carcinoma yields groups of squamoid cells with intranuclear cytoplasmic inclusions (arrow). **D:** Histologic sections of papillary carcinoma show thick bubble-gum colloid, nuclear enlargement, crowding, and the so-called "orphan Annie" nuclear clearing. It may have follicular architecture (shown here) or classic branching papillary architecture.

> e. Papillary thyroid carcinomas are associated with several oncogenic pathways, including **RET,** *BRAF,* and *NTRK1* mutations.
> f. **Prognosis** is most closely related to patient **age** (<45 years old is favorable) and **gender** (female is favorable).
> *(1)* Stage 1: <2 cm in size and limited to the thyroid
> *(2)* Stage 2: <4 cm in size and limited to the thyroid
> *(3)* Stage 3: minimal extra-thyroid extension
> *(4)* Stage 4: vascular invasion or metastases
> 4. **Medullary thyroid carcinoma** is a neuroendocrine neoplasm that may be sporadic or associated with MEN IIA or IIB.
> a. It arises from the **parafollicular** or **C cells.**
> b. The C cell secretes **calcitonin,** which can be measured in the serum by clinical assay or used as an immunohistochemical marker on paraffin-embedded tissue sections.

c. It can be solitary or multifocal.

    d. Familial versions of medullary thyroid carcinoma are associated with **multifocal C cell hyperplasia,** prior to development of carcinoma.

    e. Histologic sections of the neoplasm show neuroendocrine plasmacytoid and spindle cells with "salt and pepper" chromatin, which are arranged in sheets and nests.

    f. There may be Congo red positive **amyloid** deposits that show characteristic **apple-green birefringence with polarization.**

    g. Tumor cells immunostain for **calcitonin.**

  5. Anaplastic carcinoma is a poorly differentiated thyroid malignancy with an extremely poor prognosis.

    a. Mortality is essentially 100% within a year of diagnosis.

    b. The tumor aggressively invades adjacent structures in the neck, and it is composed of **highly anaplastic cells,** including tumor giant cells and sarcomatous spindle cells.

    c. No effective therapy is currently available.

FINE-NEEDLE ASPIRATION OF THYROID NODULES

CLINICAL
CORRELATION

- *Fifteen percent of people have a detectable nodule in the thyroid, either by palpation, or by ultrasound imaging.*
- *Fine-needle aspiration is a minimally invasive method to biopsy nodules and screen for rare cases of carcinoma.*

III. Parathyroid

  A. Primary Hyperparathyroidism

    1. Increased levels of circulating parathyroid hormone (PTH) leads to hypercalcemia and hypophosphatemia (Table 11–2).

      a. PTH enhances calcium reabsorption from the distal tubules and the thick ascending limb of the nephron.

      b. It stimulates osteoclast precursors and bone resorption.

      c. PTH promotes activation and absorption of vitamin D.

    2. **Adenomas** are common, benign, and usually solitary.

      a. Adenomas may be associated with MEN type I.

      b. Parathyroid carcinoma is exceedingly rare.

Table 11–2. Disorders of calcium homeostasis.

Condition	PTH	Calcium	Phosphate
Primary hyperparathyroidism	↑	↑	↓
Secondary hyperparathyroidism	↑	↓	↑
Primary hypoparathyroidism	↓	↓	↑
Pseudohypoparathyroidism	↑	↓	↑
Vitamin D deficiency	↑	↓	↓

PTH, parathyroid hormone.

3. **Hyperplasia** is diffuse enlargement of multiple parathyroid glands.
4. The diagnosis of primary hyperparathyroidism is made by determination of serum calcium and PTH.
   a. PTH is measured by clinical immunoassay.
   b. **Elevated** serum calcium levels with inappropriately elevated PTH levels indicate primary hyperparathyroidism.

LOCATING THE PARATHYROIDS

CLINICAL CORRELATION

- *The inferior parathyroid glands arise from the dorsal wing of the third pharyngeal pouch and migrate caudally with the thymus.*
- *The superior parathyroids originate from the dorsal wing of the fourth pharyngeal pouch and migrate a shorter distance to arrive at a position more posterior and medial to the inferior parathyroids.*
- *Altered or arrested migration may leave parathyroid tissue anywhere from the carotid bifurcation to the aortopulmonary window.*
- *Failure of the third and fourth brachial pouches to differentiate results in congenital thymic aplasia and absent parathyroid glands are characteristic of DiGeorge syndrome.*

   B. **Secondary Hyperparathyroidism**
      1. **Chronic renal insufficiency** is the most common cause of secondary hyperparathyroidism and leads to decreased phosphate excretion, hyperphosphatemia, decreased vitamin D and calcium, which in turn induces compensatory PTH hypersecretion and hyperplasia.
      2. Likewise, any condition with resistance to the metabolic effects of parathyroid hormone, or increased calcium liberation, can lead to secondary hyperparathyroidism.
         a. Prostatic carcinoma may induce hypocalcemia with osteoblastic metastases that sequester calcium.
         b. Conversely, **multiple myeloma,** breast, and lung cancer drive increased osteoclastic activity that liberates calcium.
      3. Elevated levels of PTH can lead to **osteitis fibrosa cystica,** a disorder of increased bone resorption.

   C. **Primary Hypoparathyroidism**
      1. Primary hypoparathyroidism is an absolute reduction in secretion of PTH leading to hypocalcemia (Table 11–2).
      2. There are several etiologies that can lead to hypoparathyroidism.
         a. **DiGeorge syndrome** is associated with the congenital absence of the parathyroids.
         b. **Chronic mucocutaneous candidiasis** is an immunodeficiency that is associated with hypoparathyroidism and adrenal insufficiency.
         c. **Autoimmune hypoparathyroidism** has autoantibodies to parathyroid antigens including calcium-sensing receptors.
         d. **Inadvertent removal of parathyroids,** grossly mistaken for lymph nodes, may occur during thyroid surgery.
      3. The laboratory profile includes low serum PTH with accompanying low levels of serum calcium and elevated levels of phosphate.

   D. **Pseudohypoparathyroidism,** also known as **Albright hereditary osteodystrophy,** is due to an end-organ resistance to the effects of circulating PTH.
      1. The G-protein family, important in mediating the actions of PTH, is an important factor in the pathophysiology.

2. Unlike true hypoparathyroidism, this condition is associated with low serum calcium, elevated levels of phosphate but high levels of PTH due to end-organ resistance to the effects of PTH.

IV. Pancreas

A. Diabetes Mellitus

1. Type 1 diabetes is due to immune-mediated destruction of the beta-islet cells, leading to absolute insulin reduction.
  a. Type 1 presents in **childhood** and requires **insulin therapy.**
  b. Autoantibodies to **glutamic acid decarboxylase,** insulin, and islet cell antigens can be detected in the serum.
  c. There are genetic risk factors.
  d. **C-peptide** levels are low or undetectable.
   (1) C-peptide, a metabolite of endogenous pro-insulin, is not present in exogenously administered insulin.
   (2) This helps discriminate an insulinoma from factitious insulin abuse.
  e. Diabetic **ketoacidosis** and coma can develop.

2. Type 2 diabetes is an insulin-resistant syndrome with some degree of relative insulin reduction.
  a. It is much more common than type 1 diabetes, accounting for **>95%** of cases.
  b. The incidence is skyrocketing due to the increased prevalence of **obesity** and subsequent insulin resistance.
  c. Although it typically presents in **adults,** there is an increasing proportion of affected children.
  d. Risk factors include obesity, ethnicity, and genetic factors.
  e. Treatment includes weight loss and medication (eg, **metformin**).
  f. Insulin may be required as insulin deficiency develops.

3. Mature onset diabetes of the young (MODY), also called "type one-and-a-half," stems from **genetic defects** in the beta-islet cells.
  a. The clinical presentation is different than type 1 diabetes.
   (1) Ketoacidosis can be presenting manifestation.
   (2) There are no circulating autoantibodies, and MODY presents later in the patient's life than type 1 diabetes.
  b. Treatment is insulin therapy.

4. Endocrinopathies can lead to diabetes mellitus, Cushing syndrome, pheochromocytoma, glucagonoma, and hyperthyroidism.

5. Destructive diseases of the exocrine pancreas that lead to secondary diabetes include **hereditary hemochromatosis,** cystic fibrosis, and chronic pancreatitis.

6. Laboratory diagnosis of diabetes is based on assessment of glucose levels, both fasting and after a glucose challenge.
  a. A **fasting plasma glucose** greater than or equal to 126 mg/dL is the standard limit for the diagnosis of diabetes mellitus.
  b. Two hours after a 75-gram oral glucose load, the plasma glucose will be 200 mg/dL or higher in a diabetic patient.
  c. **Gestational diabetes** has different cutoffs (the fasting cutoff value is 95 mg/dL, the 2-hour cutoff is 155 mg/dL).

7. Long-term glycemic control in diabetic patients can be assessed with several laboratory studies.

a. **Hemoglobin A_{1C}** is a measurement of glycosylated hemoglobin, normal hemoglobin A_{1C} levels are <7%.

b. The **fructosamine** assay measures glycosylation of albumin; the shorter half-life of albumin (14–20 days) yields a more short-term determination of glycemic control.

c. Both the hemoglobin A_{1C} and fructosamine tests can be confounded by factors such as hemoglobinopathies, blood loss and transfusion, hemolytic anemia, fluctuations in protein levels from illness, and loss of albumin due to diabetic nephropathy.

8. Measurement of albumin in the urine provides an assessment of diabetic-related nephropathy (**microalbuminuria**).

9. The presence of glucose in the urine, or **glycosuria,** indicates that blood glucose levels exceed the renal threshold of glucose reabsorption (usually **180 mg/dL**).

10. **Ketone testing** is an important tool in monitoring patients with type 1 diabetes mellitus who are at risk for **diabetic ketoacidosis,** since early detection can often prevent serious complications.

   a. Ketones derive from the metabolism of fatty acids and include **acetoacetate** and **β-hydroxybutyrate.**

   b. During insulin deficiency, ketone production increases.

   c. Elevated ketone levels can be measured in blood or urine.

11. The complications of diabetes mellitus are legion and beyond the scope of this outline, but they can be divided by time course.

   a. **Acute complications** include both diabetic ketoacidosis and non-ketotic hyperosmolar coma.

   b. **Chronic complications** account for the majority of morbidity and mortality, especially due to the toxic effects of persistent hyperglycemia on blood vessels and nerves.

   (1) **Macrovascular** disease is characterized by accelerated atherogenesis and atherosclerosis of the coronary, cerebral, and peripheral arteries; it results in myocardial infarction (the most common cause of death in persons with diabetes), stroke, and ischemic gangrene of the distal lower extremities.

   (2) **Microvascular** disease involves concentric thickening of vessels due to hyaline deposition.

   (3) **Diabetic nephropathy** encompasses several lesions, including nodular glomerulosclerosis (**Kimmelstiel-Wilson disease**), renovascular arteriosclerosis, and necrotic papillary structures/pyelonephritis.

   (4) **Peripheral neuropathies** are extremely common, affecting distal nerves with sensory and motor deficits, and are likely due to toxicity from hyperglycemia and ischemia.

   (5) **Ocular complications** include **retinopathy** and **cataracts.**

B. Hypoglycemia

   1. **Drugs** are the most common cause of hypoglycemia, especially insulin and sulfonylureas used to treat diabetes.

      a. Sulfonylurea derivatives prod the pancreatic beta cells to release insulin.

      b. The release of insulin increases levels of C-peptide.

      c. Administration of insulin would result in high insulin levels, but a low or undetectable C-peptide level.

d. Some drugs can cause hypoglycemia by either altering glucose metabolism (alcohol and β-blockers) or by directly damaging beta cells (pentamidine, an antimicrobial).

BLOOD SUGAR

- *Acute hypoglycemia manifests as tremors, seizure, coma, and death.*
- *Chronic hyperglycemia encourages glycosylation of various proteins and is toxic to blood vessels.*
- *While four hormones (cortisol, epinephrine, glucagon, and growth hormone) raise blood glucose levels, only insulin lowers it.*
- *Insulin resistance is the failure of target organs to respond normally to the action of insulin.*

    2. Severe illness, such as sepsis, renal failure, liver failure, or malnutrition can lead to hypoglycemia due to increased utilization of glucose, decreased production, or decreased intake of glucose.

    3. Autoimmune insulin syndrome is autoantibody-mediated interference with insulin or the insulin receptor.

    4. Hereditary metabolic diseases should be included in the clinical differential diagnosis in children with hypoglycemia (eg, glycogen storage diseases, galactosemia, and carnitine deficiency).

C. Acute Pancreatitis

    1. Acute pancreatitis is a life-threatening, but reversible disease caused by acute inflammation of the pancreas.

    2. It presents with severe abdominal pain.

    3. Possible causes vary and include the following:

      a. Metabolic (**alcoholism,** hyperlipoproteinemia, hypercalcemia)

      b. Drugs (thiazides, furosemide, estrogen, azathioprine, sulfonamides, methyldopa, pentamide, procainamide)

      c. Mechanical (**gallstones,** iatrogenic injury, occlusion of ducts with *Ascaris lumbricoides* or *Clonorchis*)

      d. Vascular (shock, atheroembolism, polyarteritis nodosa)

      e. Infectious (mumps, coxsackievirus, *Mycoplasma pneumoniae*)

      f. **Idiopathic** (10–20% of cases)

      g. **Hereditary pancreatitis,** which is an autosomal dominant disease caused by the cationic trypsinogen (*PRSS1*) gene.

    4. The pathologic changes are secondary to the release of activated **pancreatic enzymes** leading to edema, fat necrosis, acute inflammation, and hemorrhage.

    5. The diagnosis is made by detecting elevated **amylase** during the first 24 hours and elevated **lipase** within 72–96 hours.

      a. **Glycosuria** occurs in 10% of cases.

      b. **Hypocalcemia** may occur secondary to saponification.

      c. Imaging studies show a diffusely enlarged pancreas.

      d. Needle biopsy shows acute inflammation and fat necrosis.

    6. The prognosis is poor (20% mortality rate) if not treated.

      a. Poor prognostic factors include systemic organ failure, disseminated intravascular coagulation (DIC), peripheral vascular collapse and shock with acute tubular necrosis and acute respiratory distress syndrome.

      b. Pancreatic pseudocysts, sterile pancreatic abscesses, or secondary infection may develop in patients who recover from acute pancreatitis.

D. **Chronic Pancreatitis**
1. Chronic pancreatitis leads to **irreversible** impairment of pancreatic function with destruction of the exocrine pancreas, fibrosis, and destruction of the endocrine pancreas.
2. It presents as recurrent bouts of acute pancreatitis or as a silent process until significant pancreatic dysfunction is detected.
3. Pancreatic exocrine insufficiency will cause weight loss and hypoalbuminemic edema secondary to malabsorption.
4. Causes of chronic pancreatitis include the following:
   a. Alcohol abuse
   b. Long-standing **obstruction** of the pancreatic duct (calculi, trauma, pseudocysts, neoplasms, pancreatic divisum)
   c. Tropical pancreatitis (associated with malnutrition)
   d. Hereditary pancreatitis (germline mutations in *PRSS1* or *SPINK1* genes)
   e. **Cystic fibrosis**
   f. Idiopathic
5. The diagnosis may be difficult.
   a. There may be mild fever, **pain,** and mildly elevated **amylase.**
   b. Gallstone obstruction may lead to elevated alkaline phosphatase and **jaundice.**
   c. Radiologic imaging may reveal **calcifications.**
   d. Needle biopsy shows diffuse fibrosis and rare ductal cells with loss of acini (Figure 11–3A inset).
6. Chronic pancreatitis leads to pancreatic exocrine insufficiency with **chronic malabsorption.**
   a. Diabetes mellitus may eventually develop.
   b. Pancreatic **pseudocysts** develop in 10% of patients.
   c. There may be an increased risk of cancer.
E. **Congenital Cysts**
1. Benign congenital cysts are associated with polycystic disease and von Hippel-Lindau disease.
2. They are usually 3–5 cm in diameter and are lined by benign ductal type epithelium.
F. **Pancreatic Endocrine Neoplasia (Islet Cell Tumors)**
1. Islet cell tumors of the neuroendocrine pancreas all have metastatic potential despite size and differentiation; many are functional with hypersecretion of specific hormones that can result in clinical symptoms (eg, insulinoma, gastrinoma, glucagonoma).
   a. **Insulinoma** shows beta-islet cell differentiation and clinical symptoms of hypoglycemia due to hypersecretion of insulin.
   b. **Gastrinoma** causes clinical symptoms related to hypersecretion of gastrin, including **diarrhea** (due to high acid secretion neutralizing pancreatic enzymes), duodenal ulcer(s), and gastroesophageal reflux.
   c. **Glucagonomas** show alpha-islet cell differentiation with clinical symptoms related to elevated glucagon levels, including mild diabetes mellitus, weight loss, and a characteristic skin rash called **necrolytic migratory erythema.**
   d. Somatostatinomas show delta-islet cell differentiation and clinical manifestations, including diabetes, hypochlorhydria, cholelithiasis (due to

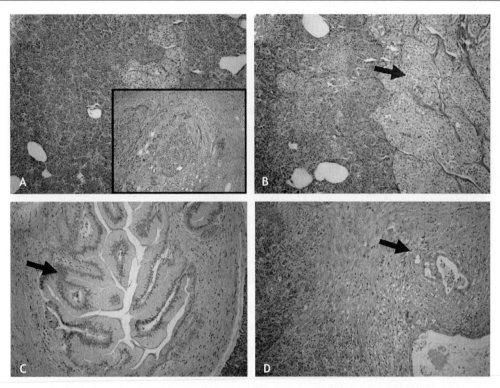

Figure 11–3. Pancreatic pathology. A: Normal pancreas is predominantly acinar cells with a few scattered islets. Pancreatitis leads to fibrosis and loss of acini (inset). **B:** Islet cell tumors (endocrine tumors) usually occur in the tail of the pancreas, they stain for chromogranin, and have metastatic potential despite relatively bland features. **C:** Intraductal papillary mucinous neoplasms are a common premalignant ductal proliferation within large ducts that progress to invasive ductal carcinoma (**D**) in approximately 30% of cases.

suppression of cholecystokinin), diarrhea, and weight loss, which are thought to arise from high somatostatin secretion.

2. Pancreatic neuroendocrine neoplasms typically arise in the **tail of the pancreas** and are well circumscribed and solitary.

3. Features that predict increased metastatic potential include **angioinvasion, necrosis, perineural invasion,** and many **mitoses.**

4. Needle biopsy findings reveal a neoplasm with various growth patterns, including **solid nests** (Figure 11–3B) and **glands.**

    a. Tumor cells have a plasmacytoid or spindle cell morphology with round nuclei; **salt-n-pepper** chromatin; and delicate cytoplasm, which may contain red neuroendocrine granules.

    b. Islet cell tumors immunostain for chromogranin.

    c. Functioning tumors may be immunostained for insulin and so on, but this is rarely required given serologic studies.

G. **Pancreatic Ductal Adenocarcinoma**
1. Intraductal papillary mucinous neoplasms (**IPMN**) appear to be a precursor lesion to invasive ductal carcinoma.
   a. Approximately **30%** of IPMNs are associated with **carcinoma.**
   b. These tumors present with pancreatic duct obstruction symptoms (jaundice, elevated amylase) due to a mass lesion.
   c. Needle biopsy reveals a **papillary tumor** with mild to moderate nuclear atypia in a background of abundant **mucin** (Figure 11–3C).
   d. Duct fluid may show significantly elevated carcinoembryonic antigen (CEA) levels.
   e. Treatment is often **surgery** to completely remove the neoplasm, because of the risk of associated ductal adenocarcinoma.
2. Pancreatic ductal adenocarcinoma is usually discovered after it has already invaded outside the pancreas and has metastasized.
   a. It presents with abdominal pain (boring into the back) and obstructive jaundice.
   b. **Trousseau sign** (migratory thrombophlebitis) occurs in 10% of patients.
   c. Risk factors include **smoking, alcoholism,** chronic **pancreatitis,** point mutations of **K-*ras*** and *p53*, and toxin exposures (**B-napthylamine,** benzidine).
   d. The diagnosis is confirmed by needle biopsy showing desmoplastic stroma invaded by malignant glands with variably sized nuclei, irregular nuclear membranes, nucleoli, and conspicuous mitoses (Figure 11–3D).
   e. Treatment is surgical resection (Whipple) and chemotherapy.
   f. Prognosis depends on tumor stage, but is poor; survival is usually only months:
      (1) **Stage 1:** Carcinoma is limited to the pancreas.
      (2) **Stage 2:** Carcinoma is invading outside pancreas.
      (3) **Stage 3:** Carcinoma is unresectable.
      (4) **Stage 4:** Distant metastases (eg, liver) are present.
3. Solid pseudopapillary tumor is a rare neoplasm occurring in the **tail** of the pancreas, primarily in **young women.**
   a. Needle biopsy reveals a cytologically bland papillary neoplasm with prominent fibrovascular cores.
   b. **Beta-catenin** mutations are common in these tumors.
   c. Surgical excision is usually curative.
4. Acinar cell carcinoma is rare.
   a. Needle biopsy reveals bland tumor cells arranged in solid, trabecular, or acinar patterns, similar to islet cell tumors.
   b. Tumor cells have abundant red granular cytoplasm.
   c. Metastatic potential is similar to islet cell tumors, but data suggest acinar cell carcinoma may be more aggressive.
5. Pancreatoblastoma is a rare tumor primarily occurring in **children.**
   a. Needle biopsy reveals a hypercellular small round blue cell tumor arranged in well-formed glands and solid nests; squamoid corpuscles may be present.
   b. The prognosis is favorable.

V. Adrenal

A. Congenital Adrenal Hyperplasia

1. Adrenal hyperplasia represents a common pathway for multiple disorders, which lead to bilateral nodular enlargement.
2. Clinical symptoms are due to decreased production of aldosterone and cortisol, leading to **hypotension, salt wasting, shock,** and increased production of androgens leading to **sexual ambiguity, virilization, hirsutism,** and **infertility.**
3. Hyperplasia is due to increased levels of ACTH and corticotropin-releasing hormone (CRH) that are stimulated due to the blockade of corticosteroid hormone synthesis.
4. Most cases (over **90%**) arise from **21-hydroxylase deficiency.**
   a. The 21-hydroxylase enzyme is responsible for synthesis of both mineralocorticoids and cortisol, so a block in this enzyme results in **decreased synthesis** of aldosterone and cortisol.
   b. Increased concentrations of precursors are shunted to the androgen pathway, leading to increased production of androgens with **ambiguous genitalia** in females.
   c. The degree of enzyme deficiency is variable from case to case; lesser deficiencies, predictably, have less severe clinical presentations with early menarche or virilization, but no salt wasting.
5. The second most common form of congenital adrenal insufficiency (about **7%**) is **11B-hydroxylase deficiency.**
   a. This enzyme defect prevents synthesis of cortisol and corticosterone; however, salt wasting does not develop since precursors also possess mineralocorticoid properties leading to hypertension and hypokalemia.
   b. Increased androgen production induces virilization.

B. Cushing Syndrome

1. Adrenal **Cushing syndrome** arises from an adrenal cortical adenoma or carcinoma that drives autonomous production of cortisol and suppression of CRH and ACTH (ACTH-independent).
2. Diagnosis is made by detecting cortisol hyperproduction, then determining the cause of production (ACTH-independent or dependent).
   a. **24-hour urine for free cortisol** should be done along with serum and urinary creatinine to make sure the glomerular filtration rate (GFR)is normal and collection is adequate since decreased GFR will lead to decreased excretion of cortisol and a false-negative result.
      (1) This test is not affected by fluctuations in cortisol binding globulin or daily serum fluctuations.
      (2) Borderline high values may be observed with pregnancy, depression, anxiety disorders, alcoholism, and obesity.
   b. The **overnight dexamethasone suppression test** is another common screening test for Cushing syndrome.
      (1) A dose of dexamethasone is given at night.
      (2) Plasma cortisol is then measured the following morning.
      (3) Lack of suppression of the cortisol level is evidence of Cushing syndrome.

c. **Confirmatory testing** includes a midnight plasma cortisol measurement and the low-dose dexamethasone suppression test.
  (1) Once hypercortisolism is confirmed, ACTH is measured.
  (2) Elevated levels of serum ACTH indicate Cushing disease, or ectopic ACTH production.

d. **High-dose dexamethasone test** differentiates Cushing disease from Cushing syndrome because suppression occurs in Cushing disease but not Cushing syndrome.

C. Adrenal Insufficiency

1. It may be primary adrenal insufficiency or secondary adrenal insufficiency at the pituitary level.

2. Clinically, it is associated with nausea, vomiting, diarrhea, weight loss, hypoglycemia, salt-wasting, and hyperpigmentation of mucosal surfaces caused by cross-stimulation of **melanin production** due to elevated ACTH levels.

KENNEDY'S TAN

CLINICAL CORRELATION

- *During the first televised presidential debates of 1960, many viewers noted how healthy and tan John F. Kennedy appeared compared to the pale sweating Richard M. Nixon.*
- *President Kennedy was wholly dependent on cortisone therapy, similar to patients with Addison disease, which often presents with increased skin pigmentation.*

3. **Primary adrenal insufficiency** is caused by destruction of the adrenal gland tissue.
  a. It is associated with cortisol and mineralocorticoid deficiency
  b. Common causes include autoimmune destruction (80-90%), **tuberculosis,** Addison disease, HIV/AIDS, metastatic disease, granulomatous diseases, and hemorrhage (related to meningococcal sepsis).

4. **Central adrenal insufficiency** results from chronic hypothalamic-pituitary axis suppression by corticosteroid administration and less commonly by pituitary diseases.

5. Laboratory tests are available to confirm adrenal hypofunction.
  a. **Basal hormone levels,** such as an early morning plasma cortisol level, help establish the diagnosis if they are low.
  b. The **ACTH stimulation test** involves administering synthetic ACTH to stimulate the adrenals then measuring cortisol levels.
  c. With **overnight metyrapone testing,** an inhibitor of 11B-hydroxylase (metyrapone) results in accumulation of 11-deoxycortisol among normal persons whereas low or absent 11-deoxycortisol levels occurs among patients with insufficiency.

D. Neoplasia

1. **Adrenal cortical adenoma** is a benign neoplasm.
  a. They are common (7% of people) and are usually detected as "incidentalomas" during abdominal imaging for other indications.
  b. Most are nonfunctional but about 20% secrete hormones derived from the different cortical cells types (glomerulosa = aldosterone "salt"; fasciculata = cortisol "sugar"; reticularis = androgens "sex").

c. Most cases are unilateral.

   d. **Cortisol**-secreting adenomas may cause **Cushing syndrome.**

   e. **Aldosterone**-secreting adenomas may present with hypertension and hypokalemia, also known as **Conn syndrome,** a rare type of secondary hypertension.

   f. **Androgen**-secreting adrenal adenomas are quite **rare** but present with symptoms attributable to increased androgens in females (hirsutism, amenorrhea, virilization), or increased estrogens in males (gynecomastia, sexual dysfunction).

2. **Adrenal cortical carcinoma** is malignant and may be distinguished from its adenomatous counterpart in several ways.

   a. **Size:** Adrenal cortical carcinomas are typically larger (often greater than 5 cm) and are **>100 g.**

   b. **Necrosis:** Malignancies more likely feature areas of hemorrhage and necrosis, which may be apparent by imaging.

   c. **Invasion:** Carcinomas invade surrounding structures, including blood vessels, culminating in distant metastases.

3. **Pheochromocytoma** is an exceedingly rare neoplasm arising from the adrenal medulla.

   a. The term "pheochromocytoma" is derived from a color change that happens when samples of the neoplasm are exposed to oxidizers (**chromaffin reaction**).

   b. Recall the "**rule of 10s**" for pheochromocytoma, which will serve a great purpose on internal medicine rounds.

     (1) 10% of pheochromocytomas are bilateral.

     (2) 10% are extra-adrenal (paraganglioma).

     (3) 10% are malignant.

     (4) 10% are syndromic or familial.

     (5) 10% are "incidentalomas."

     (6) 10% are clinically nonfunctional.

     (7) 10% present in the pediatric age group.

   c. Symptoms derive from **excess circulating catecholamines** and are sporadic and episodic (headache, hypertension, diaphoresis, palpitations, chest pain, abdominal pain, and anxiety).

   d. **Genetic syndromes** associated with pheochromocytoma include von Hippel-Lindau syndrome, neurofibromatosis type 1, and multiple endocrine neoplasia type 2 (**MEN II**).

   e. In patients with a familial or genetic syndrome, there is often concurrent diffuse adrenal medullary hyperplasia.

   f. Similar to adrenal cortical neoplasms, metastatic potential is a function of size, necrosis, and invasion.

   g. Histologic sections reveal a "**zellballen**" **architecture,** which is characterized by nests of cells surrounded by a framework of stroma (Figure 11–4A), similar to paraganglioma (Figure 11–4B).

   h. Similar to other neuroendocrine neoplasms, these tumors immunostain for **chromogranin** (adrenal cortical tumors are negative); moreover, S100 will stain sustentacular cells rimming the zellballen nests.

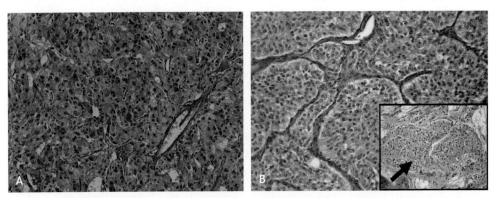

Figure 11–4. Pheochromocytoma and extra-adrenal paraganglioma. A: Pheochromocytoma is very rare, arising from the adrenal medulla. The tumor secretes catecholamine and stains for chromogranin. **B:** About 10% of cases are extra-adrenal pheochromocytomas, which are called paragangliomas that often arise in the organ of Zuckerkandl (inset), located at the aortic bifurcation.

CLINICAL
CORRELATION

PHEOCHROMOCYTOMA AND HYPERTENSION

- *When pheochromocytoma is clinically suspected, the first step is to measure plasma metanephrines and normetanephrines **(catecholamines).***
- *If both are normal, a pheochromocytoma is very unlikely.*
- *Pheochromocytoma and adrenal cortical adenoma (Conn syndrome) are two of three causes of hypertension (renal artery stenosis is the third) that are treated surgically.*

    4. Paragangliomas are extra-adrenal pheochromocytoma-like neoplasms derived from the parasympathetic or sympathetic nervous system.
        a. Common sites for **parasympathetic paragangliomas** are the head, neck, and mediastinum.
        b. **Sympathetic paragangliomas** follow the distribution of the sympathetic nervous system, so para-aortic and paravertebral locations are more common.
        c. Clinical symptoms are usually due to compression of surrounding structures due to mass effects.
        d. Biopsy reveals the same "zellballen" pattern and immunostaining profile as adrenal pheochromocytomas (Figure 11–4).
    5. Metastases are more common than primary adrenal neoplasia.
        a. The incidence increases with advancing patient age.
        b. **Lung,** gastric, esophagus, biliary, and **breast** carcinomas are among the most frequent sources of metastases to the adrenals.
        c. **Renal cell carcinoma** is the most common neoplasm to directly invade the adrenal, which sometimes presents a diagnostic challenge since renal cell and adrenal cortical neoplasms are nearly morphologically identical.
        d. Adrenal insufficiency develops only rarely.

VI. Inherited Tumor Syndromes of the Endocrine System

    A. Multiple Endocrine Neoplasia
        1. Type I MEN (Wermer syndrome) arises from a germline mutation and is characterized by *p*ituitary, *p*ancreatic islet cell, and *p*arathyroid neoplasia (the 3 Ps) (Table 11–3).

Table 11–3. Characteristics of multiple endocrine neoplasia (MEN).

Type	Characteristics
I (Wermer syndrome)	Parathyroid adenoma Pancreatic neoplasms Pituitary adenomas
IIA (Sipple syndrome)	Parathyroid disease Pheochromocytomas Medullary thyroid carcinoma (*ret* oncogene)
IIB	Parathyroid disease Pheochromocytomas Medullary thyroid carcinoma Mucocutaneous ganglioneuromas (*ret* oncogene)

    2. Type IIA MEN (Sipple syndrome) features medullary thyroid carcinoma, pheochromocytoma, and hyperparathyroidism secondary to parathyroid gland hyperplasia.
        a. MEN IIA is linked to mutations within the ***ret*** proto-oncogene.
        b. By the "rule of 10s," 10% of phcochromocytomas are MEN IIA.
    3. Type IIB MEN (also known as MEN III), includes medullary thyroid carcinoma and pheochromocytoma.
        a. There are associated mucosal ganglioneuromas.
        b. The mutations of the *ret* oncogene observed in MEN IIB are distinct from those of MEN IIA.
    4. Carney complex (distinct from **Carney triad**) is a rare MEN variant with cardiac myxomas, lentigines, and endocrine hyperactivity.
  B. von Hippel-Lindau syndrome
    1. This syndrome is a rare, progressive multisystemic disorder involving angiomatous hamartomas.
    2. It arises from a mutation of the ***VHL*** tumor suppressor gene.
    3. The clinical presentation varies with the location of the tumor.
        a. Retinal capillary hemangiomas are present in 50% of patients.
        b. Some patients have **cerebellar hemangiomas.**
    4. Like MEN II, *VHL* is also associated with **pheochromocytoma,** but the clinical and biochemical profiles differ (eg, the MEN II-related pheochromocytoma is more likely to induce paroxysmal hypertension, and has lower total plasma catecholamine levels than *VHL*).
    5. These patients are at greater risk for other types of neoplasia, especially **renal cell carcinoma.**
VII. Nutritional Pathology
  A. Obesity
    1. Approximately **two-thirds of adults** and an increasing proportion of children and adolescents are overweight or obese.
        a. Body mass index (BMI) is calculated from weight and height.

b. Adults with a BMI ranging from 25 kg/m² to 30 kg/m² are considered overweight.

c. Adults with a BMI >30 kg/m² are considered obese.

2. Obesity is predominantly due to **high calorie diets** and lack of **exercise,** a sedentary lifestyle.

a. Each pound of fat is the product of 3500 kilocalories of energy not used to meet metabolic demands.

b. Excess adiposity, particularly involving the waist (an increased "gut-to-butt" ratio), is associated with the complex of insulin resistance, hypertension, dyslipidemia, and a proinflammatory drive known as the **metabolic syndrome.**

c. Despite commonly cited concerns about hypothyroid-induced weight gain, thyroid dysfunction is rarely causative (<1%).

3. Adipocytes are an **endocrine organ.**

a. Adipocytokines are released, which include adiponectin and **leptin.**

b. Fat cells also produce estrogens and cortisol that may lead to **endometrial hyperplasia, polycystic ovary syndrome,** and **infertility.**

4. Obesity creates several other strains on the body aside from diabetes and heart disease.

a. Increased fatty tissue about the oropharynx predisposes patients to **obstructive sleep apnea.**

b. Higher body mass is a risk factor for orthopedic pathology.

(1) Adults are prone to osteoarthritis and back injury.

(2) Childhood obesity is associated with a higher incidence of **slipped capital femoral epiphysis,** which initially presents as a painful limp.

c. Alterations in abdominal mechanics favor herniation, and lessened esophageal tone causes **gastrointestinal reflux disease.**

d. Obesity is also an independent risk factor for multiple types of neoplasia, including esophageal adenocarcinoma, colon, breast, endometrial, and renal cancer.

B. Vitamin Deficiencies and Toxicities

1. **Fat-soluble vitamins** (vitamins A, D, E, and K) require lipids for intestinal absorption and undergo relatively slower excretion.

a. **Vitamin A** (both retinol and related retinoids) is essential to vision and gene transcription (Table 11–4).

(1) Deficiency results in impaired vision, especially in low light conditions (**night blindness**).

(2) Ongoing deficiency promotes the replacement of lacrimal and moisturizing tissues with keratinized epithelium, clinically noted as **Bitot spots.**

(3) If left untreated, the entire cornea may be affected (**keratomalacia**), leading to blindness.

(4) Acute toxicity manifests as headache, altered vision, ataxia, nausea, and vomiting.

b. **Vitamin D** (both D₂ (ergocalciferol) and D₃ (cholecalciferol), plays a critical role in calcium homeostasis.

(1) Vitamin D may be ingested or **synthesized from 7-dehydrocholesterol under UV exposure,** so deficiency may result from either

Table 11–4. Nutrient deficiencies.

Nutrient	Solubility	Dietary sources	Deficiency
Vitamin A	Fat	Liver, carrots	Impaired night vision
Vitamin B$_1$	Water	Enriched grains, animal tissues, seeds, sprouts	Beriberi Wernicke-Korsakoff syndrome
Vitamin B$_2$	Water	Milk, eggs, liver, wheat germ, green vegetables	Oral-buccal lesions Dermatitis
Vitamin B$_3$	Water	Liver, meats, peanuts, legumes, whole wheat, enriched grains	Pellagra (dermatitis, diarrhea, dementia, death)
Vitamin B$_5$	Water	Ubiquitous, especially liver, meat, whole grain	Rare
Vitamin B$_6$	Water	Carrots, peas, spinach, whole grains, bananas, meat, eggs	Weakness, irritability, insomnia May lead to microcytic anemia, neural demyelination
Vitamin B$_7$	Water	Egg, milk, liver, and brewer's yeast	Rare and mild
Vitamin B$_9$	Water	Liver, leafy vegetables, yeast	Neural tube defects Megaloblastic anemia
Vitamin B$_{12}$	Water	Animal tissue	Megaloblastic anemia
Vitamin C	Water	Citrus, cabbage, strawberries, tomatoes	Scurvy
Vitamin D	Fat	Fortified dairy products	Rickets and osteomalacia
Vitamin E	Fat	Green leafy vegetables, nuts	Rare neurologic dysfunction
Vitamin K	Fat	Spinach and cruciferous vegetables	Bleeding diathesis

impaired absorption, insufficient sunlight, or compromised hepatic or kidney function that limits conversion into active metabolites.

(2) Deficiency results in multiple skeletal abnormalities, including **rickets, osteomalacia,** and **osteoporosis.**

(3) Predictably, **hypervitaminosis D** leads to **hypercalcemia** with attendant constipation and irritability.

(4) Deficiency and toxicity are assessed by measuring serum 1,25-dihydroxyvitamin D.

  c. **Vitamin E** (various tocopherols) is a potent antioxidant.
   (1) Deficiency is associated with various neurologic complications, including ataxia.
   (2) Excess vitamin E may prolong prothrombin time by inhibiting vitamin K–dependent carboxylase.

  d. **Vitamin K,** originally known as the "Koagulation factor" to German and Scandinavian researchers, participates in the gamma-carboxylation of glutamate residues within specific proteins associated with coagulation, vascular activity, and metabolism.
   (1) **Factors II, VII, IX, and X** as well as **protein C** and **protein S** are vitamin K–dependent.
   (2) **Warfarin** and related coumarins inhibit vitamin K epoxide reductase that would otherwise recycle vitamin K from its oxidized state after carboxylation.
   (3) Vitamin K injections are administered to neonates as prophylaxis against **hemolytic disease of the newborn.**

2. **Water-soluble vitamins** (B complex and vitamin C) are more readily excreted and thus less prone to toxic overdosing.

  a. **Vitamin B$_1$** (thiamine or thiamin) is a component of thiamine pyrophosphate, an essential coenzyme for both carbohydrate metabolism and neural function.
   (1) Thiamine deficiency results in beriberi.
    (a) **Dry beriberi** presents with peripheral polyneuropathy, **Wernicke encephalopathy,** and finally **Korsakoff syndrome** with memory loss and confabulation.
    (b) **Wet beriberi** refers to cardiovascular involvement with initial peripheral vasodilation followed by salt retention and fluid overload.
   (2) Beriberi was once endemic in Asia where polished **white rice** milled from its thiamine-rich husk was a staple.
   (3) Recovery is often rapid with thiamine replacement.

  b. **Vitamin B$_2$** (riboflavin) is a constituent of both flavin mononucleotide (FMN) and flavin adenine dinucleotide (FAD), redox cofactors for multiple metabolic pathways.
   (1) Deficiency (**ariboflavinosis**) is marked by fissures along the corners of the mouth (angular cheilitis), glossitis, keratitis, photophobia, and scrotal dermatitis.
   (2) So named for its bright yellow-orange color (Latin "flavus" meaning yellow), riboflavin is a common colorant added to food products, so deficiency is relatively rare.
   (3) Excess is excreted by the kidneys within hours.

  c. **Vitamin B$_3$** (niacin) is a precursor of both nicotinamide adenine dinucleotide (NAD) and its phosphate (NADP) involved in electron transport, such as the pentose phosphate pathway.
   (1) **Pellagra,** characterized clinically by **dermatitis, diarrhea, dementia,** and **death** (the 4 Ds), results from severe deficiency.
   (2) Corn processed without lime is relatively low in niacin, so pellagra was once common.

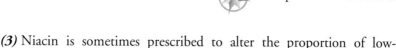

(3) Niacin is sometimes prescribed to alter the proportion of low-density to high-density cholesterol.

d. Vitamin B$_6$ (pyridoxine) is converted to pyridoxal phosphate, a cofactor in amino acid, glucose, and lipid metabolism.

(1) Deficiency leads to seborrheic dermatitis, cheilosis, glossitis, peripheral neuropathy, and rarely convulsions.

(2) Like other water-soluble vitamins, overdose is rare but associated with transient neuropathy.

e. Vitamin B$_9$, more commonly known as **folate or folic acid,** is activated as **tetrahydrofolate** (THF) and is a cofactor in methyl transfer reactions, as in the conversion of deoxyuridine monophosphate to thymidine monophosphate during DNA synthesis.

(1) Folate is absorbed in the first portion of the small intestine, and normal folate stores are equivalent to approximately 3 months.

(a) Dietary folate deficiencies are common among **alcoholics** with poor nutrition.

(b) Any condition associated with **malabsorption** such as celiac sprue may hamper folate replenishment.

(c) **Methotrexate,** an antimetabolic agent prescribed for many neoplastic and autoimmune conditions, reversibly inhibits dihydrofolate reductase.

(d) Even if dietary intake is stable and no chemotherapy is onboard, increased metabolic states, including **pregnancy** and rapid red cell turnover, may tip patients into a **folate deficiency.**

(2) A deficiency of either folate or vitamin B$_{12}$ impairs DNA synthesis and delays cell division, which may lead to neural tube defects during development and megaloblastic anemia in adults.

(a) Hemoglobin synthesis is unaffected, and the resultant red cell precursors are enlarged (**megaloblastic anemia).**

(b) Neutrophils display nuclear hypersegmentation.

f. Vitamin B$_{12}$ (cobalamin) is required to return methylated folate to active THF.

(1) Lacking vitamin B$_{12}$, methyl folate accumulates ("the methyl folate trap") and is unavailable.

(a) While folate supplementation can partially bypass this problem, other more strictly vitamin B$_{12}$–dependent reactions remain affected.

(b) In one such process, vitamin B$_{12}$ is essential for methylmal-0onyl CoA mutase to convert methylmalonyl CoA to succinyl CoA.

(i) Without adequate vitamin B$_{12}$, the excess methylmalonic acid destabilizes myelin sheaths.

(ii) To avoid irreversible neurologic complications, vitamin B$_{12}$ deficiency must be excluded before masking it with folate replacement.

(2) Gastric parietal cells secrete intrinsic factor that permits subsequent ileal absorption of vitamin B$_{12}$.

(3) The cytologic findings are similar to those noted in cases of folate deficiency.

g. **Vitamin C** (ascorbic acid) is an antioxidant.

(1) Deficiency leads to scurvy (Latin "scorbutus") in which defective collagen synthesis results in capillary fragility, mucosal bleeding, abnormal hair development, and open infected wounds.

(2) Humans lack the enzyme to produce vitamin C.

(3) Although it is present in multiple fruits and vegetables, it degrades with light and oxygen exposure; fresh produce is required for vitamin C.

C. **Malnutrition**

1. Dietary protein provides amino acids for a diverse array of biosynthetic pathways.

   a. **Compromised immunity,** including decreased production of lymphocytes, complement, and secretory IgA, as well as impaired phagocytosis, accompanies chronic protein malnutrition.

   b. Resultant severe infections exacerbate malnutrition by increasing metabolic demand (fever) while simultaneously decreasing nutrient absorption (diarrhea).

   c. **Small bowel atrophy** and **hepatic steatosis** may also be observed along with decreased intravascular volume inducing secondary hyperaldosteronism.

2. Several indices are used to evaluate protein status.

   a. A **complete blood count** with differential and a peripheral smear can help exclude anemias secondary to deficiencies of either iron, folate, or vitamin B_{12}.

   b. The quantity of specific **plasma proteins,** such as albumin, indicates nutritional status.

3. **Marasmus** is a compensated response to an overall caloric deficit.

   a. Physical findings include muscular atrophy with relative preservation of the skeleton, kidneys, and brain.

   b. Adaptation to the negative energy balance follows a pattern of progressive decrease in physical activity and basal metabolism, growth slowing, and eventual weight loss.

   c. Patients assume an increasingly wasted appearance with sunken eyes, abdominal distention, and thin extremities.

   d. In advanced cases, the metabolic machinery to handle protein, itself composed of protein, may be consumed to the point that protein re-feeding is very difficult.

4. **Kwashiorkor,** by contrast, occurs with inadequate protein intake amidst otherwise adequate caloric intake.

   a. Derived from an African dialect meaning "rejected one," kwashiorkor arises when a child is weaned and the diet shifts from protein-rich milk to starch.

   b. As plasma proteins decrease, osmotic shifts result in **peripheral edema** that often masks the underlying wasting.

   c. Other findings include **marked ascites** and hair with **alternating bands of pigmentation** (flag sign).

5. **Cachexia** is wasting, particularly muscle atrophy, associated with chronic illness (eg, neoplasia, AIDS).

6. **Psychiatric causes** of poor nutritional status include anorexia nervosa, bulimia, and the more recently recognized orthorexia.

CLINICAL PROBLEMS

1. A 45-year-old woman complains of anxiety, palpitations, heat intolerance, and diaphoresis. She has been taking some nutritional supplements to aid in weight loss. Which of the following laboratory profiles is the most likely?

   A. Elevated thyroid-stimulating hormone (TSH), low free T_4

   B. Elevated TSH, high free T_4

   C. Suppressed TSH, low free T_4

   D. Suppressed TSH, high free T_4

   E. Normal TSH, high free T_4

2. A patient arrives at the emergency department with serum glucose of 28 mg/dL (normal is 80–100 mg/dL). He has no history of diabetes and is not taking any medications. Which of the following statements is **FALSE**?

   A. Elevated C-peptide level would be consistent with an insulinoma.

   B. Surreptitious use of insulin should have a low C-peptide level.

   C. Surreptitious use of sulfonylureas have an elevated C-peptide.

   D. Use of β-blockers may mask symptoms of hypoglycemia.

   E. Most insulinomas are in the head of the pancreas.

3. A patient has fatigue and some gradual weight gain. She has no other symptoms and has no other medical history. Her physical examination is normal, including examination of the thyroid gland. A complete blood count (CBC) shows a hemoglobin level of 8.2 g/dL, otherwise the rest of her routine laboratory tests are normal. Thyroid function tests show a thyroid-stimulating hormone (TSH) level that is slightly increased over normal and a free thyroxine level that is normal. Which of the following statements is **TRUE**?

   A. The elevated TSH is diagnostic of overt clinical hypothyroidism.

   B. The patient's thyroid is likely contributing to her symptoms.

   C. Anti-microsomal antibodies could indicate autoimmune thyroiditis.

   D. Elevated TSH and normal free thyroxine indicate Graves disease.

   E. A thyroid scan and uptake would likely be abnormal.

4. A 35-year-old man has a 3-cm nodule in the left lobe of the thyroid. There is no associated cervical lymphadenopathy. Which of the following statements is **FALSE**?

   A. A fine-needle aspiration biopsy is the best screening test.

   B. Thyroid function studies are likely to be normal.

   C. The presence of a cystic lymph node may indicate metastasis.

   D. Abundant colloid with bland epithelium suggests a benign nodule.

   E. A cystic nodule rules out the possibility of malignancy.

5. A 25-year-old man complains of erectile dysfunction. A CT scan of the head is normal. A serum prolactin level is markedly elevated. Which of the following statements is **TRUE**?

   A. A normal CT of the head rules out a macroprolactinoma.

   B. An elevated prolactin level confirms a prolactinoma.

   C. Histology can differentiate a secretory and nonsecretory adenoma

   D. Patients with MEN type I do not have an increased risk of parathyroid adenomas.

   E. Patients with MEN type IIB do not have an increased risk of pituitary adenomas.

6. An 82-year-old patient undergoes an endoscopic ultrasound-guided fine-needle aspiration biopsy of a pancreatic tail mass. Which of the following statements is **TRUE**?

   A. The most likely diagnosis is ductal adenocarcioma.

   B. The most likely diagnosis is solid pseudopapillary tumor.

   C. The most likely diagnosis is a pancreatic endocrine tumor.

   D. Immunohistochemical markers will be negative for chromogranin.

   E. Accessory splenic tissue does not mimic islet cell tumors.

7. Which of the following statements about pheochromocytoma is **TRUE**?

   A. Marked nuclear pleomorphism does not indicate malignancy.

   B. Vascular invasion increases metastatic potential.

   C. Tumor cells will stain positively with chromogranin.

   D. Necrosis, mitoses, and invasion are indicators of malignancy.

   E. All of the above statements are true.

8. Which of the following statements about autoimmune thyroiditis is **FALSE**?

   A. Autoimmune thyroiditis increases the risk of papillary carcinoma.

   B. Oncocytic (Hürthle cell) metaplasia is common in thyroiditis.

   C. Autoimmune thyroiditis increases the risk of follicular carcinoma.

   D. These patients may have goiter and discrete nodules.

   E. Thyroiditis has a smaller goiter than iodine deficiency.

9. A fine-needle aspiration is performed on a solitary thyroid nodule in a 60-year-old woman. Which feature is **NOT** associated with papillary thyroid carcinoma?

   A. High cellularity with papillary architecture

   B. Intranuclear cytoplasmic pseudo-inclusions

   C. Dense squamoid cytoplasm

   D. Hürthle cell metaplasia

   E. Psammoma bodies

10. Which of the following statements regarding pheochromocytoma is **FALSE**?

   A. They are associated with von Hippel-Lindau disease.

   B. They are associated with neurofibromatosis type I.

C. There is immunohistochemical staining for tyrosine hydroxylase.

D. They are associated with MEN type I.

E. None of the above

ANSWERS

1. The answer is D. The patient has a clinical presentation suggestive of thyrotoxicosis. She is likely taking nutritional supplements containing thyroid hormone. The elevated free thyroxine and suppressed TSH is diagnostic of thyrotoxicosis.

2. The answer is E. Most insulinomas are in the tail of the pancreas.

3. The answer is C. Her symptoms are likely due to the anemia and not the thyroid function abnormality. A slightly elevated TSH and free thyroxine level is indicative of subclinical hypothyroidism. These patients can have circulating titers of anti-microsomal or anti-thyroid antibodies, usually indicative of early autoimmune thyroiditis. Progression to clinical hypothyroidism will certainly be a concern. Graves disease will usually present with features of hyperthyroidism with a suppressed TSH and elevated free thyroxine. The thyroid scan and uptake study will likely be normal in this clinical scenario.

4. The answer is E. Papillary thyroid carcinoma can be cystic, so a cystic nodule does not rule out malignancy.

5. The answer is E. Patients with MEN type IIB do not have an increased risk for pituitary adenomas—that is MEN type I.

6. The answer is C. This is a neuroendocrine neoplasm, which usually presents in the tail of the pancreas. Ductal carcinoma usually occurs in the head. Solid pseudopapillary tumors occur in the tail of the pancreas in young women. Accessory spleen in the tail may indeed mimic islet cell tumor in imaging studies. Neuroendocrine tumors are positive for chromogranin.

7. The answer is E. All the statements are true.

8. The answer is C. Autoimmune thyroiditis is not a risk factor for follicular carcinoma.

9. The answer is D. Hürthle cell metaplasia is not associated with papillary carcinoma; although the rare tall cell variant of papillary carcinoma may be oncocytic, it has other papillary carcinoma features.

10. The answer is D. Patients with MEN type I are at increased risk for pituitary adenomas, parathyroid neoplasia, and pancreatic neuroendocrine neoplasms. Patients with von Hippel-Lindau can have pheochromocytoma and pancreatic islet cell neoplasia.

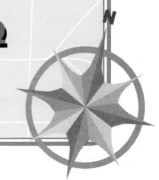

CHAPTER 12
BREAST

There is a passion for hunting something
deeply implanted in the human breast.
—Charles Dickens

I. Normal Breast

A. Embryology-Anatomy
1. The breast originates as a modified skin appendage.
2. Six to twelve major ducts meet the skin at the nipple, and distally branch into small caliber ducts, terminating at the secretory units and lobules (terminal duct lobular units-TDLU).

B. Histology
1. Ducts and lobules are lined by a two-layer epithelium, including **luminal cells,** and the surrounding contractile **myoepithelial cells.**
2. Luminal cells are the functional secretory cells in the breast.
3. Interlobular stroma and adipose tissue surround these structures.
4. Pathologic changes may affect any of these structures, but the **epithelial cells** are most commonly affected, giving rise to carcinoma (Figure 12–1).

C. Lactation
1. Lobules increase in size and number during pregnancy.
2. They may form a benign mass lesion called a lactional adenoma.

II. Inflammatory and Reactive Changes

A. Acute Mastitis
1. Mastitis occurs most commonly during lactation, as *Staphylococcus aureus* or *Streptococcus* species gain access to breast tissue especially via fissures in the nipple.
2. Symptoms begin as redness, tenderness, fever.
3. Mastitis is rarely biopsied but will show neutrophilic inflammation or **abscess** formation.
4. Mastitis is treated with antibiotics and drainage of milk; if untreated, the infection may spread to involve the entire breast.

B. Fat Necrosis
1. Fat necrosis is typically associated with ruptured ducts, prior surgery, or trauma, though the patient may not recall trauma.

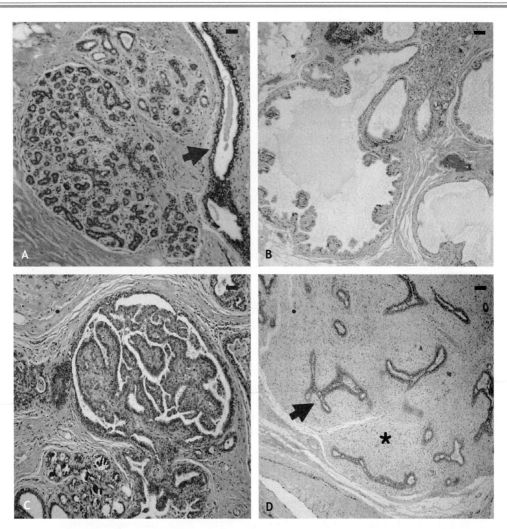

Figure 12–1. Benign breast lesions. A: Normal breast parenchyma is composed of lobules that secrete into larger duct (arrow), which eventually connects to the nipple. **B:** Cysts and apocrine change are characteristic of "fibrocystic change," a process that is likely hormonally related. **C:** Intraductal papilloma has branching tree-like architecture with fibrovascular cores. Most are benign lesions, but they may develop ductal hyperplasia or carcinoma. **D:** A fibroadenoma is a distinct "marble" in the breast composed of benign branching ducts that may have a staghorn appearance (arrow) and hypocellular stroma (asterisk). In contrast, a phyllodes tumor would have hypercellular stroma and invade surrounding breast tissue (not shown). Bar is 100 mcm.

2. Microscopic examination shows foamy histiocytes infiltrating partially necrotic fibroadipose tissue.

3. Fat necrosis can produce a mass lesion, skin retraction, or calcification on imaging studies, each mimicking carcinoma.

C. **Duct Ectasia**

  1. Patients with duct ectasia may have microcalcifications, nipple retraction/inversion, or nipple discharge.

  2. Histologic studies show large duct dilatation with thickened, fibrotic walls and necrobiotic material within the lumen.

III. Fibrocystic Changes

A. **Clinical Presentation**

  1. Patients are most commonly young to middle age (25–45 years old) and characteristically may experience cyclical breast pain.

  2. Fibrocystic change is a diffuse process, the so-called "lumpy bumpy breast," although its uneven distribution can often produce palpable mass-like irregularities discovered on physical examination, or appear as a mammographic asymmetry.

B. **Nonproliferative**

  1. Cysts can be microscopic to grossly visible (grossly, the "**blue dome cyst**"); the cyst fluid contents range from clear to amber.

  2. Some of the cysts and ducts are lined by cells showing **apocrine metaplasia,** characterized by abundant granular eosinophilic cytoplasm, a low nuclear cytoplasmic ratio, and round nuclei with prominent nucleoli (Figure 12–1B).

  3. Fibrocystic change confers no increased risk of carcinoma.

C. **Proliferative**

  1. Fibrocystic change may be accompanied by proliferative lesions, involving the epithelium, stroma, or both; importantly, there is **no cytologic atypia or dysplasia.**

  2. **Epithelial hyperplasia,** by definition, is the presence of more than the normal two layers of epithelium in a ductular or lobular space; this is also known as "**usual (ductal) hyperplasia.**"

  3. **Sclerosing adenosis**, characterized by round whorling ductal proliferations, and a **radial scar (complex sclerosing lesion with desmoplastic-like stroma),** are two lesions that may mimic carcinoma on clinical, radiographic, and histologic appearance.

  4. Proliferative fibrocystic change, or usual ductal hyperplasia, confers a slightly increased (two-fold) risk of carcinoma.

D. **Intraductal Papilloma**

  1. Intraductal papilloma usually presents as **bloody** nipple discharge.

  2. Physical examination usually reveals a nodule deep to the nipple.

  3. Mammogram may show a solid lesion associated with cystic changes.

  4. Biopsy shows a papillary (tree-like) neoplasm with ductal cells lining fibroepithelial cores within a cystic space (Figure 12–1C).

  5. Papillomas may be involved by any epithelial lesion such as usual ductal hyperplasia or ductal carcinoma in situ (DCIS).

MAMMOGRAPHY

- *Mammograms are essentially radiographs of breast tissue and are most useful in detecting calcifications and mass lesions.*
- *Mammographic screening is recommended yearly after age 40; screening may begin earlier in high-risk women.*
- *Radiologists may be able to distinguish "benign" calcifications from "malignant" calcifications; however, if there is uncertainty, biopsy specimens should be obtained.*
- *Other imaging modalities, such as ultrasound and MRI, are not used for screening, but for targeted evaluations to rule out multifocal disease or to screen very high-risk patients.*

IV. Fibroepithelial Lesions

A. Fibroadenoma
1. Fibroadenomas occur most commonly in young women (age 20–35) and are characteristically round and mobile with palpation.
2. This correlates well with the **well-circumscribed** lesion that is seen grossly and under the microscope.
3. Fibroadenomas are biphasic composed of ductal epithelium compressed into slit-like "staghorn" arrangements within benign hypocellular stroma (Figure 12–1D).
4. Fibroadenomas are **benign** with a low recurrence risk.

B. Phyllodes Tumors
1. Phyllodes tumors are also biphasic with broad leaf-like ductal arrangements within hypercellular stroma.
2. Unlike fibroadenomas, phyllodes tumors may recur and metastasize depending on whether they invade surrounding breast tissue, are cytologically malignant, or have a high mitotic rate.

V. Atypical Hyperplasia

A. Atypical Ductal Hyperplasia (ADH)
1. ADH is diagnosed by worrisome cytologic features (atypical nuclei), or worrisome architecture (solid or cribriform) but not enough to warrant a diagnosis of carcinoma.
2. Patients with **ADH** have a 4- to 5-fold relative risk of cancer developing in the future (Table 12-1).

B. Atypical Lobular Hyperplasia (ALH)
1. ALH is a proliferation of lobular cells that does not meet the diagnostic criteria for lobular carcinoma (see below).
2. Patients with ALH have a 4- to 5-fold risk of developing invasive lobular carcinoma in the future.

VI. Breast Carcinoma

A. Epidemiology
1. Breast cancer is the most common malignancy among women in the United States, affecting 13% (1/8) of women.
2. Breast cancer is the second most common cause of cancer death among women in the United States (lung cancer is first).

Table 12–1. Risk of invasive carcinoma related to biopsy findings.

Lesion	Clinical Features	Pathologic Features	Cancer Risk
Nonproliferative fibrocystic change	'Lumpy-bumpy' cyclical pain	Cysts, apocrine metaplasia, fibrotic stroma	0
Duct ectasia	Nodule with calcification	Inflammatory lesion	0
Fat necrosis	Traumatic, firm mass	Foreign body giant cell reaction	0
Fibroadenoma	Mobile, marble-like	Stromal-epithelial benign neoplasm	0
Proliferative fibrocystic change	'Lumpy-bumpy' cyclical, calcification	Epithelial hyperplasia, sclerosing adenosis	2-fold
Papilloma	Bloody nipple discharge, subareolar mass	Tree-like branching in cystic space	2-fold
Atypical ductal hyperplasia (ADH)	Mass lesion with or without calcifications	Atypical ductal cells, not enough for DCIS	4-fold
Ductal carcinoma in situ (DCIS)	Mass lesion with or without calcifications	Cribriform, papillary or solid with atypical nuclei	8-fold

  3. Overall mortality from breast cancer is ~20%.
  4. Cancer usually occurs in the upper-outer quadrant of the breast.
 B. Risk Factors
  1. One of the strongest risk factors for breast cancer is **family history,** specifically **first-degree relatives (mother, sister, or daughter)** with carcinoma.
  2. Several tumor suppressor genes commonly mutated in breast cancer have been identified.
   a. *BRCA1* mutation also confers risk of ovarian cancer.
   b. *BRCA2* mutation confers a different cancer risk profile, although it is part of a common DNA repair pathway with *BRCA1* (**Fanconi anemia pathway**).
  3. Lifetime hormonal exposure seems to increase risk of breast cancer, especially estrogen exposure.
   a. Breast cancer risk increases with **age, early menarche, late menopause, and nulliparity.**
   b. Risk also increases with obesity and insulin resistance.
   c. Data suggest postmenopausal hormone replacement therapy (HRT) may also have a role in estrogen-driven breast cancers.

EVALUATING BREAST LESIONS: THE TRIPLE TEST

- *The triple test evaluates breast lesions using **clinical data** (physical examination), **radiologic** findings, and **tissue** sampling (fine-needle aspiration or needle biopsy).*
- *Correlation of these three features in each patient significantly improves sensitivity and specificity for detection of breast cancer.*

VII. In Situ Breast Carcinoma

A. Ductal Carcinoma In Situ

1. **DCIS** is a clonal proliferation of **neoplastic ductal cells** that remain bound by the **basement membrane** and has an intact surrounding layer of myoepithelial cells.
2. **Comedonecrosis** is necrotic tumor cells in the center of a duct containing DCIS; this will often calcify, allowing mammographic detection (Figure 12–2A).
3. By definition, DCIS is not invasive, and tumor cells have no access to lymphatics, so pure **DCIS cannot metastasize.**
4. However, DCIS is considered a direct precursor of invasive carcinoma, so it must be treated.
5. Treatment for DCIS is complete surgical excision; patients are often given radiotherapy to prevent recurrence.

B. Lobular Carcinoma In Situ (LCIS)

1. It is a clonal proliferation of neoplastic lobular cells with characteristic cytologic features, including eccentrically placed small round nuclei (Figure 12–2B).
2. Similar to DCIS, it is bound by the basement membrane and surrounding myoepithelial cells, making it an *in situ* lesion.

VIII. Invasive Breast Carcinoma

A. Invasive Ductal Carcinoma

1. Invasive ductal carcinoma is the classic "breast carcinoma," comprising approximately 80% of cases.
2. It is composed of **invasive malignant ductal cells forming glands.**
3. By definition, tumor cells have broken through the basement membrane; they often invoke stromal change, the characteristic **desmoplastic stroma** (Figure 12-2C) that results in a **stellate gross** and **radiographic appearance.**
4. **Grading** of invasive breast carcinoma, like all carcinomas, is based on the **nuclear** and **architectural features** of the tumor; the grading system is based on three key features: tubule formation, nuclei, and mitotic rate.
5. **Staging** of invasive breast carcinoma, like all carcinomas, is based on the **size and extent of tumor spread;** staging is performed according to the **Tumor, Nodes, Metastasis (TNM)** system (Table 12–2).

B. Invasive Lobular Carcinoma

1. Invasive lobular carcinoma accounts for ~10% of breast cancers; since it typically does not form a mass lesion, it is more clinically and radiographically silent.
2. Invasive lobular carcinoma has distinct cytologic and architectural features, characteristically small, relatively round uniform cells, growing in **single file arrangements** (Figure 12–2D).

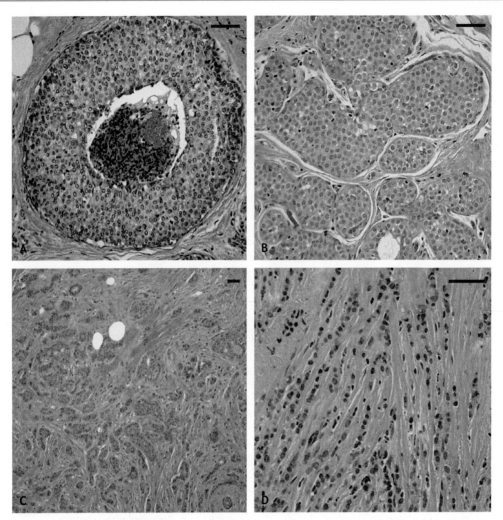

Figure 12–2. Mammary carcinoma. A: Ductal carcinoma in situ has not broken out of the basement membrane, or surrounding myoepithelial cells, and may show comedo necrosis as shown here. **B:** Lobular carcinoma in situ expands the lobules with tumor cells, but they do not invade surrounding stroma. **C:** Invasive ductal carcinoma forms glands that infiltrate the stroma inducing a host reaction called "desmoplasia." **D:** Invasive lobular carcinoma does not form glands, instead it may form single files of predominantly dyscohesive tumor cells. Bar is 100 mcm.

Table 12–2. Breast carcinoma staging by "TNM."

T: Tumor size	
Tis: in situ carcinoma	Stage 0
T1: 2 cm or less	Stage I if N0M0
T2: 2-5cm	Stage II if N0,1, M0
T3: > 5cm	Stage III if N1, or N2, M0
T4: invading chest wall	
N: Nodal spread (axillary lymph nodes; simplified)	
N1: Metastasis to 1–3 lymph nodes	
N2: Metastasis to 4–9 lymph nodes	
N3: Metastasis to > 10 lymph nodes	
M: Metastasis (distant)	
M1: Distant metastasis	Stage IV

PAGET DISEASE

- *The main presenting symptom is a red scaly nipple, which may be itchy and mimic eczema.*
- *It is caused by underlying adenocarcinoma colonizing the skin.*

  C. **Invasive Carcinoma: Special Types**
  1. Pure **tubular and mucinous carcinomas** tend to have an excellent prognosis; they are very low-grade carcinomas.
  2. **Medullary carcinoma** may clinically mimic benign lesions like a fibroadenoma, since it is well circumscribed; although the cells are high grade, patient prognosis is relatively good.
  3. **Micropapillary carcinoma** has a propensity for metastasis.

INFLAMMATORY CARCINOMA

- *Patients with "peau de orange" skin changes (skin looks like the thickened and textured skin of an orange) often have inflammatory carcinoma.*
- *Inflammatory carcinoma is tumor emboli within lymphatics.*
- *Inflammatory carcinoma has a poor prognosis.*

  D. **Prognostic and Predictive Factors**
  1. Prognostic factors help forecast patient outcome.
  2. **Stage is the number one prognostic factor for breast cancer.**
     a. 60% overall 5-year survival for node-negative disease
     b. 30% overall 5-year survival for node-positive disease
  3. Other minor prognostic factors include grade, angiolymphatic invasion, histologic subtype, hormone receptor status.
     a. **Estrogen receptor (ER)–positive** tumors have better prognosis than ER-negative tumors; further, ER positivity predicts response to hormonal therapy (anti-estrogen).
     b. *HER2/neu* **positive tumors** have a worse prognosis compared with *HER2/neu*–negative tumors, but *HER2/neu* positivity predicts response to targeted antibody therapy (**trastuzumab**).

SENTINEL LYMPH NODE BIOPSY

- *Since stage is such an important prognostic factor in breast cancer, and the first sites of breast cancer spread is axillary lymph nodes, these nodes must be pathologically evaluated in patients with invasive cancer to determine N stage.*
- *Sentinel lymph node biopsy is a technique to identify the first lymph node to drain the breast; if this node is negative, the patient does not need a full axillary dissection.*
- *Preferential sites for distant metastasis of breast carcinoma include lungs, bones, liver, brain, and adrenals. Lobular carcinoma also has a predilection for ovaries.*

IX. Male Breast Lesions

- **A. Gynecomastia**
  - **1.** Gynecomastia is commonly associated with increased estrogens and decreased androgens (eg, alcoholism and obesity).
  - **2.** Physical examination reveals a firm painful disc-like lesion deep to the nipple (in contrast to excessive subcutaneous fat).
  - **3.** Histologically, gynecomastia is a benign proliferation of ducts and surrounding edematous stroma; lobules are absent.
- **B.** Male breast **carcinoma** comprises 1% of breast carcinomas, and there is an increased incidence in Klinefelter syndrome.

X. Nonepithelial Breast Malignancies

- **A. Angiosarcoma** is a malignant vascular tumor; malignant cells recapitulate blood vessels. It sometimes occurs post surgery and radiation, specially if there is lymphedema.
- **B.** Lymphoma may present in cutaneous sites, including breast (see Chapter 17).
- **C.** Melanoma may present on the breast skin (see Chapter 3).

CLINICAL PROBLEMS

1. Which of the following is **NOT** part of the initial workup of a woman with a breast abnormality?

   A. Mammography

   B. Mastectomy

   C. Fine-needle aspiration biopsy (or core biopsy)

   D. Clinical examination

   E. All the above

2. Identify the malignant breast lesion.

   A. Fibroadenoma

   B. Papilloma

   C. Paget disease of the nipple

   D. Fibrocystic disease

   E. Radial scar

3. Which of the following confers a **DECREASED** risk of breast cancer?

   A. Multiparity

   B. Hormone replacement therapy

   C. Obesity

   D. *BRCA1* mutation

   E. Early menarche

4. Select the most important prognostic factor for breast carcinoma.

   A. E-cadherin status

   B. Proliferative rate

   C. Grade

   D. Number of positive lymph nodes

   E. Estrogen receptor status

5. A young woman comes to the office in her fourth week of breastfeeding. Her right breast is locally painful, warm and red. What is the **MOST** likely diagnosis?

   A. Inflammatory carcinoma

   B. Paget disease

   C. Ductal carcinoma in situ

   D. Papilloma

   E. Acute mastitis

6. What is the best estimate for the rate of nodal metastasis for ductal carcinoma in situ?

   A. 0%

   B. 10%

   C. 25%

   D. 50%

   E. 100%

7. Which of these breast lesions is **LEAST** frequently associated with the presence of invasive carcinoma in the breast?

   A. Fibrocystic change

   B. Atypical ductal hyperplasia

   C. Lobular carcinoma in situ (LCIS)

   D. Ductal carcinoma in situ (DCIS)

   E. None of the above

8. According to the most recent recommendations of the Public Health Service, at what age should screening mammograms be started?

   A. 30 years old

   B. 35 years old

   C. 40 years old

D. 45 years old

E. 50 years old

9. Which one of these lesions does not require treatment?

A. Paget disease

B. Tubular carcinoma

C. Proliferative fibrocystic change

D. Medullary carcinoma

E. Ductal carcinoma in situ

10. What is the triple test?

A. Mammography, ultrasound examination, and impedance imaging

B. Physical examination, mammography, and needle biopsy of lesion

C. Mammography, ultrasound examination, and fine-needle biopsy

D. Physical examination, needle biopsy, and excisional biopsy

E. All the above

ANSWERS

1. The answer is B. Mammography, tissue sampling, and clinical examination are the triple test and should be part of the initial workup of a breast abnormality. Mastectomy is a treatment, not a diagnostic test.

2. The answer is C. Paget disease of the nipple is essentially adenocarcinoma of the skin. Fibroadenoma is a benign fibroepithelial lesion. Fibrocystic change/disease is a common, diffuse, benign breast finding. Papilloma and radial scar are proliferative lesions that often accompany fibrocystic change.

3. The answer is A. Multiparity is associated with a lower risk of breast cancer, probably related to hormonal effects. Early menarche has the opposite effect on hormonal exposure. Postmenopausal hormone replacement therapy is becoming better characterized as a risk factor. *BRCA1* mutations are identified in familial cancer.

4. The answer is D. Stage is the most important breast cancer prognostic factor, and the number of involved lymph nodes is an important component of the TNM stage. Grade is a weaker prognostic factor. Estrogen receptor status is a prognostic and predictive factor, but not as important as stage. E-cadherin loss may help identify lobular carcinomas.

5. The answer is E. Acute mastitis commonly occurs early in breastfeeding. Pregnancy-associated breast cancers occur rarely.

6. The answer is A. Ductal carcinoma in situ (DCIS) by definition has not breached the basement membrane, so it cannot gain access to lymphatics.

7. The answer is A. Fibrocystic change is not associated with an increased risk of invasive cancer. Hyperplastic fibrocystic change, the so-called proliferative or usual hyperplasia, has a 2-fold increased risk; ADH, a 4-fold risk; DCIS and LCIS, an 8-fold risk.

8. The answer is C. Screening mammograms should begin after age 40. Patients with a significant family history or at very high risk may begin before 40 years old, but the general population recommendation is 40.

9. The answer is C. Fibrocystic change is benign. Paget disease of the breast is involvement of the skin or nipple (or both) by underlying adenocarcinoma. Tubular, medullary, and DCIS are all cancer.

10. The answer is B. The sensitivity and specificity provided by combining the results of *clinical impression* (firm indistinct mass), *imaging* (stellate with microcalcifications), and *needle biopsy* (atypical ductal cells with irregular nuclei, lacking associated myoepithelial cells) is powerful. This triple test is the standard of care.

A night with Venus (or Mars), a lifetime with Mercury
— Oscar Wilde

I. Vulva and Vagina

A. Infection

1. **Candidiasis** is a persistent or recurrent superficial infection of the skin or mucous membranes by *Candida* species, most often *Candida albicans*, and it is the most frequently observed form of **vaginitis.**

   a. Infection is accompanied by vulvovaginal pruritus and a thick, white ("cottage cheese") discharge.

   b. The **long, thin hyphae** may be demonstrated with a potassium hydroxide (KOH) preparation, or they may be seen in a Papanicolaou (Pap) smear "skewering" or "spearing" sloughed squamous cells (Figure 13–1).

2. **Herpes simplex virus** (HSV) types 1 and 2 are members of a highly infectious family of neurotropic DNA viruses.

   a. Patients complain of painful vesicles and ulcers.

   b. HSV-infected cells show a diagnostic pattern of multinucleation, nuclear molding, and marginating chromatin.

   (1) The **Tzanck smear** is obtained by unroofing and scraping of the base of a lesion to recover multinucleated giant cells for light microscopy.

   (2) The **polymerase chain reaction** (PCR) is more rapid than viral culture and may eventually supplant viral culture as the preferred assay, but this technique cannot distinguish actively replicating from latent viral DNA.

3. **Syphilis** is an infection by the **spirochete** *Treponema pallidum.*

   a. It may present as a painless ulcer "chancre," or as a wart "**condyloma latum**" (in contrast to condyloma acuminatum).

   b. It is also one of the pathogens that may cross the placenta to induce fetal complications (eg, TORCHs: *t*oxoplasmosis, *o*ther, *r*ubella, *c*ytomegalovirus (CMV), *h*erpes, *s*yphilis).

   c. Pathologic diagnosis is made by serologic tests, dark-field microscopy, or biopsy.

   d. Biopsy shows spirochetes in a background of plasma cells.

4. ***Chlamydia trachomatis*** is an obligate intracellular **bacterium** associated with multiple gynecologic complications.

228

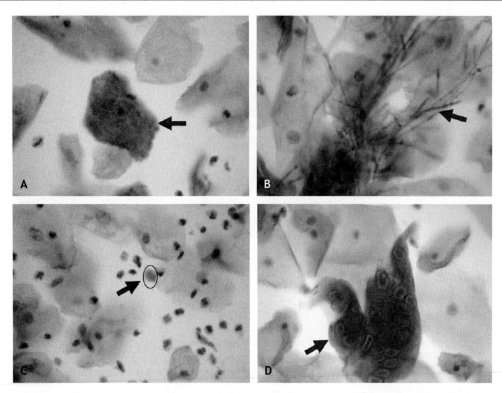

Figure 13–1. Common gynecologic infections. A: Bacterial vaginosis is coccobacilli coating squamous "clue cells" and presents as "fishy smelling" *white* discharge. **B:** *Candida albicans* is a fungus leading to "cottage cheese" like discharge that may be painful. **C:** *Trichomonas vaginalis* is a protozoan (in circle) with red neuroendocrine-like granules. It causes a "fishy smelling" *green* discharge. **D:** Herpes simplex virus is a sexually transmitted disease with characteristic multinucleated, molding nuclei with marginating chromatin.

    a. **Pelvic inflammatory disease** (PID) involving the fallopian tubes is a sexually transmitted disease.
    b. Lymphogranuloma venereum is inguinal lymph node hyperplasia with necrotizing granulomas caused by *C. trachomatis.*
    c. DNA-based PCR assays improve detection sensitivity.

PELVIC INFLAMMATORY DISEASE

- C. trachomatis and N. gonorrhoeae are *common causes of PID.*
- *The signs and symptoms include lower quadrant pain (simulating appendicitis in some cases), cervical motion tenderness, and a mucopurulent cervical discharge.*
- *There is an increased risk of infertility and ectopic pregnancy.*

CLINICAL CORRELATION

5. **Human papillomavirus** (HPV) is a DNA virus that causes warts and is a leading cause of cancer.

    a. **HPV types 6 and 11** are the most common cause of genital warts, the so-called **"low-grade dysplasia,"** which is usually transient and self-resolving.

    b. **HPV types 16 and 18** are the most common cause of HPV-related neoplastic transformation, the so-called **"high-grade dysplasia,"** which is usually progressive and requires surgery.

    c. HPV infection is characterized by enlarged dark irregular nuclei with sharp perinuclear cytoplasmic clearing, the so-called **koilocytes,** on Pap smears and surgical biopsies (Figure 13–2).

B. **Reactive Changes**

  1. **Lichen sclerosus et atrophicus** is an itchy white vulvar plaque that **mimics carcinoma,** prompting biopsy to exclude malignancy.

    a. Biopsy shows benign epithelium overlying homogenized stroma.

    b. The associated atrophy of the vulvar epithelium increases the risk of secondary infection.

  2. **Vestibulitis** is a common and painful disease of the vestibular tissue that is between the vulva and vagina.

    a. The cause is unknown.

    b. Diagnosis is clinical, but tissue shows neural hyperplasia, which persists unless completely excised.

  3. **Adenosis** is müllerian glandular cells in the epithelium of the upper third of the vagina.

    a. Although asymptomatic, oral contraceptives may induce adenosis detected on Pap smears.

    b. **Diethylstilbestrol** (DES) exposure in utero, which was a synthetic nonsteroidal estrogen previously prescribed for vaginitis, menopausal symptoms, and lactation suppression, increases the risk of developing **carcinoma** in vaginal adenosis in the offspring of women treated with DES.

MÜLLERIAN DUCTS

- *The two müllerian ducts fuse caudally to the urogenital sinus. Unfused ducts form the fallopian tubes and the fused segment becomes the uterine cavity and upper one-third of the vagina.*

- *Carcinoma arising from müllerian duct resembles cervix (mucinous), endometrium (endometrioid), fallopian tube (serous), renal pelvis (urothelial), and renal cortex (clear cell carcinoma).*

- *These types of müllerian carcinomas are encountered in the endocervix, uterus, ovary, and female pelvic peritoneum.*

C. **Benign Neoplasms**

  1. Fibroepithelial polyps are **benign skin tags** (acrochordon).

  2. **Condyloma acuminatum** (genital wart) is a form of **low-grade** dysplasia caused by the "low-risk" HPV types 6 and 11.

    a. Low-grade dysplasia is diagnosed by the presence of enlarged, hyperchromatic nuclei and rare mitotic figures restricted to the lower half of the mucosa (Figure 13–2).

    b. Low-grade dysplasia almost never progresses to cancer.

  3. **Melanocytic nevus** (mole) may be atypical if large, dark, irregular, and asymmetric (see Chapter 3).

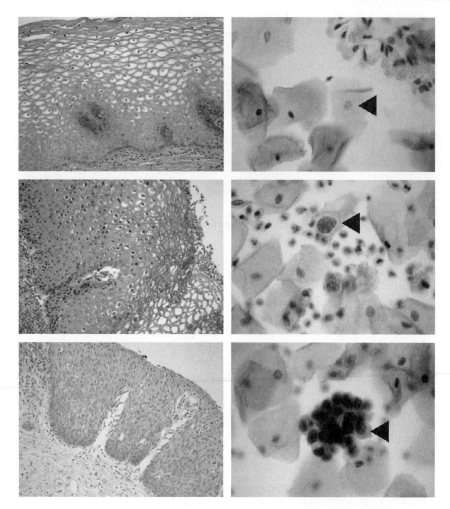

Figure 13–2. Human papillomavirus–related dysplasia and carcinoma. Characteristic histologic features (left column) and corresponding cytology in Pap smears (right column). Compared with normal squamous mucosa (top), dysplasia is characterized first by enlarged dark nuclei (low-grade dysplasia, LSIL, CIN-1), followed by increasing nuclear cytoplasmic ratios due to increased proliferation in high-grade dysplasia (HSIL, CIN2-3).

4. **Endometriosis** may present as a vulvar mass; biopsy findings will reveal bland endometrial glands and stroma and blood.
5. Ectopic breast tissue may arise within the ventral remnants of the mammalian milk lines from the axilla to the vulva and is subject to the same potential for neoplastic transformation as the breast.
6. Papillary hidradenoma is a benign sweat gland tumor.
   a. It mimics carcinoma clinically.
   b. Biopsy reveals a well-circumscribed neoplasm with papillary (tree-like) architecture and bland uniform nuclei.

D. **Malignant Neoplasms**
1. **Vulvar intraepithelial neoplasia** (VIN) results from HPV infection and is considered a graded continuum of intraepithelial dysplasia from the basal third (VIN 1) to full thickness involvement (VIN 3).
    a. **Low-grade** (VIN 1) is unlikely to progress to carcinoma.
    b. **High-grade** (VIN 2-3) is likely to progress if untreated.
2. **Vaginal intraepithelial neoplasia** (VAIN) is also due to HPV infection with the same diagnostic features and prognosis as VIN.

THE PAPANICOLAOU SMEAR

CLINICAL
CORRELATION

- *Since its introduction, the Pap smear is credited with decreasing the mortality associated with cervical, vaginal, and anal carcinoma.*
- *Although the conventional Pap smear is easier and less expensive, blood and inflammatory cells may obscure dysplastic cells.*
- *More recent liquid-based preparations have greater sensitivity for detecting clinically significant (high-grade) dysplasia.*
- *Sensitivity is significantly enhanced by HPV testing, but the specificity of HPV testing is poor in young, sexually active women because most have positive results for high-risk HPV infection, while high-grade dysplasia develops in less than 0.5%.*

3. **Invasive squamous cell carcinoma** of vulva and vagina most often arises from untreated HPV-related high-grade dysplasia.
    a. The risk of **metastasis** increases with the depth of invasion.
    b. Metastasis is usually first to inguinal lymph nodes.
    c. Staging guides treatment decisions and provides prognosis.
        (1) Stage 1: Confined to vulva (excellent survival)
        (2) Stage 2: Local spread
        (3) Stage 3: Regional spread
        (4) Stage 4: Invades organs or metastasizes (poor survival)
4. **Extramammary Paget** disease is de novo **adenocarcinoma** resembling pagetoid spread of breast ductal carcinoma to the skin.
    a. However, extramammary Paget disease arises from the epidermis and is usually confined to the epidermis (**in situ lesion**) without an ectopic breast ductal component, or invasion.
    b. Extramammary Paget disease manifests as a pruritic, scaly, erythematous lesion.
    c. Diagnosis is made by biopsy; results show mucin-secreting adenocarcinoma cells populating the vulvar epidermis.
    d. While it is indolent and rarely metastasizes, there is a high potential for **recurrence.**
5. **Melanoma** accounts for **10% of malignant vulvar neoplasia.**
    a. Invasion is associated with metastatic potential.
    b. It metastasizes to inguinal lymph nodes that drain the vulva.
6. There are also a few rare and unusual tumors.
    a. **Rhabdomyosarcoma** is a rapidly progressive, malignant skeletal muscle neoplasm. Although rare in adults, it is among the most common of pediatric soft tissue sarcomas (see Chapter 19).
    b. **Breast-like adenocarcinoma** arises from milk line, and these lesions are staged and treated in the same manner as carcinomas originating in the breast.

c. **Aggressive angiomyxoma** is a **low-grade** soft tissue tumor in the vulva of young women that contains characteristic vascular proliferation (angio-) within a gelatinous (myxoid) matrix; although it is classified as low grade, these lesions have a high **potential for recurrence.**

II. Cervix

A. Reactive Cervicitis

1. Infections are common, but usually not clinically significant unless the patient is symptomatic.
   a. *Gardnerella vaginalis* causes a "shift in flora" from lactobacilli to cocci (**clue cells**) (Figure 13–1).
   b. **Candidiasis** is common, especially during pregnancy.
   c. **Trichomoniasis** is a sexually transmitted infection by the flagellated protozoan ***Trichomonas vaginalis.***
      (1) Presenting signs and symptoms include pruritus, dysuria, and a malodorous green frothy vaginal discharge.
      (2) Inflamed "strawberry cervix" is a sign of infection.
      (3) Diagnosis is often made by Pap smear showing characteristic protozoan with flagella (Figure 13-1).
   d. **HSV** is a sexually transmitted virus.
      (1) Most cases of genital herpes are caused by HSV type 2.
      (2) An estimated 10–15% of cases result from HSV type 1 infection from oral-genital contact.
2. **Atrophic cervicitis** occurs in postmenopausal women because low estrogen leads to loss of squamous mucosa maturation.
3. Endocervical polyps cause inflammation and bleeding.

THE TRANSFORMATION ZONE

- *The cervix, penis, and anus, bridging the transition between the external environment and internal organs develop a transformation zone between external squamous cells and internal glandular cells.*
- *Immature stem cells from this zone are susceptible to HPV infection, especially in persons who smoke or who are immunosuppressed.*

B. Squamous Dysplasia and Carcinoma

1. Low-grade dysplasia (mild dysplasia, CIN-1) is usually a **transient HPV infection** of squamous cells by **types 6 or 11.**
   a. **20%** of low-grade dysplasia cases **progress** to high-grade dysplasia (Figure 13–2).
   b. However, **80%** of cases are transient infections and are **cleared** by the patient's immune system.
2. High-grade dysplasia (moderate CIN-2, or severe CIN-3) is **neoplastic transformation** of squamous cells, usually induced by **HPV 16 or 18,** and **80%** of high-grade cases **progress** to invasive squamous cell carcinoma if untreated.
3. **Invasive** squamous cell carcinoma has **metastatic potential.**
   a. **Deeper** invasion is more likely to **metastasize.**
   b. Staging guides treatment and provides prognosis.
      (1) Stage 1: Confined to the cervix (excellent survival)
      (2) Stage 2: Local spread
      (3) Stage 3: Regional spread
      (4) Stage 4: Metastases beyond pelvis (poor survival)

HUMAN PAPILLOMAVIRUS VACCINE

- *Outcome studies suggest the vaccine may effectively prevent dysplasia in two-thirds of young women if administered before HPV infection.*
- *Since dysplasia may develop in the remaining one-third, all females should continue to be screened by cervical Pap smears.*
- *Males are common carriers but at the time of writing this text they are not vaccinated.*

    C. **Endocervical Adenocarcinoma**

      1. Endocervical adenocarcinoma is caused by **HPV** infection.

      2. Adenocarcinoma in situ is not invasive.

        a. Squamous dysplasia is much more common.

        b. It is detected by Pap smear or surgical biopsy.

        c. It is characterized by endocervical glands with dark nuclei, increased nuclear:cytoplasmic ratios, and mitotic figures.

        d. Prognosis is good if excised by cone biopsy or hysterectomy.

      3. Invasive endocervical adenocarcinoma is rare and deadly.

        a. High metastatic potential prompts **radical hysterectomy.**

        b. Prognosis is most closely associated with tumor stage, which is the same as for squamous cervical cancer.

    D. **Unusual Neoplastic Variants**

      1. Adenofibroma presents as an endocervical polyp.

        a. It has stroma that is more cellular than a benign polyp.

        b. Complete excision (usually hysterectomy) is required to prove there is no invasion, which distinguishes it from adenosarcoma.

      2. Adenosarcoma looks like adenofibroma, but is **invasive.**

        a. This very rare malignant neoplasm may present as a polyp.

        b. It is a **low-grade sarcoma** with recurrent potential and low metastatic potential.

      3. Small cell neuroendocrine carcinoma manifests as a **highly malignant** rapidly growing mass with high metastatic potential and has a similar appearance to **small cell carcinoma** of the lung.

III. Uterine Corpus

    A. **Abnormal Uterine Bleeding**

      1. Abnormal uterine bleeding is defined as irregular or excessive uterine bleeding out of cycle phase (eg, at mid-cycle, weeks after missed menses, or post-menopausal).

      2. Common causes of abnormal uterine bleeding are **usually benign.**

        a. **Pregnancy** is a common cause of irregular uterine bleeding.

          (1) Miscarriage may occur weeks after expected menses.

          (2) Diagnosis is made by serum hCG, ultrasound, and biopsy.

          (3) Retained placenta postpartum may cause bleeding.

        b. **Infection** is an uncommon cause of uterine bleeding.

          (1) **Pyometra** is an abscess in the uterine cavity caused by **streptococci** or **clostridia** sometimes after instrumentation.

          (2) **Intrauterine device** for birth control may cause endometrial inflammation and infection by ***Actinomyces.***

          (3) **Chronic endometritis** has diagnostic plasma cell infiltration.

(a) Endometritis may be a sign of **PID (salpingitis)** but is more commonly identified postpartum, associated with instrumentation, or associated with postmenopausal cervical stenosis.

(b) Tuberculosis may cause granulomatous endometritis.

c. **Anovulation** is a common cause of abnormal uterine bleeding.

(1) At the beginning of menarche and at the beginning of menopause, there are periods of anovulation that lead to irregular cycles and abnormal uterine bleeding.

(2) Excessive unopposed estrogen (in the absence of progesterone made by the corpus luteum) leads to hyperplasia and mucosal breakdown.

(3) Common causes of excessive estrogen include obesity, polycystic ovary syndrome, and medications.

(4) The diagnosis is made by **endometrial biopsy.**

(5) Biopsy results usually reveal disordered proliferative endometrium with stromal breakdown, sometimes hyperplasia, but rarely cancer.

d. **Endometrial polyps** may be detected by endometrial biopsy, but usually require curettage and **ultrasound guidance.**

(1) Endometrial polyps are usually benign.

(2) They are characterized by variably dilated simple glands composed of various müllerian types in a background of fibrous stroma and thick-walled blood vessels.

(3) They are sometimes associated with simple hyperplasia.

e. **Cystic atrophy** in postmenopausal women leads to thickening of the endometrium by dilated simple glands and breakdown of the mucosa, which causes abnormal uterine bleeding.

3. Endometrial hyperplasia is stimulated by estrogen and increases the risk of developing adenocarcinoma (Figure 13–3).

a. **Simple hyperplasia,** characterized by "ring-like" glands, is almost always benign.

b. **Complex hyperplasia** is usually benign, but risk for cancer is increased.

(1) It is characterized by "pretzel or tree-like" shapes.

(2) If the nuclei are uniform and bland, it is usually benign.

(3) If the nuclei have prominent nucleoli, the risk of cancer is increased.

(4) **Atypical polypoid adenomyoma** mimics invasive carcinoma.

(a) It occurs in young women as an endometrial polyp in the lower uterus, but histology looks like complex glands invading muscle.

(b) The penalty of over-diagnosing cancer in this context is hysterectomy.

4. Endometrial metaplasia mimics the appearance of adenocarcinoma.

a. **Ciliary metaplasia** often presents as complex glandular hyperplasia with prominent nucleoli (worrisome for cancer).

b. **Papillary syncytial metaplasia** has complex tree-like architecture and dark nuclei, mimicking uterine papillary serous carcinoma, but they lack mitotic activity.

c. **Mucinous metaplasia** has simple architecture associated with neutrophils; if the architecture is complex, there is an increased risk of cancer despite the absence of nuclear atypia.

d. **Squamous metaplasia,** also known as "morules," mimics clear cell and squamous cell carcinoma.

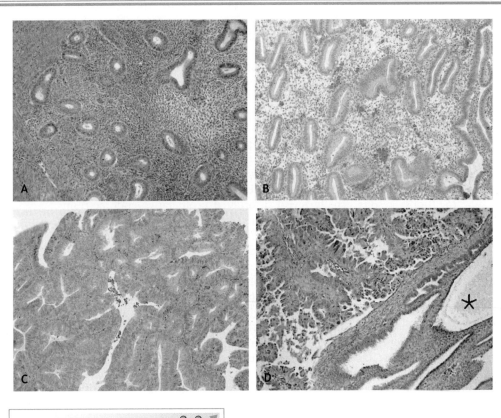

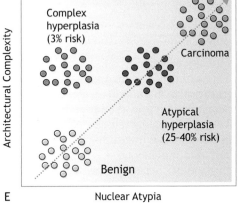

Figure 13–3. Endometrial carcinoma. A: Proliferative phase endometrium with scattered simple glands in abundant stroma. **B:** Secretory phase endometrium showing crowding of vacuolated glands. **C:** Complex hyperplasia with atypia shows branching glands with minimal stroma and mild nuclear atypia. **D:** Adenocarcinoma with large pleomorphic dark nuclei arranged in complex papillary and macroglandular architecture (compare to benign dilated cystic glands (asterisk). **E:** Malignancy is a function of architectural complexity and nuclear atypia. Atypical complex hyperplasia has a 25–40% risk of developing cancer.

B. **Endometrial Adenocarcinoma**
1. Uterine cancer usually presents as abnormal uterine bleeding, but may be incidentally detected by Pap smear screening.
2. **Hyperestrogenic** states (eg, obesity) and age are the most common risk factors for endometrial cancer.
3. The diagnosis is confirmed by endometrial biopsy; the results reveal complex "**macroglandular architecture**" and nuclear atypia.
4. **Grading** tumor differentiation guides surgery and prognosis.
   a. Well differentiated (grade 1) has mild nuclear atypia.
      (1) It is unlikely to be metastatic unless deeply invasive.
      (2) It is often cured by hysterectomy.
   b. Poorly differentiated (grade 3) has marked nuclear atypia.
      (1) It is often metastatic.
      (2) It requires chemotherapy and often radiation.
5. **Staging** provides prognostic information.
   a. Stage 1: Confined to the uterus (excellent survival)
   b. Stage 2: Local spread (eg, cervix)
   c. Stage 3: Regional spread (pelvis)
   d. Stage 4: Metastases beyond pelvis (poor survival)
6. **Carcinosarcoma** (also called *malignant mixed müllerian tumor*) is a poorly differentiated carcinoma with a very poor prognosis.
   a. It is characterized by a spindle cell component resembling sarcoma that shows at least patchy immunostaining for cytokeratin (epithelial).
   b. It may have "heterologous elements" (eg, rhabdomyosarcoma, chondrosarcoma) that behave like sarcoma rather than carcinoma.

ESTROGEN AND ENDOMETRIAL CANCER

- *Benign polyps are the most common endometrial lesions associated with estrogen therapy.*
- *However, estrogen may also lead to endometrial hyperplasia or adenocarcinoma, although these "hyperestrogenic" carcinomas are most often well differentiated and effectively treated by hysterectomy.*
- *Progestin therapy effectively treats hyperplasia, including atypical hyperplasia.*

C. **Endometrial Stromal Neoplasia**
1. It usually presents as uterine bleeding in middle-aged women.
   a. Imaging studies may show a distinct uterine mass.
   b. Endometrial curettage shows **stromal proliferation.**
2. **Stromal nodule,** like cervical fibroma, is **not invasive.**
   a. It is a rare benign neoplasm.
   b. Nuclei are uniform and bland with rare mitotic figures.
   c. Diagnosis requires hysterectomy to rule out invasion.
3. **Endometrial stromal sarcoma** is *invasive.*
   a. Histology is deceptively bland with few mitotic figures.
   b. It is a **low-grade sarcoma** with low metastatic potential.
      (1) Angiolymphatic invasion increases metastatic potential.
      (2) Metastases are uncommon but usually go to the lungs.
4. **Adenosarcoma** is a mixture of benign glands and stromal sarcoma.
   a. Periglandular stromal "condensation" is characteristic.
   b. Like stromal sarcoma, it has low metastatic potential.

5. Uterine tumor resembling sex-cord ovarian tumor resembles ovarian sertoli cell tumor or granulosa cell tumor and is thought to be **low grade** and behave like endometrial stromal sarcoma.

6. **Undifferentiated high-grade uterine sarcoma** is an "anaplastic" sarcoma with **high metastatic potential.**

D. Myometrial Neoplasia

1. **Adenomatoid tumor** is a benign mesothelial proliferation leading to an intramural mass lesion in the myometrium, and it is similar to tumors in the fallopian tube and spermatic cord.

2. **Adenomyosis** is **endometriosis** of the myometrium.
   a. It may present as uterine bleeding or pain.
   b. It grossly resembles a leiomyoma.
   c. Histologically, it is identical to endometriosis.

3. **Leiomyoma** is a **benign** smooth muscle tumor of the myometrium.
   a. It may present as uterine enlargement or bleeding.
   b. It is grossly a solid **well-circumscribed** submucosal, intramural, or subserosal mass within the myometrium.
   c. Histologically, tumor cells are **uniform** and **bland** with a low mitotic rate and without acute tumor cell necrosis.
   d. Intravenous leiomyomatosis, characterized by a "worm-like" growth of leiomyomata into veins, is not a sign of malignancy.
   e. Benign "metastasizing" leiomyoma, which sometimes presents after hysterectomy for fibroids, is not a sign of malignancy.

4. **Leiomyosarcoma** is a **malignant** high-grade smooth muscle sarcoma.
   a. It presents as an enlarging uterine mass, often with gross invasion and necrosis.
   b. It is a **rare sarcoma** and almost never arises from leiomyoma.
   c. Hysterectomy reveals a neoplasm with enlarged hyperchromatic and **irregular nuclei** (Figure 13–4) with a **high mitotic rate** and areas of acute ischemic tumor cell **necrosis.**
   d. Leiomyosarcoma has high recurrent and metastatic potential.

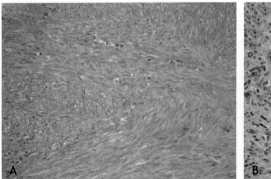
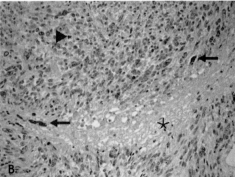

Figure 13–4. Diagnosing leiomyosarcoma. Compared to leiomyoma (**A**), which has uniform bland oval nuclei, leiomyosarcoma (**B**) has variably sized dark nuclei (arrows), necrosis (asterisk), and mitoses (arrowhead).

IV. Fallopian Tube

A. Infection, or **PID** (salpingitis), is an ascending infection usually caused by *N. gonorrhoeae* or *C. trachomatis.*

1. Chlamydial infections may be clinically silent, but they may also lead to tubal inflammation and injury, which increase the risk of ectopic pregnancy.

2. **Ectopic pregnancy** should be ruled out by hCG test and ultrasound in premenopausal women with lower quadrant pain.

3. Granulomatous salpingitis, caused by tuberculosis, is rare.

B. Adenomatoid tumor is a benign mesothelial cell proliferation.

C. Malignant fallopian tube neoplasia is rare, and the diagnosis requires exclusion of a more common ovarian primary.

1. **Papillary serous carcinoma** is the most common fallopian tube primary.

2. Although müllerian sex-cord stromal tumors may arise at any point along the müllerian tract, they are very rare within the tubes.

V. Ovary

A. **Benign Functional Cysts**

1. **Follicular** cysts and **hemorrhagic corpus luteal** cysts arising during the ovulatory cycle may grossly mimic malignancy.

a. Patients may complain of acute abdomen due to cyst rupture and bleeding into the peritoneal cavity (very painful).

b. Cyst formation is stimulated in patients taking fertility drugs, or in obese women with polycystic ovary disease (PCOD)**.**

c. In PCOD, follicular cysts produce androgens that are converted to estrogen**,** which suppresses follicle-stimulating hormone (FSH), leading to infertility, endometrial hyperplasia, and uterine bleeding.

B. **Endometriosis**

1. Endometriosis is an extrauterine proliferation of benign **endometrial glands and stroma** that undergoes monthly apoptosis and breakdown, leading to cyclical hemorrhage and growth.

2. **Endometriosis** is common (affecting almost 1 of every 10 women) and is associated with **infertility** (30% of cases) and **cyclical pain.**

a. The cause is unknown, but hypotheses include ectopic implantation versus de novo growth in müllerian peritoneum.

b. The ovary is the most common site of endometriosis.

c. "**Chocolate cyst**" is a hemorrhagic cyst of menstrual-like blood that mimics gross malignancy.

(1) It may rupture causing pain.

(2) It may adhere to surrounding structures causing **ovarian torsion,** producing acute hemorrhagic infarction and pain.

3. Endosalpingiosis is an extra-fallopian tube proliferation of benign ciliated mucosa, which is usually an incidental finding.

ENDOMETRIOSIS AND INFERTILITY

· *Endometriosis may manifest as pain and infertility.*

· *Laparoscopic examination reveals multiple black "burn-like" spots throughout the abdomen.*

· *Studies have demonstrated a transient improvement in fertility following treatment of endometriosis.*

C. Metastatic disease
1. Gastrointestinal mucinous adenocarcinoma (Krukenberg tumor) is a malignant implant that usually seeds both ovaries with myxomatous stroma and scattered mucin-secreting signet cells; this pattern may be histologically indistinguishable from ovarian carcinoma.
2. Breast cancer, especially lobular carcinoma, may also metastasize to the ovaries and may present as ascites.

D. Primary Ovarian Neoplasia
1. Ovarian cancer is **rare,** but it is usually not detected until later stages when survival is limited.
   a. Currently, there are no effective screening tests.
   b. **CA-125** is sensitive, but not specific, rising due to many causes, including irritation of the peritoneal lining.
2. **Risk factors** are similar to breast cancer, including numerous **ovulatory cycles** (early menarche, nulligravida, late menopause), **patient age** (>50% of malignant ovarian carcinomas present after age 50), genetic predisposition (*BRCA* **mutation** increases risk of breast and ovarian carcinoma).
3. Ovarian neoplasia may be classified into three broad categories that are often a function of the patient's age (Figure 13–5).

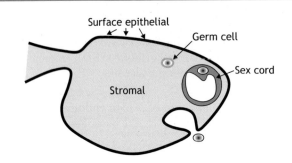

	Epithelial	Germ Cell	Sex cord Stromal
Patient Age	Older	Younger	All Ages
Diagnostic Types	Serous	Teratoma	Granulosa Cell
	Mucinous	Dermoid	Sertoli-Leydig
	Endometrioid	Immature	
	Clear Cell	Yolk sac	Fibroma
	Brenner	Dysgerminoma	Leiomyoma

Figure 13–5. Primary ovarian neoplasia. Epithelial cells most commonly lead to cancer; therefore, most ovarian neoplasms are surface epithelial. Germ cell neoplasms occur in children and young adults. Granulosa and Sertoli cells rarely become neoplastic.

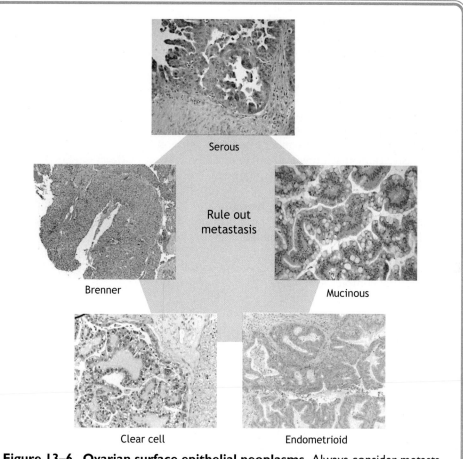

Figure 13–6. Ovarian surface epithelial neoplasms. Always consider metastasis, especially if the neoplasm is mucinous and bilateral. Papillary serous carcinoma is the most common primary ovarian neoplasm with slit-like spaces and areas that resemble fallopian tube mucosa. Mucinous tumors commonly have goblet cells or resemble endocervical mucosa. Endometrioid tumors are similar to endometrial adenocarcinoma. Brenner tumors are usually benign but may be malignant with features similar to bladder cancer. Clear cell carcinoma looks similar to kidney cancer.

    a. **Germ cell tumors** usually present in children and adolescents.
    b. **Sex-cord stromal tumors** present at any age.
    c. **Malignant epithelial tumors** usually present in older women.
  4. All three broad categories are staged similarly.
    a. Stage 1: Confined to the ovary (good survival)
    b. Stage 2: Local spread (eg, pelvis)
    c. Stage 3: Regional spread (eg, abdomen)
    d. Stage 4: Metastases beyond abdomen (poor survival)

5. Surface epithelial neoplasms represent 90% of all malignant primary ovarian tumors (Figure 13–6).

  a. They usually present in late stage with low survival.

  b. Clinical symptoms are **vague** and not specific (eg, constipation, diarrhea, discomfort).

  c. Pathophysiology is uncertain.

    (1) Tumors may arise from surface müllerian epithelium.

    (2) They may arise from entrapped inclusions.

      (a) Entrapped cyst(s) could grow into cystadenoma.

      (b) Hyperplasia within cyst could be borderline tumor.

      (c) Invasive clone may grow into carcinoma.

  d. Papillary serous tumors make up the **majority** of ovarian surface epithelial neoplasms.

    (1) Most papillary serous tumors are **benign.**

      (a) Cystadenoma is diagnosed by a uniform single layer of ciliated epithelium lining cysts in a fibrous stromal background.

      (b) Surgery is curative.

    (2) In **borderline tumors** (low malignant potential), there is increased architectural complexity.

      (a) Nuclei are bland with rare to absent mitoses.

      (b) In contrast to carcinoma, there is no invasion.

    (3) 20% of primary ovarian serous tumors are **malignant.**

      (a) There is nuclear atypia, mitoses, and **invasion.**

      (b) If tumors are present in the upper abdomen, mesothelioma must be ruled out.

        (i) The pattern of antigen expression provides a clue (mesothelioma expresses cytokeratin (CK) 5/6 while ovarian serous tumors usually express CK7 and estrogen receptor (ER).

        (ii) The treatment of mesothelioma is different.

  e. Mucinous tumors are the next most common and are usually **unilateral.**

    (1) Most ovarian mucinous tumors are **benign;** cystadenoma has cysts lined by bland simple mucinous epithelium that is either **intestinal type** (rule out metastasis from appendix) or **müllerian** (looks like cervical mucosa).

    (2) Borderline tumors have increased architectural complexity; although there is no invasion, pseudomyxoma peritonei ("jelly belly") may occur rarely if there is a recurrence in the abdomen.

    (3) 5% of primary ovarian mucinous tumors are **malignant.**

      (a) It has sheet-like expansile growth or **invasion.**

      (b) It is difficult to distinguish from metastasis.

  f. Endometrioid ovarian tumors are less common.

    (1) They resemble uterine endometrial mucosal tumors.

    (2) Most coexist with **endometriosis** although neoplasia arising from endometriosis is very rare.

    (3) Malignancy requires expansile growth or invasion.

    (4) Most are stage 1 and well-differentiated (grade 1).

  g. Clear cell carcinoma is unusual but **malignant.**

    (1) It resembles clear cell carcinoma of the kidney with clear cytoplasm, but they usually have large dark pleomorphic 'hobnail' nuclei.

(2) Notably, histology is also similar to yolk sac tumor.
- *(a)* Young women (30 years old) may have either.
- *(b)* Therapy is different than yolk sac tumors.

h. **Brenner** tumors are rare but almost always **benign.**
- *(1)* They resemble renal pelvis tumors (bladder urothelium).
- *(2)* **Benign** is a cystadenofibroma with urothelium.
- *(3)* **Borderline** resembles low-grade bladder carcinoma.
- *(4)* **Malignant** variants may resemble either invasive high-grade bladder cancer or squamous cell carcinoma, which raises the possibility of carcinoma arising in a mature teratoma.

6. Germ cell tumors (Figure 13–7) comprise 20% of ovarian neoplasia.
- a. Most are diagnosed in children and young adults.
- b. 95% are benign mature teratomas.
- c. 5% are malignant (yolk sac or dysgerminoma).
- d. **Mature teratoma** is a benign germ cell tumor composed of all three of the germ cell layers (endoderm, mesoderm, and ectoderm), commonly containing skin, hair, cartilage, and elements of the gastrointestinal tract.
  - *(1)* **Struma ovarii** is a mature teratoma composed of thyroid.
  - *(2)* **Squamous cell carcinoma** may arise in mature teratomas.
  - *(3)* **Thyroid carcinoma** may arise in struma ovarii.
- e. **Immature teratoma** is usually primitive neural tubes (small round blue cell tumor) that if present in more than one 5-mm field has significant metastatic potential requiring postoperative chemotherapy.
- f. **Yolk-sac** carcinoma (also called **endodermal sinus tumor**) is characterized by elevated serum **alpha-fetoprotein** levels and histologically by **Schiller-Duval** bodies, which are papillary structures with fibrovascular cores, lined by tumor cells with clear cytoplasm and dark malignant-appearing nuclei (similar to clear cell carcinoma).
  - *(1)* It is sometimes mixed with embryonal carcinoma (hCG).
  - *(2)* Survival is excellent with chemotherapy.
- g. **Dysgerminoma,** the ovarian counterpart of **seminoma,** is characterized by nests of immature germ cells with large round nuclei, prominent nucleoli, and abundant glycogenated cytoplasm.
  - *(1)* There may be intermixed syncytiotrophoblasts (hCG) and numerous small normal lymphocytes.
  - *(2)* Survival is excellent with chemotherapy.

7. Sex-cord stromal tumors (Figure 13–7) are rare.
- a. They may present at any age, but different types of sex-cord tumors are associated with different patient symptoms and ages.
  - *(1)* **Sertoli cell tumor** is seen in young patients.
  - *(2)* **Granulosa cell tumor** is seen in **postmenopausal** women.
- b. **Sertoli-Leydig cell tumor** usually occurs in young women (aged 20-40 years) with associated androgen effects (eg, **virilization**).
  - *(1)* Histologically, there are tubule-like glands lined by Sertoli cells that immunostain for **inhibin.**
  - *(2)* Ovarian hilus cell tumor is a virilizing **Leydig cell** tumor with **Reinke crystals** that also stains for inhibin.

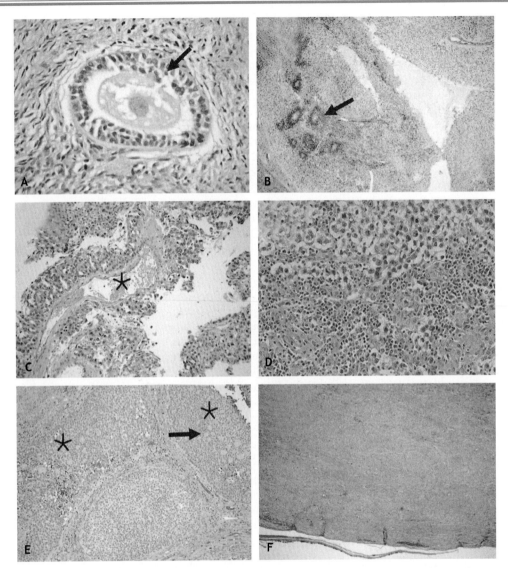

Figure 13–7. Germ cell and sex-cord stromal tumors. The most common germ cell tumor is mature teratoma (dermoid) with skin and hair (image not shown). **A:** Sex-cord stromal tumors arise from the cells supporting the oocytes (arrow). **B:** Immature teratomas are usually identified as primitive neural tubes (arrow). **C:** Yolk sac tumor (also called endodermal sinus tumor) has characteristic clear cytoplasm and fibrovascular cores (Schiller-Duval bodies, asterisk). **D:** Dysgerminoma is characterized by tumor cells with large round nuclei, abundant glycogenated cytoplasm, and conspicuous intermixed small lymphocytes. **E:** Granulosa cell tumor (sex cord) usually occurs in older women and may have characteristic Call-Exner bodies (asterisk) with hyalinized globules (arrow). **F:** Fibroma is a benign stromal tumor that may lead to Meigs syndrome. Fibrothecoma and leiomyoma are other common stromal tumors (not shown).

(3) Sex cord tumor with annular tubules (SCTAT) is an esoteric variant of Sertoli cell tumor that is associated with **Peutz-Jeghers syndrome.**

(4) Prognosis is usually related to tumor size and grade.

c. **Granulosa cell tumor** usually occurs in postmenopausal women with associated hyperestrogenic effects (eg, uterine bleeding).

(1) Histologically, there are sheets of uniform bland spindle cells with coffee-bean grooved nuclei that immunostain for **inhibin** and WT-1.

(2) **Call-Exner bodies** (complex glandular-appearing structure with red hyaline in the lumens) are rare and difficult to identify but are characteristic.

(3) Prognosis is usually related to tumor size.

d. Both fibroma/thecoma (benign stromal proliferation) and leiomyoma (benign smooth muscle proliferation) have malignant counterparts (ovarian fibrosarcoma and leiomyosarcoma, respectively) that are very rare.

MEIGS SYNDROME

* *Patients with Meigs syndrome may have a solid ovarian mass and pleural effusion. The cytology of the pleural effusion, however, is benign serous fluid.*
* *Microscopic evaluation of resected mass will reveal a benign fibroma rather than suspected malignancy.*
* *The clinical significance of Meigs syndrome is that ascites, pleural effusion, and elevated CA-125 may complicate the evaluation of a benign ovarian neoplasm.*

VI. Placenta

A. Abnormal Placentation

1. Ectopic pregnancy is usually in the fallopian tube.

a. It is a confined space without protective decidual lining, leading to invasion and rupture of the fallopian tube.

b. Diagnosis is made by hCG, ultrasound, and absence of placental chorionic villi in endometrial curettage.

2. Placentation site pathology leads to perinatal bleeding.

a. **Placenta previa** is abnormal placentation over the cervix associated with increased risk of both life-threatening hemorrhage and placenta accreta.

b. Placenta *accreta* is chorionic villi *a*ttached to myometrium.

(1) Placenta accreta requires manual extraction.

(2) It is rare (1/70,000 deliveries), but there is an increased risk with lower transverse cesarean section.

c. Placenta *increta* features villi *i*nvading myometrium, most often into a previous cesarean section scar (Figure 13–8).

d. In placenta *percreta*, the villi *p*erforate through myometrium.

(1) Again, the placenta usually pushes through scar tissue.

(2) It may invade into surrounding organs.

e. **Retroplacental abruption** is a hematoma between the placenta and uterus that obstructs maternal blood flow to the fetus, and it is associated with both preeclampsia and trauma.

B. Infection

1. **Chorioamnionitis** is a sensitive **maternal response** to an ascending amnionic infection, such those caused by group B streptococcus or *Escherichia coli.*

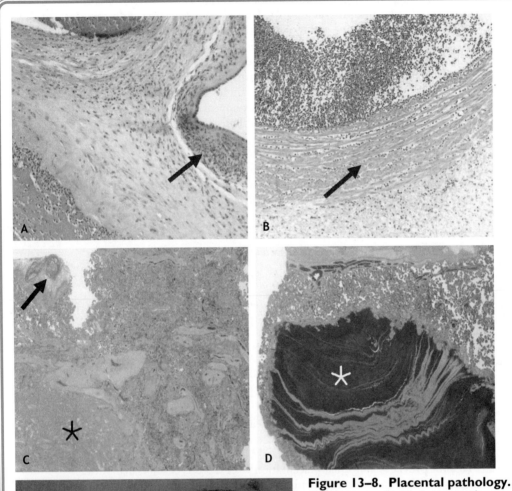

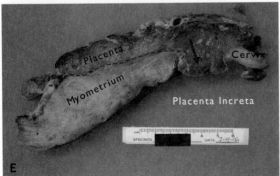

Figure 13–8. Placental pathology.
A: Chorioamnionitis is maternal neutrophils marginating toward intra-amnionic infection (arrow). **B:** Funisitis is fetal neutrophils marginating in umbilical vein (most specific sign of infection). **C:** Decreased blood flow to the placenta leads to infarction (asterisk), perhaps due to sick maternal blood vessels (arrow). **D:** Retroplacental abruption with lines of Zahn (asterisk). **E:** Abnormal placental attachment to prior lower transverse cesarean section scar, leading to placenta increta (shown in sagittal section).

a. It presents as **preterm labor** or premature rupture of membranes and may lead to fetal demise either from sepsis or morbidity associated with preterm birth.
   b. Currently, there is no reliable early detection method.
   c. The presence of chorioamnionitis is highly sensitive for amnionic infection (>95% negative predictive value).
2. **Funisitis** is a specific **fetal response** to amnionic infection.
   a. Because the fetus is less capable of mounting an adequate immune response, the presence of any inflammation from the fetus is highly specific for infection.
   b. The presence of neutrophils marginating into the umbilical cord is diagnostic.
3. **Chronic villitis** is a relatively nonspecific maternal response to a hematogenous infection by TORCHs.

C. Uteroplacental Insufficiency
1. Uteroplacental insufficiency is relatively decreased **blood flow** to the placenta.
2. The mismatch between vascular supply and placental demand manifests in several ways.
   a. The **placenta adapts** by accelerating maturation of the villi, leading to increased tree-like arborization of the placental architecture that increases the **surface area** available for **nutrient** exchange.
   b. Chorangiosis, a type of angiogenesis, enhances exchange.
   c. Decreased blood flow may lead to ischemic **infarctions.**
   d. Chronically decreased blood flow may result in a placenta that is small for gestational age (**SGA**).
3. Uteroplacental insufficiency is associated with multiple common pregnancy complications.
   a. Pregnancy-induced hypertension with proteinuria (**preeclampsia**) is a multifactorial disease, but placental insufficiency is a leading contributor.
   b. Intrauterine growth retardation (**IUGR**) is associated with small placentas, consistent with placental insufficiency.
   c. **Cerebral palsy** may be a consequence of perinatal hypoxia.
   d. "Idiopathic" preterm labor (not caused by infection) may be the fetal response to placental insufficiency, similar to early delivery commonly encountered with multiple gestations (eg, twins are often delivered at 36 weeks', triplets at 32 weeks').

D. Fetal Meconium
1. Fetal stool (meconium) into the amnion may be acute or chronic.
2. Acute release at the time of delivery may be insignificant.
3. Chronic release may be associated with fetal distress.
   a. Meconium may be a cause or effect of fetal distress.
   b. There are legal implications if **distress** is "prolonged."

E. Hydatidiform Mole
1. **Partial mole** (69 XXY) has low risk of persistent disease (<5%).
   a. It is a **triploid** placenta, and the fetus is often present.
   b. Grossly, it is a mixture of normal and hydropic villi.
   c. Histologic sections show characteristic **hydropic villi,** circumferential **trophoblastic proliferation,** and islands of trophoblasts in the villous stroma, the so-called **scalloping.**

2. Complete mole (46 XX) has moderate risk of persistence (33%).
   a. It is a **diploid** placenta with **no fetus.**
   b. It has an entirely paternal genome (uniparental disomy).
      (1) Paternally imprinted genes help make the placenta.
      (2) Maternally imprinted genes help make the fetus.
   c. It usually presents as uterine enlargement for gestational dates with a "**snow-storm**" of villi seen by ultrasound and relatively elevated serum **hCG levels.**
   d. A complete mole is characterized by diffusely hydropic villi, pronounced trophoblastic proliferation, and no fetal vessels.
   e. Without molecular testing, pathologists cannot reliably distinguish complete from partial mole in the first trimester.

F. **Choriocarcinoma**
   1. Choriocarcinoma is a very **rare malignant** primitive carcinoma affecting 1/100,000 pregnancies.
   2. It may present after a complete mole or, less often, after a miscarriage or term pregnancy.
   3. Choriocarcinoma is characterized by a **biphasic proliferation** of immature placental mononuclear **trophoblasts** and multinucleated **syncytiotrophoblasts** with numerous **mitotic figures** in a background of **hemorrhage** and **necrosis.**
   4. The presence of chorionic villi usually excludes the diagnosis of choriocarcinoma and favors persistent mole.
   5. Hematogenous metastases to vagina, lungs, and brain lead to hemorrhage and may be life-threatening; the prognosis, however, is usually good with **chemotherapy.**
   6. Choriocarcinoma must be distinguished from the more common placental site trophoblastic tumor (PSTT).
      a. PSTT does not respond to chemotherapy and requires hysterectomy.
      b. PSTT has a low mitotic count and low metastatic potential.

AUTOPSY OF THE PREGNANCY

• *The evaluation of the placenta is an autopsy of the pregnancy.*
• *Complicated pregnancies often are associated with characteristic placental findings.*
• *These findings may have medicolegal implications for both sides in an obstetric malpractice case.*

CLINICAL PROBLEMS

1. Which one of the following statements regarding extramammary Paget disease is **not** correct?
   A. Extramammary Paget disease has a good prognosis
   B. It originates from primitive progenitor cells in the epidermis
   C. It is a type of melanoma
   D. It is often not associated with underlying adenocarcinoma
   E. Tumor cells are positive for mucin stains

2. Which one of the following statements about the cervical-vaginal (Pap) smear is **not** correct?

    A. Regular Pap smears can prevent most cervical cancers

    B. Endometrial adenocarcinoma may be detected by Pap smear

    C. The sensitivity of a Pap smear is approximately 80%

    D. Human papillomavirus testing has replaced the Pap smear

    E. Pap smear is the most effective cancer screening program for women

3. Which one of the following statements about cervical carcinoma is **not** correct?

    A. It is strongly associated with infection by human papillomavirus

    B. Invasive carcinoma has a worse prognosis than high-grade dysplasia

    C. Smoking is a risk factor

    D. Radiation is the preferred method of treating high-grade dysplasia

    E. Risk of cervical dysplasia increases during pregnancy

4. Endometrial adenocarcinoma is **not** associated with which of the following?

    A. Age

    B. Polycystic ovary disease

    C. Infection by herpes virus

    D. Ovarian granulosa cell tumor

    E. Obesity

5. Which of the following characteristics of uterine leiomyosarcoma is false?

    A. Histologic features include necrosis, mitoses, and pleomorphism

    B. Clinically may present with metastases to lungs

    C. Arises from leiomyoma (fibroids)

    D. Type of malignant smooth muscle neoplasm

    E. Immunostains for smooth muscle actin and desmin

6. Which of the following associations are **incorrectly** paired?

    A. Stein-Leventhal syndrome and endometrial adenocarcinoma

    B. Choriocarcinoma and elevated serum hCG

    C. Endodermal sinus tumor and elevated serum alpha-fetoprotein

    D. Meigs syndrome and endometriosis

    E. None of the above

7. Which of the following statements about dysgerminomas is true?

    A. Common ovarian tumor of older women

    B. Chemotherapy resistant with a poor prognosis

    C. Schiller-Duval bodies are characteristic

    D. Testicular homolog is a seminoma

    E. No listed option is correct

8. Which of the following statements about ovarian surface epithelial neoplasms is correct?

   A. Most are benign

   B. Papillary serous carcinoma is the most common malignant tumor

   C. Borderline tumors have low recurrent potential

   D. Mucinous borderline tumors may cause pseudomyxoma peritonei

   E. All the above

9. Choriocarcinoma is most closely associated with which of the following?

   A. Complete mole

   B. Partial mole

   C. Term placenta

   D. Elective abortion

   E. Ectopic tubal pregnancy

10. Which of the following choices are correct?

   A. Placenta previa is preterm delivery

   B. Placenta accreta means abruption (hematoma)

   C. Placenta increta means placenta invades the bladder

   D. Placenta percreta means placenta is overlying the cervix

   E. None of the above

ANSWERS

1. The answer is C. Paget disease is not a type of melanoma. It is a de novo adenocarcinoma in situ of the vulva that is rarely invasive.

2. The answer is D. Human papillomavirus (HPV) testing has not replaced the Pap smear. Although testing for high-risk HPV provides excellent sensitivity and negative predictive value (>95%), the positive predictive value is low in young, sexually active women, leading to many false-positive results. Cervical dysplasia rarely develops in most young women who have HPV (75%) because their immune system clears the virus.

3. The answer is D. High-grade dysplasia is treated by surgical excision not radiation. Cervical cancer is strongly associated with infection by human papillomavirus, usually genotypes 16 and 18 (so-called high risk). Persistent infection leads to neoplastic transformation of immature epithelial cells at the transformation zone. If left untreated, high-grade dysplasia will usually progress to invasive carcinoma with metastatic potential. The risk increases with smoking history and immunosuppression.

4. The answer is C. Herpes simplex virus is not associated with adenocarcinoma. Major risk factors for endometrial cancer are age and hyperestrogenic states, including granulose cell tumor.

5. The answer is C. Leiomyosarcoma does not appear to arise from leiomyomas (fibroids). They are malignant smooth muscle neoplasms that immunostain for actin and desmin. They arise de novo with characteristic nuclear pleomorphism, numerous mitotic figures, and acute tumor cell necrosis. Lungs are a common site of metastasis for sarcomas.

6. The answer is D. Meigs syndrome is ascites and pleural effusion associated with benign ovarian fibroma *not* endometriosis. Polycystic ovary disease leads to elevated estrogen levels and increased risk of endometrial carcinoma. Choriocarcinoma (malignant germ cell tumor or placental neoplasm) often has markedly elevated hCG levels. Yolk sac tumor has elevated serum alpha-fetoprotein.

7. The answer is D. Dysgerminoma is a seminoma of the ovary that has a good prognosis. Germ cell tumors are uncommon and happen in young women. Schiller-Duval body is a papillary structure with a fibrovascular core characteristic of yolk sac tumor.

8. The answer is E. Ovarian surface epithelial tumors are most often benign, especially in women younger than 50 years. Borderline tumors recur in approximately 10% of cases; mucinous borderline tumors may recur as "jelly belly." Papillary serous carcinoma is the most common malignant primary ovarian neoplasm.

9. The answer is A. Choriocarcinoma is most closely associated with a complete mole (50% of cases). They may arise from partial moles, after term pregnancy, or miscarriage.

10. The answer is E. Placenta previa overlies the cervix; accreta is attached to the myometrium, increta invades, and percreta perforates and may invade the bladder.

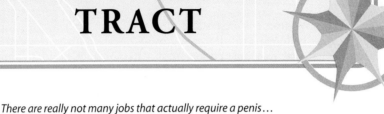

CHAPTER 14
MALE GENITAL TRACT

There are really not many jobs that actually require a penis…
—Gloria Steinem

I. Prostate

A. Anatomy

1. The prostate is similar to breast tissue, salivary glands, and the pancreas, composed of acinar glands feeding into larger ducts.
2. It encircles the bladder neck and proximal urethra.
3. It secretes prostatic fluid into the semen.
4. The anatomy is divided into **three zones:** outer **peripheral zone** (where **cancer** usually occurs), **transitional zone** (where benign **nodular hyperplasia** usually occurs), and the **central zone** (urethra).
5. It makes prostate-specific antigen (**PSA**) (<4 ng/mL).
6. Histologic sections reveal lobules of cytologically bland simple glands, lacking nuclear enlargement or prominent nucleoli.
7. Benign acinar glands are rimmed by a second **basal epithelial layer** (similar to the myoepithelial layer in breast).
8. Testosterone and its metabolite dihydrotestosterone (DHT) stimulate prostatic growth.
9. Castration (physical or chemical) leads to atrophy.

B. Inflammation and Infection

1. **Acute prostatitis** is usually caused by *Escherichia coli* and other organisms commonly responsible for urinary tract infections (UTIs).
   a. It presents with fever, dysuria, and a tender boggy prostate.
   b. Note that the patient's PSA may be elevated due to inflammation and destruction of the acinar glands.
   c. Treatment is antibiotics.

DIGITAL RECTAL EXAMINATION

- *Rectal examination should be a routine part of the physical examination in middle-aged (>40 years old) and elderly men.*
- *It is a means of screening for rectal cancer and prostatic disease.*
- *The prostate is palpated on the ventral aspect of the rectum.*

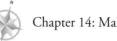

- *It is bilobed and should feel like your chin; if it feels like the tip of your nose, it is too boggy (prostatitis); if it feels like your forehead, it is too hard (cancer).*

    2. Chronic prostatitis may occur in patients with chronic UTIs but is usually asymptomatic.

    3. Granulomatous prostatitis is usually associated with **bacille Calmette-Guérin (BCG)** therapy for bladder cancer (injection of an attenuated tuberculosis strain).

        a. Biopsy reveals caseating granulomas similar to those seen in patients with tuberculosis.

        b. It has no clinical significance other than to recognize it is most likely a consequence of therapy rather than disease.

C. Prostatic Nodular Hyperplasia (Benign Nodular Hyperplasia)

    1. Nodular hyperplasia is very common with an incidence of approximately 20% of men at 40 years and 90% by 75 years of age.

        a. Urethral **obstructive symptoms** are seen in 25% of patients, which means most men are usually asymptomatic.

        b. Nonetheless, because it is so common, symptoms will develop in 33% of men during their lifetime.

        c. Symptoms generally include urinary frequency, dysuria, nocturia, difficulty with urination, urinary retention leading to bladder hypertrophy (trabeculation), and more UTIs.

        d. Prostatic smooth muscle tension is mediated by α_1-adrenoreceptors; therefore, α_1-**antagonists** are sometimes used to relieve obstructive symptoms.

    2. DHT stimulates prostatic growth.

        a. It is made from testosterone by **5α-reductase,** which is synthesized in prostatic stromal cells.

        b. DHT is 10 times more potent than testosterone; therefore local stromal DHT production leads to **stromal hyperplasia.**

        c. In turn, blocking 5α-reductase (eg, finasteride) is one method to treat nodular hyperplasia.

    3. Nodular hyperplasia is **not a premalignant condition.**

    4. Mild cases are treated medically.

    5. More severe cases are treated by transurethral resection of the prostate (**TURP**) or prostatectomy if necessary.

D. Prostatic Intraepithelial Neoplasia (PIN)

    1. High-grade PIN is the likely **precursor lesion** to invasive adenocarcinoma (similar to breast ductal carcinoma in situ [DCIS]).

        a. It is characterized by nuclear features resembling cancer (enlarged nuclei with **prominent nucleoli**), but the glands remain bound by the second basal epithelial layer (Figure 14–1).

        b. Unlike most cases of prostatic adenocarcinoma, PIN also shows increased architectural complexity (resembling ductal hyperplasia or DCIS of the breast).

        c. Approximately 80% of adenocarcinoma cases are associated with high-grade PIN, while most cases of PIN lack carcinoma.

        d. High-grade PIN occurs in the peripheral zone, like carcinoma.

        e. Unlike DCIS of the breast, the **risk** of tumor progression from high-grade PIN to invasive adenocarcinoma is **unknown.**

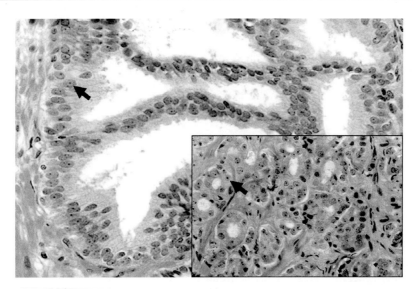

Figure 14–1. Prostatic adenocarcinoma. Similar to the breast, there is in situ high-grade dysplasia (prostatic intraepithelial neoplasia) with enlarged nuclei and prominent nucleoli, but tumor cells are bound by a basal layer and are not invasive. In contrast, invasive carcinoma lacks a basal layer and architecturally appears as crowded simple glands (inset, Gleason grade 3) or cribriform glands within glands (Gleason grade 4).

  2. Low-grade PIN is also characterized by complex hyperplastic architecture, but the nuclei are small and lack nucleoli; it is currently thought to have no clinical consequence.

E. **Prostatic Adenocarcinoma**
  1. Adenocarcinoma of the prostate is the **most common** cancer in men and is the second leading cause of cancer death.
     a. 20% of men have at least focal prostatic cancer by age 50.
     b. 70% of men have prostatic cancer by age 70.
     c. Screening men by serum PSA levels and digital rectal examination are effective means of detecting cancer early.
     d. Most cases of adenocarcinoma (>75%) occur in the posterior peripheral zone.

PSA LEVELS AND PROSTATIC ADENOCARCINOMA

- *Serum prostate-specific antigen (PSA) levels greater than 4 ng/mL are considered abnormal.*
- *False-positive levels are commonly encountered in cases of acute prostatitis, nodular hyperplasia, and rectal trauma.*
- *False-negative levels (<4 ng/mL) may be seen in cases of high-grade cancer or insufficient tumor volume to significantly raise PSA.*

CLINICAL CORRELATION

2. Risk factors include, age, race, diet, and genetic associations.
    a. Prostatic cancer shows a race bias with an increased frequency in blacks compared with whites.
    b. High-fat diet increases the risk, while **lycopenes** and anti-oxidant supplements may decrease the risk.
    c. There is *no association* between testosterone levels and cancer risk, but the number of CAG trinucleotide repeats in the androgen receptor gene may play a role.
        (1) An **androgen receptor gene** with **shorter CAG repeats** makes receptors that are more **sensitive to androgen** stimulation.
        (2) Blacks have shorter CAG repeats than whites, which are shorter than Asians.
    d. **Hypermethylation** of the **glutathione S-transferase** (*GSTP*) gene is seen in nearly all prostatic adenocarcinomas (>90%).
        (1) *GSTP-1* is a tumor suppressor gene that prevents damage caused by various carcinogens.
        (2) Hypermethylation may represent DNA modifications arising from the patient's diet, or during **carcinogenesis**, but there is also accumulating evidence that prostatic cancer may be driven by epigenetic modifications in utero, the so-called **fetal programming.**
3. Prostatic adenocarcinoma is diagnosed by tissue biopsy revealing infiltrating small acinar glands with enlarged nuclei and prominent nucleoli, lacking the second basal epithelial layer (unlike PIN).
    a. Other histologic clues include conspicuous blue mucin or red rhomboid crystals in tumor glands.
    b. Immunostaining for basal cells (eg, high-molecular-weight cytokeratin) is performed in diagnostically challenging cases.
4. Grading is by architecture rather than nuclear atypia.
    a. **Gleason grade 3** is **well-differentiated** carcinoma composed of simple "donut-like" tumor glands (Figure 14–2).
    b. **Gleason grade 4** is moderately differentiated carcinoma composed of "pretzel-like" glands within glands (cribriform).
    c. **Gleason grade 5** is poorly differentiated carcinoma composed of single tumor cells and sheets of tumor cells, lacking glandular architecture.
5. A final score is the combination of the predominant and minor architectural patterns (eg, Gleason grade 3 plus minor component of grade 4 = **3 + 4**).
    a. Small foci of 3+3 develop in most men in later life, which is often clinically insignificant.
    b. Larger tumor volume and higher grade are associated with increased metastatic potential (eg, lymph nodes, or **osteoblastic bony metastases).**
6. Treatment is radical prostatectomy with radiotherapy and hormonal therapy as indicated.
    a. Metastases to the spine may lead to cord compression.
    b. Radiotherapy is an effective means to palliate metastases.
7. Prognosis is related to stage.
    a. **Stage 1** is an incidental small focus of low-grade cancer.
    b. **Stage 2** is confined to the prostate.
    c. **Stage 3** is carcinoma invading outside the prostate.
    d. **Stage 4** is regional spread or any metastatic disease.

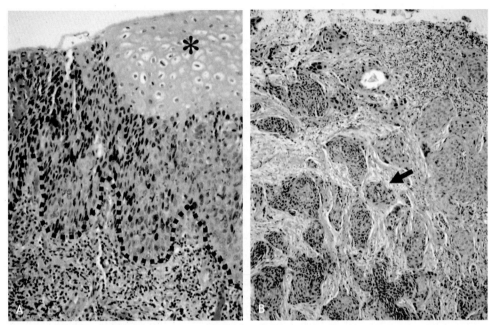

Figure 14–2. Penile cancer. Similar to the cervix, penile dysplasia is usually caused by the HPV virus (**A**). Low-risk types (6, 11) cause low-grade dysplasia (condyloma, usually occurring on the glans penis) and high-grade types (16, 18) may cause carcinoma (**B**). Low-grade dysplasia has low nuclear to cytoplasmic ratios (asterisk), while high-grade dysplasia has high N:C ratios and an intact basement membrane (dotted line), which distinguishes in situ carcinoma (on the left) from invasive squamous cell carcinoma (on the right) that has islands of tumor cells infiltrating desmoplastic stroma (arrow).

   F. Prostatic Stromal Proliferations
      1. These are very rare.
      2. However, there are reports of "*p*rostatic *s*tromal *p*roliferations of *u*ncertain *m*alignant *p*otential (PS-PUMP)."

   G. Seminal Vesicles
      1. Seminal vesicle epithelium is composed of cells with enlarged atypical nuclei and **brown-pigmented** cytoplasm.
      2. Biopsy findings may **mimic** prostatic adenocarcinoma, because of the nuclear atypia.
      3. Surprisingly, seminal vesicle carcinoma is extremely uncommon.

II. Penis

   A. Congenital Anomalies
      1. Hypospadias is a common birth defect of the urethral opening that may arise anywhere along the **ventral** urethral groove from the distal tip of the penis (mild) to the scrotum and perineum (severe).

a. It is the second most common male genital birth defect (after cryptorchidism) occurring in nearly 1% of births.

       b. Most cases are isolated and sporadic.

       c. Most cases are mild and adequately repaired by surgery.

    2. Epispadias is uncommon and is defined as openings along the **dorsal** shaft; they are usually associated with penile malformations.

B. Inflammation and Infection

    1. The glans and urethra (the distal penis) are the most common sites of inflammation and infection.

    2. Balanoposthitis is defined as the inflammation of the foreskin and glans, usually in uncircumcised males with poor hygiene.

       a. Multiple fungal and bacterial organisms may be involved.

       b. Candidal infection appears to be most common; although *Gardnerella* and *Streptococcus* have also been implicated.

    3. Phimosis is a common condition (1% of males) where the foreskin cannot be fully retracted from the head of the penis.

       a. Infantile phimosis may represent congenital fusion of the foreskin to the glans or may arise from chronic balanitis.

       b. Most acquired cases are caused by chronic inflammation.

       c. Balanitis xerotica obliterans is an esoteric skin condition that leads to loss of distal foreskin elasticity and phimosis.

       d. Circumcision is usually the treatment of choice.

    4. Chlamydial infection is the most prevalent sexually transmitted disease (STD) in the United States.

       a. Approximately 20% of sexually active adults are infected.

       b. Males are common **carriers** and are usually asymptomatic.

       c. Symptoms include dysuria (pain) and mucus discharge.

       d. Infected females may develop **pelvic inflammatory disease.**

    5. Gonorrhea is also one of the most prevalent STDs.

       a. It is caused by *Neisseria gonorrhoeae* and is treated with antibiotics.

       b. Symptoms usually present within 1 week of infection with dysuria and urethral **pus** (gleet).

       c. It may spread from the urethra to the testes, leading to abscess, scarring, and **infertility.**

    6. Syphilis is less common, but remains a significant STD because of the severe clinical consequences.

       a. It is caused by the bacterium *Treponema pallidum.*

       b. It is spread by contact with an open sore, or it may be spread vertically from the mother to child.

       c. The **primary** symptom is a hard painless ulcer (**chancre**) at the site of infection, which develops within a month of exposure.

       d. Secondary symptoms including fever, lymphadenopathy, and rash develop shortly thereafter.

       e. In the **tertiary** stage, which may occur years after infection, there may be widespread mass lesions (**gummas**), cardiovascular involvement, and neurosyphilis with psychological effects, **tabes dorsalis** (sensory nerve destruction), and blindness.

       f. Penicillin is usually curative if administered in the early stages of infection.

C. Squamous Cell Dysplasia
1. **Condyloma acuminata (low-grade dysplasia)** is an STD presenting as a penile wart, usually on the glans, and is caused by the human papillomavirus (HPV).
    a. Similar to low-grade dysplasia in the cervix, these lesions are usually caused by low-risk types of **HPV 6 and 11.**
    b. Risk factors include the number of sexual partners, **tobacco** use, age, stress, and **immunosuppression.**
    c. It rarely progresses to high-grade dysplasia (carcinoma in situ) and is treated by surgical resection.
2. **High-grade dysplasia (Bowen disease)** is surprisingly **rare** in men compared with cervical dysplasia but shows similar histologic features, including full epithelial-thickness atypia (Figure 14–2).
    a. However, similar to high-grade dysplasia in the cervix, these lesions are usually caused by high-risk types of **HPV 16 and 18.**
    b. Interestingly, Bowen disease usually involves the shaft of the penis rather than the glans or urethra.
    c. It progresses to **invasive carcinoma** in about 10% of cases if untreated (compared with 40–60% in females) and complete surgical resection is recommended.
3. **Invasive squamous cell carcinoma** is very rare in men in the United States (<0.02% of male cancers) but not uncommon in Africa and South America (10% of male cancers).
    a. Invasion is characterized by infiltration of the underlying stroma by islands of tumor cells with associated desmoplastic (scarring) host response (Figure 14–2).
    b. It is treated by wide local excision (often penile **amputation**) and chemoradiation as indicated.
    c. Prognosis is based on stage, but the overall 5-year survival is favorable in the absence of metastatic disease.
        (1) **Stage 1** is superficially invasive.
        (2) **Stage 2** invades the corpus spongiosum or cavernosum.
        (3) **Stage 3** invades the **urethra** or multiple positive nodes.
        (4) **Stage 4** invades pelvis or distant **metastases.**
4. Melanoma occurs on the penis similar to other skin.

III. Testicle

A. Congenital Anomalies
1. Normally, the testicles descend from the abdomen through the inguinal canal into the scrotal sac.
    a. They are encased by a white fibrous tunica (Figure 14–3).
    b. Germ cells mature into spermatids within tubules lined by Sertoli cells.
    c. Leydig cells populate the spaces between tubules.

TESTICULAR TORSION

CLINICAL CORRELATION

• *Twisting the spermatic cord cuts off the blood supply to the testicle, culminating in irreversible infarction within hours.*
• *It is a medical emergency and must be reduced within 6 hours of the event to salvage the affected testicle.*
• *Torsion typically presents in adolescents who have an anomalous testicular suspension defect, so-called "bell-clapper anomaly," related to increased testicular mobility within the scrotum.*
• *It presents as a sudden onset of severe pain associated with trauma, or with no clear inciting event.*

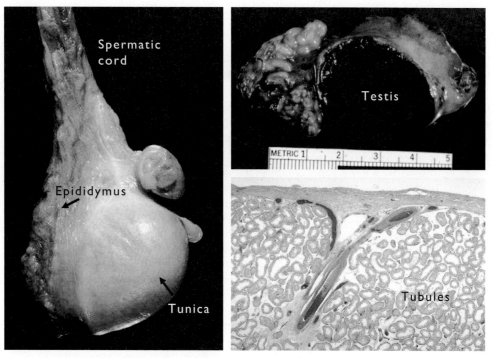

Figure 14–3. Normal testis. Gross and microscopic images of a normal testis with seminiferous tubules encased in a thick white fibrous tunica.

2. **Cryptorchidism**, undescended testis, is the most common congenital anomaly of the male genital tract (1% of newborn males).
   a. Most cases (>90%) are a failure to transverse the inguinal canal into the scrotal sac.
   b. It is usually unilateral.
   c. Usually, the entrapped testicle regresses into a fibrous **calcified remnant.**
   d. Surgical removal is indicated because of the increased risk of developing **testicular cancer**, inguinal **hernia**, and **infertility** associated with germ cell hypoplasia in the contralateral (descended) testis.
3. **Klinefelter** syndrome is male **hypogonadism** associated with sex chromosome aneuploidy (>80% of cases are **47XXY**).
   a. The incidence is 1/500 males.
   b. Presenting symptoms and signs include the following:
       (1) Small atrophic testes
       (2) Elongated body habitus
       (3) Lack of typical male features (facial hair)
       (4) Decreased IQ
       (5) Infertility
   c. It is also associated with an increased risk of breast cancer and **autoimmune disease** (eg, systemic lupus erythematosus).
   d. The diagnosis is usually made during puberty.

e. Follicle-stimulating hormone levels are elevated and testosterone is decreased; karyotype is diagnostic.

MALE INFERTILITY

CLINICAL
CORRELATION

- *Male infertility is nearly as common as female infertility and has a multifactorial etiology, including cryptorchidism, Klinefelter syndrome, germ cell hypoplasia (associated with varicocele), germ cell arrest, germ cell aplasia (after chemotherapy), and obstruction.*
- *Testicular needle core biopsies are used at times to distinguish hypospermatogenesis from obstruction.*
- *Tubules lined only by Sertoli cells with Leydig cell hyperplasia support germ cell pathology, while active spermatogenesis supports obstruction (eg, scarring from gonorrhea).*

   B. Inflammation and Infection
- **1. Epididymitis** is much more common than orchitis.
    - a. It is usually associated with a **urinary tract infection.**
    - b. Pediatric cases may be related to genitourinary anomaly.
    - c. *Chlamydia* and *N gonorrhoeae* occur in sexually active males.
    - d. *E coli* and other UTI organisms are more common in elderly.
    - e. Infection may lead to scarring and **infertility.**
- **2.** Orchitis may follow epididymitis or present as a primary site.
    - a. **Gonorrhea** is transmitted from the urethra to the prostate, seminal vesicles, epididymis, and finally to the testicles, where it may cause suppurative orchitis.
    - b. **Mumps** virus may cause orchitis in **adults,** causing sterility; it is uncommon in children.
    - c. **Syphilis** may cause orchitis, producing diffuse edema associated with a characteristic **plasmacytic** infiltrate.

   C. Germ Cell Tumors
- **1.** Testicular germ cell tumors are the leading cause of cancer in young men (**15–35 years old**).
    - a. There are nearly 10,000 cases each year in the United States, with **5% mortality.**
    - b. Whites are affected 5 times more often than blacks.
    - c. Other risk factors include cryptorchidism, Klinefelter syndrome, and genetic factors (eg, **isochromosome of 12p**).
- **2.** Most testicular germ cell tumors are a mixture of multiple types (eg, teratoma mixed with embryonal carcinoma and seminoma).
- **3.** Although most are **mixed germ cell tumors**, many are pure seminomas, which is a clinically significant distinction (**seminomatous versus nonseminomatous**) because seminoma is less likely to metastasize and is more susceptible to radiotherapy.
- **4.** The precursor lesion of most germ cell tumors is **intratubular germ cell neoplasia**, a type of germ cell carcinoma in situ that immunostains for placental alkaline phosphatase (PLAP) like seminoma (Table 14–1).
- **5. Seminoma** is the most common type of pure testicular germ cell tumor in males (homologue of **dysgerminoma** in females).
    - a. Seminoma is characterized by sheets of polygonal tumor cells with enlarged round nuclei, prominent nucleoli, and abundant glycogenated cytoplasm (**fried eggs**), in a background of numerous small **lymphocytes** (Figure 14–4).

Table 14–1. Laboratory results of germ cell tumors.

Testicular Tumor	AFP	hCG	Immunostain
Teratoma	—	—	None
Seminoma	—	Low levels	PLAP and CD117
Embryonal carcinoma	—	Low levels	Cytokeratin and CD30
Yolk sac tumor	High levels	—	AFP
Choriocarcinoma	—	High levels	Chorionic gonadotropin

AFP, alpha-fetoprotein; hCG, human chorionic gonadotropin; PLAP, placental alkaline phosphatase.

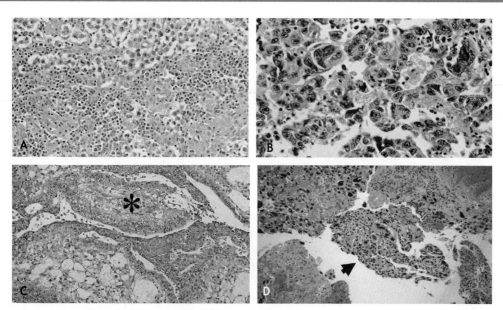

Figure 14–4. Malignant germ cell tumors. Unlike the ovary, mature teratoma is uncommon in the testicles. Germ cell tumors are often mixed, composed of a combination of teratoma (not shown), seminoma (**A**, fried eggs and lymphocytes), embryonal carcinoma (**B**, ugly pleomorphic nuclei), yolk sac tumor (**C**, papillary Schiller-Duval bodies with fibrovascular cores, asterisk), and bloody choriocarcinoma with trophoblasts and syncytiotrophoblasts (**D**).

b. There may be occasional intermixed syncytiotrophoblasts that synthesize low levels of human chorionic gonadotropin (**hCG**).

c. **Spermatocytic seminoma** is a distinct variant that occurs in older males (>65 years old) and typically arises de novo (without ITGCN) and only **rarely metastasizes.**

6. **Embryonal carcinoma** is histologically malignant with variably pleomorphic and hyperchromatic nuclei (Figure 14–4).

a. It is usually part of a mixed tumor.

b. It is more aggressive and has increased metastatic potential.

c. Tumor cells immunostain for cytokeratin and CD30.

7. **Yolk sac tumor** (endodermal sinus tumor) is the most common germ cell tumor in **infants** (<3 years old).

a. Serologic studies show elevated alpha-fetoprotein levels.

b. Histologic sections reveal a poorly differentiated **clear cell** neoplasm arranged in sheets, glands, and papilla with prominent fibrovascular cores (**Schiller-Duval bodies**).

c. It is also aggressive and has increased metastatic potential.

8. **Choriocarcinoma** is a bloody, highly malignant, germ cell tumor identical to the *much less common* **placenta** derived malignancy.

a. Serum studies show markedly elevated **hCG** levels.

b. Histologic sections reveal a characteristic **biphasic pattern** composed of **mononuclear** malignant trophoblasts and **multinuclear** syncytiotrophoblasts (Figure 14–4).

c. It is highly **aggressive** and almost invariably mixed with other germ cell tumor types.

9. **Testicular teratoma** is most commonly mixed with other germ cell tumor types, unlike in the ovary where it is most often a pure tumor.

a. It may be composed of mature elements (eg, cartilage), or immature elements (eg, small round blue cells).

b. Notably, chemotherapy induces maturation of all germ cell tumors, leading to mature teratomatous elements affected sites (eg, retroperitoneal lymph nodes, lungs, brain).

10. Treatment is orchiectomy and chemoradiation as indicated.

11. **Germ cell tumor prognosis** is related to whether the neoplasm is seminomatous (70% are stage 1) or mixed (most are more than stage 2).

a. **Stage 1** is tumor confined to the testis.

b. **Stage 2** has lymph node metastases.

c. **Stage 3** has distant metastases.

D. **Sertoli-Leydig Cell Tumors**

1. **Sertoli cell tumors** are uncommon and usually **benign.**

a. They secrete **estrogen** and androgens that may lead to **precocious feminization** or masculization.

b. Sections reveal well-formed glands or sheets of cytologically bland Sertoli cells that immunostain for **inhibin.**

2. **Leydig cell tumors** are also uncommon and are usually **benign.**

a. They may also secrete androgens and estrogens leading to **gynecomastia** in adults and **precocious puberty** in children.

b. Sections reveal a grossly distinct brown nodule within the testicle (Figure 14–5) composed of Leydig cells with characteristic **Reinke crystals.**

c. Leydig cell tumors also stain strongly for **inhibin.**

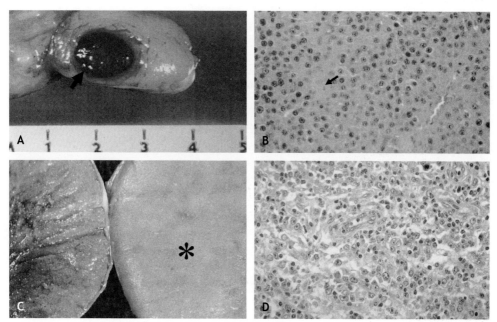

Figure 14–5. Unusual testicular neoplasms include sex-cord stromal tumors similar to the ovary (eg, Leydig cell tumor, **A**), which may have characteristic red Reinke crystals (**B**) and immunostain for inhibin. Lymphoma may be primary or systemic showing grossly solid fish-flesh appearance (**C**) and sheets of discohesive large lymphocytes (**D**) with vesicular nuclei and prominent nucleoli, which immunostain for B-cell markers (eg, CD20).

E. Lymphoma and Metastases

1. **Primary lymphoma** accounts for 5% of testicular neoplasms and is the most common testicular neoplasm in **older men** (>60-years-old).
   a. Most cases are diffuse large B-cell lymphoma (Figure 14–5).
   b. Most cases are associated with systemic disease.
   c. The prognosis is usually poor.
2. **Metastases** to the testicle are uncommon, but are most often from the kidney (renal cell carcinoma) or melanoma.

CLINICAL PROBLEMS

1. A great American bicycle racer complains of hemoptysis and fatigue. Workup revealed metastatic testicular cancer to the lungs and brain. Serum human chorionic gonadotropin (hCG) and alpha-fetoprotein levels were elevated. Which is the **MOST LIKELY** diagnosis?

   A. Mixed germ cell tumor

   B. Pure seminoma

C. Teratoma

D. Yolk sac tumor

E. Embryonal carcinoma

2. Which of the findings has the worst prognosis?

A. Serum PSA 4 ng/mL; Gleason 3+3 adenocarcinoma on biopsy

B. Serum PSA 8 ng/mL; Gleason 4+5 adenocarcinoma on biopsy

C. Serum PSA 12 ng/mL; Gleason 4+3 adenocarcinoma on biopsy

D. All the above

E. None of the above

3. A 45-year-old male prostitute complains of dysuria and hematuria. Examination reveals a mass on the distal urethra. What is the most likely diagnosis?

A. Transitional cell carcinoma

B. Embryonal carcinoma

C. Sertoli cell tumor

D. Human papillomavirus-related squamous cell carcinoma

E. Ectopic neuroganglioma

4. Which of the following statements regarding seminoma is false?

A. It is not a type of sex cord stromal tumor

B. It rarely presents in pure form

C. It is frequently infiltrated by lymphocytes

D. It may express human chorionic gonadotropin

E. None of the above

5. Which of the following regarding high-grade prostatic intraepithelial neoplasia (PIN) is true?

A. It is uncommon in the presence of invasive adenocarcinoma

B. It is a precursor to benign prostatic hyperplasia (BPH)

C. It shares nuclear features with invasive adenocarcinoma

D. It is uncommon in the prostate of men over age 65 years

E. All the above

6. Treatment of benign prostatic hyperplasia (BPH) with a 5α-reductase inhibitor (finasteride) is effective because:

A. The drug is a potent androgen

B. The drug blocks conversion of dihydrotestosterone to testosterone

C. The drug blocks conversion of cortisol to dihydrocortisol

D. The drug blocks conversion of estrone to estradiol

E. The drug blocks conversion of testosterone to dihydrotestosterone

7. A 26-year-old medical student notices a 1-cm nodule on his left testicle during his monthly self examination. The testicle is removed revealing a pure population of large tumor cells with round nuclei, prominent nucleoli, and abundant clear cytoplasm (resembling fried eggs) in a background of numerous small lymphocytes. The correct diagnosis is:

    A. Choriocarcinoma

    B. Chronic orchitis

    C. Teratoma

    D. Seminoma

    E. Mixed large and small cell lymphoma (intermediate grade)

8. A mother notices that her 3-month-old infant son has an enlarging left testicle. A serum hCG-β is normal, but alpha-fetoprotein is markedly elevated. What is the **MOST LIKELY** diagnosis?

    A. Yolk sac tumor

    B. Choriocarcinoma

    C. Seminoma

    D. Sertoli cell tumor

    E. Hepatoblastoma

9. A teenage boy arrives at the emergency department after suffering severe right testicular pain for the past 24 hours. His testis is enlarged, warm, and tender. What is the best treatment?

    A. Surgery is necessary but will probably not save the testis

    B. He has testicular cancer and requires immediate chemotherapy

    C. Antibiotics will be started for presumptive epididymitis

    D. A venogram is necessary to look for a varicocele

    E. He should take two aspirin and call you in the morning

10. A 52-year-old man with a history of benign prostatic hyperplasia (BPH) complains of fever and dysuria. His prostate is enlarged and tender to palpation. What is the **LEAST LIKELY** cause of his symptoms?

    A. *Escherichia coli*

    B. Human papillomavirus

    C. *Klebsiella*

    D. *Enterococcus*

    E. *Enterobacter*

ANSWERS

1. The answer is A. Elevated hCG (choriocarcinoma, but may be mildly elevated in seminoma and embryonal carcinoma) and AFP (yolk sac tumor) support a mixed germ cell tumor, which is also the most common aggressive male testicular neoplasm.

2. The answer is B. Gleason grade 4+5 means there is a minor component of poorly differentiated grade 5 cancer, which implies increased malignant potential.

3. The answer is D. Similar to cervical cancer, males are at risk for HPV-mediated squamous dysplasia leading to invasive carcinoma. Risk factors include multiple sex partners, smoking, and immunosuppression.

4. The answer is B. Seminoma in males often presents in pure form and imparts a favorable prognosis.

5. The answer is C. High-grade PIN is similar to ductal carcinoma in situ in breast. It has enlarged nuclei with prominent nucleoli, exactly like invasive adenocarcinoma. Pathologists sometimes use immunostains to highlight basal cells (eg, cytokeratin) to distinguish PIN from invasion.

6. The answer is E. Finasteride blocks production of dihydrotestosterone, which in turn decreases hormonal stimulation of prostatic tissue and reduces benign prostatic hyperplasia.

7. The answer is D. Classic description of pure seminoma; note serologic studies may show mildly elevated hCG because some cases have a few syncytiotrophoblasts intermixed with the pure seminoma.

8. The answer is A. The testicular mass and elevated alpha-fetoprotein (AFP) support a diagnosis of yolk sac tumor. Notably, fetal hepatoblastoma of the liver may also present with elevated AFP.

9. The answer is A. The history suggests the patient suffers from testicular torsion and subacute infarction. Torsion must be reduced within hours to save the testicle.

10. The answer is B. Human papillomavirus causes penile, cervical, anal, and oral epithelial dysplasia but not acute prostatitis.

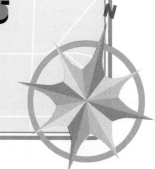

CHAPTER 15
BONE AND
SOFT TISSUE

I have no history, but the length of my bones.
—Robin Skelton

I. Bone

A. Genetic Disease

1. Achondroplasia is the most common disease of the growth plate and a major cause of dwarfism.

  a. Clinical characteristics include short stature with short limbs and normal-sized head and trunk.

  b. It is usually autosomal dominant and has a point mutation in the fibroblast growth factor receptor 3 (***FGFR3***) gene.

  c. This leads to a reduction in chondrocyte proliferation, resulting in early growth plate closure.

2. Osteogenesis imperfecta is caused by a deficiency in synthesis of type I collagen, leading to decreased bone formation with prominent osteoporosis and extreme skeletal fragility.

  a. This condition presents in childhood with **fractures.**

  b. It also affects joints, eyes (**translucent blue sclerae**), ears (hearing loss), skin, and teeth (dental imperfections).

  c. It is usually autosomal dominant.

B. Metabolic Disease

1. Osteo*petro*sis (marble bone disease, Albers-Schönberg disease) is caused by a failure of osteoclastic activity, leading to reduced bone reabsorption and increased skeletal density.

  a. Patients have **sclerotic** brittle bones that fracture.

  b. The autosomal recessive variant is fatal in infancy.

  c. The autosomal dominant variant is less severe.

2. Osteo*poro*sis is the common bone disease characterized by decreased bone mass due to either impaired synthesis or increased reabsorption of bone matrix.

  a. Patients have increased **porosity** of the skeleton and are predisposed to fracture, especially in weight-bearing bones (eg, compression fracture of vertebral body).

  b. An important radiologic finding is **diffuse radiolucency.**

c. Osteoporosis is more common in **postmenopausal** women as well as persons with reduced physical activity, hyperthyroidism, and calcium deficiency.

3. **Paget disease** (osteitis deformans) is characterized by mixed osteoblastic and osteoclastic activity.
    a. It begins with an osteolytic stage.
    b. There is then a mixed osteolytic-osteoblastic stage.
    c. It ends with an osteoblastic stage followed by quiescence.
    d. Paget disease is most often multifocal, but there is data suggesting it may be related to a slow virus infection.
    e. The axial skeleton and femur are most commonly involved.
    f. The hallmark finding is the **mosaic pattern of lamellar bone,** similar to a jigsaw puzzle.

4. **Scurvy** is caused by vitamin C deficiency, which leads to reduced collagen synthesis and impaired osteoid matrix formation.
    a. Subperiostial and joint hemorrhage can occur due to vascular wall defects and periosteal adhesion defects.
    b. Cartilaginous overgrowth may ensue due to insufficient osteoid matrix deposition and slowed reabsorption, leading to epiphyseal widening and other skeletal abnormalities.

5. **Rickets** is caused by vitamin D deficiency in children.
    a. Decreased calcification and excess accumulation of osteoid matrix results in thickening of the epiphyseal growth plates and other skeletal deformities.
    b. Clinical manifestations include classic bowing of the legs, protrusion of the sternum (pigeon breast), lumbar lordosis, late closure of fontanelles, softening of the occipital and parietal bones (craniotabes), and overgrowth of cartilage and osteoid at the costochondral junction (rachitic rosary).

6. **Osteomalacia** is caused by vitamin D deficiency in adults; it shows diffuse radiolucency, mimicking osteoporosis.

7. **von Recklinghausen disease** (osteitis fibrosa cystica) is caused by hyperparathyroidism (both primary and secondary) and is characterized by widespread osteolytic lesions that result from increased osteoclastic activity.
    a. Bone loss predisposes these patients to microfractures.
    b. **Brown tumors** in this disease are characterized by osteoclast-lined cystic spaces within bone, filled by vascular fibrous stroma, that often have a brown color from resultant hemorrhage.

8. **Avascular necrosis** (osteonecrosis) most often results from arterial disruption, resulting in infarction.
    a. The most common etiologies for avascular necrosis include trauma, embolism, thrombosis and long-term corticosteroid use.
    b. Avascular necrosis can occur in children in the head of the femur (**Legg-Calvé-Perthes disease**), tibial tubercle (Osgood-Schlatter disease), and the navicular bone (Köhler disease).

SCURVY

- *Vitamin C deficiency is more common in the poor, elderly, and drug and alcohol abusers, leading to reduced collagen synthesis and scurvy, which usually presents with bleeding and difficulty healing.*
- *The British Navy was the first to realize that eating citrus fruits during long sea voyages would prevent scurvy, the so-called "limey."*

CLINICAL CORRELATION

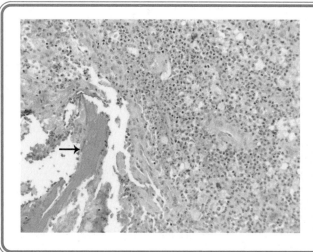

Figure 15–1. Osteomyelitis. Acute osteomyelitis (Brodie abscess) is characterized by devitalized bone (arrow) and neutrophilic infiltrate.

C. Infection
1. **Pyogenic osteomyelitis** is nearly always caused by bacteria from either hematogenous spread or direct extension.
   a. ***Staphylococcus aureus*** is the most common cause.
   b. *Pseudomonas* infection is seen in injection drug users.
   c. *Salmonella* is more common in sickle cell anemia.
   d. Pyogenic osteomyelitis most often involves the metaphysis.
   e. The feet (diabetes, peripheral artery disease), upper arm (humerus), and knee (distal femur, proximal tibia) are the most common sites of acute osteomyelitis.
   f. It is diagnosed by histologic confirmation of nonviable bone associated with acute inflammatory infiltrate (Figure 15–1).
   g. **Brodie abscess** is a small intraosseous abscess frequently involving the cortex that is walled off by granulation tissue.
2. **Tuberculous osteomyelitis** is caused by *Mycobacterium tuberculosis.*
   a. The bone may be infected by hematogenous spread from a nidus elsewhere in the body (eg, lungs).
   b. **Pott disease** is involvement of the vertebrae.

D. Neoplasia
1. **Osteochondroma** is an **exostosis** of mature bone and cartilage.
   a. It is the most common benign tumor of bone.
   b. It originates from the metaphysis of long bones as a bony stalk covered by a cartilage cap.
   c. Malignant transformation is very rare but may occur in patients with multiple hereditary osteochondromatosis.
2. **Osteomas** are likely hamartomas.
   a. They are well-circumscribed, arising from the bony cortex.
   b. They are usually solitary, slow-growing, and most often arise within the skull and facial bones of middle-aged adults.
3. Osteoid osteomas are benign bone tumors that arise in cortical bone and are painful but the pain responds to aspirin.

4. **Osteoblastomas** are larger and usually present in the axial skeleton; although benign, they may be destructive and recur.

GARDNER SYNDROME

CLINICAL
CORRELATION

- *Gardner syndrome is a variant of the familial adenomatous polyposis (FAP) syndrome caused by mutations in the APC gene.*
- *Gardner syndrome is associated with **multiple osteomas**, numerous dysplastic colon **polyps**, and **fibromatosis.***

5. **Giant cell tumor** of bone is benign.
   a. It occurs in the epiphyseal area of long bones in **adults.**
   b. It has a characteristic expansile, lytic appearance by radiographic imaging (Figure 15–2).
   c. Histologic features include mononuclear stromal cells admixed with numerous multinuclear giant cells.

6. **Langerhans cell histiocytosis** (formerly called histiocytosis X) may be local (good prognosis) or diffuse (worse prognosis).
   a. It is a neoplastic proliferation of Langerhans-like cells that immunostain for S100 and CD1a.
   b. **Electron microscopy** reveals tennis racket–shaped cytoplastic structures, the so-called **Birbeck granules.**
   c. **Eosinophilic granuloma** is the solitary localized tumor, which is usually associated with numerous intermixed eosinophils.
   d. **Hand-Schüller-Christian disease** typically presents in childhood with the classic triad of skull lesions, diabetes insipidus, and exophthalmos due to orbital involvement.
   e. **Letterer-Siwe disease** (disseminated histiocytosis) is an aggressive and often fatal disease of early childhood; it is characterized by cutaneous infiltrates and systemic involvement of the liver, bone marrow, lungs, and lymph nodes.

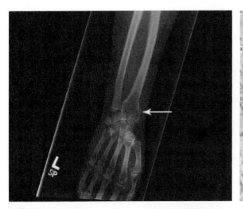
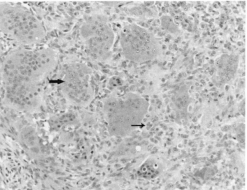

Figure 15–2. Giant cell tumor. Radiograph shows lytic lesion in the distal long bone (radius) associated with pathologic fracture (arrow). Histologic sections show neoplastic mononuclear stromal cells (thin arrow) intermixed with reactive osteoclastic giant cells (thick arrow).

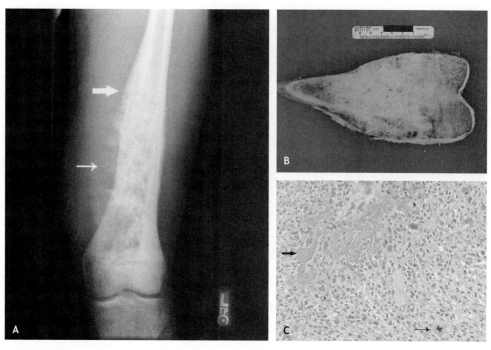

Figure 15–3. Osteosarcoma. A: Radiographic image of high-grade osteosarcoma of the distal femur showing a mixed lytic and sclerotic lesion involving the metaphysis with extension into soft tissue lifting of the periosteum (Codman triangle, arrow). There are bone spicules producing the so-called sunburst pattern (thin arrow). **B:** Gross image of osteosarcoma in metaphysis. **C:** Photomicrograph of osteosarcoma showing pleomorphic tumor cells with atypical mitoses (thin arrow) and osteoid (thick arrow).

7. **Osteosarcoma** (osteogenic sarcoma) is the most common primary malignancy of bone.
   a. It is most common in **adolescents** with a peak incidence between the ages of 10 and 20 years.
   b. It usually occurs in the metaphysis of long bones, with a preference for the **proximal tibia** and **distal femur.**
   c. Osteosarcoma presents with pain, swelling, and fracture.
   d. There are often hematogenously spread metastases to the lungs, liver, or brain at the time of diagnosis.
   e. The classic radiologic appearance is the **Codman triangle,** caused by a lifting of the periosteum by tumor expansion.
   f. Another common radiologic sign is a spiculated **sunburst pattern** of tumor growth (Figure 15–3).
   g. The diagnosis is made by identifying malignant pleomorphic tumor cells that synthesize bone (osteoid) (Figure 15–3).
8. **Ewing sarcoma** and **peripheral neuroectodermal tumors (PNETs)** are synonymous terms.

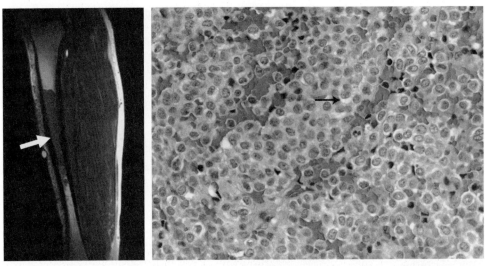

Figure 15–4. Ewing sarcoma/PNET. MRI showing diaphyseal intramedullary mass (arrow). Histologic sections reveal a monotonous population of small round blue cells with glycogen-rich cytoplasm (arrow). Diagnosis was confirmed by FISH analysis showing the characteristic t(11;22) translocation.

    a. It is a malignant "**small round blue cell**" tumor that usually presents in children and young adults.

    b. It usually arises in long bones, ribs, pelvis, and scapula.

    c. Although it is a very aggressive malignancy with early metastases, this tumor usually responds well to chemotherapy.

    d. Histologic sections show a small round blue cell tumor with delicate glycogenated cytoplasm (Figure 15–4).

    e. The diagnosis is confirmed by identifying the **t(11;22)** chromosomal translocation characteristic of Ewing sarcoma.

II. Cartilage Neoplasia

A. Enchondroma

    1. Enchondromas are benign, mature cartilage–forming neoplasms that are solitary and well demarcated.

    2. They usually present in long bones or the hands.

    3. Biopsy reveals a hypocellular hyaline blue cartilaginous matrix with minimal cytologic atypia (except for tumors in the hands where they tend to be more cellular).

B. Chondrosarcoma

    1. These malignant tumors primarily affect adults after age 50.

    2. Chondrosarcomas usually present in the pelvis with pain.

    3. Radiologically, they show an infiltrative pattern (Figure 15–5).

    4. Biopsy shows a moderately cellular blue cartilaginous matrix with moderate-to-severe cytologic atypia (Figure 15–5).

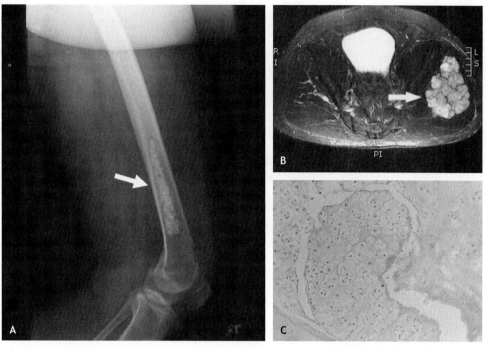

Figure 15–5. Chondrosarcoma versus enchondroma. A: Radiograph of distal femoral metaphysis shows a mineralized tumor in the medullary cavity with an intact bony cortex, consistent with a benign enchondroma. **B:** In contrast, an axial MRI of a chondrosarcoma of the left iliac bone reveals a lobulated mass invading into the gluteal musculature. **C:** Photomicrograph shows a low-grade chondrosarcoma with chondroid matrix and moderate nuclear atypia.

III. Joints

A. Arthritis

1. **Osteoarthritis,** also known as degenerative joint disease, is the most common form of arthritis.
    a. It usually affects adults after age 50.
    b. It is caused by chronic mechanical trauma of the joints ("wear and tear") and is characterized by progressive erosion of articular cartilage accompanied by new bone formation in the subchondral and peripheral areas of the articular surface.
    c. Radiographic findings include increased subchondral bone density, cystic changes in the subchondral bone, and osteophyte (bone spur) formation at the periphery of the articular surface.
    d. **Osteophytes** may fracture and float freely within the synovial fluid, which are known as "**joint mice.**"
    e. **Eburnation** refers to the polished white appearance of bone resulting from erosion of the overlying cartilage.
    f. Common clinical findings include **Bouchard nodes** (osteophytes in the proximal interphalangeal [PIP] joints of the fingers) and **Heberden**

nodes (osteophytes in the distal interphalangeal [DIP] joints of the fingers).

2. **Rheumatoid arthritis** is a chronic systemic autoimmune inflammatory disorder of the synovial joints.
   a. It usually affects adults (20–50 years of age).
   b. **Rheumatoid factor** detected in the blood is highly characteristic of this disease, although not specific.
   c. Clinically, rheumatoid arthritis presents with joint pain, fatigue, weight loss, fever, and malaise.
   d. The PIP joints as well as the metacarpophalangeal (MCP) joints of the hands are affected.
   e. Early histologic features include dense lymphocyte, macrophage, and plasma cell infiltration within the synovial joint tissue with associated synovial edema and hyperplasia.
   f. Granulation tissue (**pannus**) forms over the articular cartilage with extension into subchondral bone.
   g. Eventually, the granulation tissue bridges opposing bones and ossifies forming bony ankylosis.
   h. Tendons and ligaments around inflamed joints contract.
   i. **Rheumatoid nodules** are small, round, firm subcutaneous nodules that microscopically have a central zone of fibrinoid necrosis surrounded by a prominent rim of histiocytes.
   j. Severe cases may present with **vasculitis.**

3. **Ankylosing spondylitis** is a chronic inflammatory joint disease, likely autoimmune in nature, that is negative for rheumatoid factor.
   a. It usually occurs in young adults.
   b. 90% of affected individuals are **HLA-B27 positive.**
   c. Chronic inflammation leads to fusion of the sacroiliac joint.
   d. Patients seek medical attention complaining of chronic progressive low-back pain.

4. **Reiter syndrome** is the triad of **urethritis, conjunctivitis,** and **arthritis** associated with some intestinal and venereal infections.

5. **Psoriatic arthritis** occurs in 10% of patients with psoriasis.
   a. Histologic features are similar to rheumatoid arthritis.
   b. However, psoriatic arthritis is typically not as severe as rheumatoid arthritis and joint destruction is less frequent.

6. **Inflammatory bowel disease** may present with peripheral arthritis, or ankylosing spondylitis, but patients are usually HLA-B27 negative.

7. **Infectious arthritis** is caused by a variety of different pathogenic organisms and is clinically important because it can lead to rapid joint destruction and deformity.
   a. **Suppurative arthritis** is caused by bacterial infection through hematogenous seeding and is defined by the presence of purulent synovial fluid.
      (1) The most common form of bacterial arthritis is gonococcal arthritis and is most often monoarticular, frequently involving the knee.
      (2) The classic clinical presentation is sudden development of an acutely painful, swollen, warm joint.
      (3) Systemic symptoms may include fever and leukocytosis.

b. **Tuberculous arthritis** is a chronic monoarticular arthritis that usually develops as a complication of adjacent osteomyelitis or from hematogenous seeding.

(1) This form of arthritis can be insidious at onset and systemic symptoms may not be present.

(2) The chronic, progressive nature of this disease can result in severe joint destruction.

c. **Lyme disease–related arthritis** is caused by infection with the spirochete *Borrelia burgdorferi.*

LYME DISEASE

- *Lyme disease is transmitted from rodents to people by* Ixodes *deer ticks and is seen in the United States, Europe, and Japan.*
- *Multiple organ systems are involved.*
- *In stage 1, the spirochetes proliferate within the skin near the bite, causing the characteristic expanding erythema with pale center pattern known as* **erythema chronicum migrans.**
- *In stage 2, the early disseminated stage, the spirochetes enter the bloodstream and may cause lymphadenopathy, joint and muscle pain, cardiac arrhythmias, and meningitis.*
- *In Stage 3, or the late disseminated stage, there is chronic polyarticular arthritis, often with severe joint damage.*

8. **Gout** is caused by the massive deposition of urate crystals (tophi) in the joints and other tissues as a consequence of hyperuricemia.

a. Middle-aged adults are most often affected and acute attacks are often precipitated by a large meal or alcohol consumption.

b. **Podagra** is a term that refers to an acute attack of gout within the metatarsophalangeal joint of the large toe.

c. Diagnostic findings in the synovial fluid include the presence of urate crystals.

d. Biopsy tissue shows tophaceous deposits (urate crystals are **negatively birefringent** under polarized light).

e. Secondary gout is a less common complication of leukemia, multiple myeloma, and other myeloproliferative diseases.

f. **Lesch-Nyhan syndrome** is a rare disease with hyperuricemia and severe neurologic manifestations due to hypoxanthine-guanine phosphoribosyltransferase (HGPRT deficiency).

9. **Pseudogout** (chondrocalcinosis or calcium pyrophosphate crystal deposition disease [CPPD]) is a common disorder characterized by calcium pyrophosphate dehydrate crystal deposition within the joint.

a. Pseudogout occurs in middle-aged adults; can be polyarticular; and most commonly affects the knees, followed by the wrists, elbows, shoulders, and ankles.

b. Calcium pyrophosphate crystals are **weakly birefringent.**

B. Cysts

1. **Ganglion cysts** are nodules of connective tissue degeneration, usually around the wrist and ankle joints that may contain fluid but do not communicate with the joint space.

2. **Synovial cysts** arise from herniation of synovium through a joint capsule or from massive enlargement of a bursa.

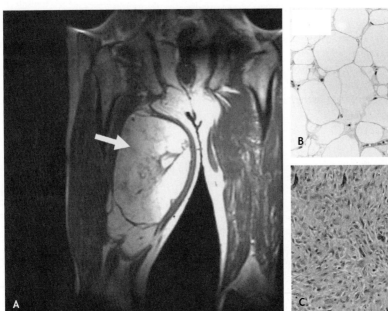
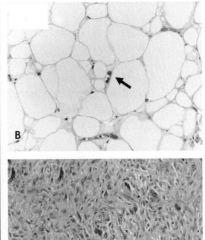

Figure 15–6. Soft-tissue sarcoma. A: MRI of sarcoma of the thigh showing an expansile mass arising within the deep soft tissue. **B:** Many sarcomas in the thigh and retroperitoneum are liposarcomas, which may be well differentiated with adipocytic differentiation and lipoblasts (arrow), or dedifferentiated into a spindle cell tumor. **C:** Pleomorphic sarcoma (also known as malignant fibrous histiocytoma [MFH]) is a high-grade neoplasm of uncertain differentiation.

    a. Synovial cysts are true cysts lined by synovium.

    b. **Baker cyst** is a synovial cyst that forms in the popliteal space in the setting of rheumatoid arthritis.

IV. Soft-Tissue Neoplasms

A. Adipocytic (Fat)

    1. Lipomas are benign mature adipose cell tumors that are the most common soft-tissue tumor in adults.

        a. Lipomas are well-demarcated nodules that are usually soft, mobile, and painless (except for the angiolipoma variant).

        b. They are usually cured by simple excision.

    2. Liposarcomas are malignant tumors of adipose tissue and are one of the most common sarcomas of adulthood.

        a. They usually arise in the deep soft tissues of the proximal extremities and retroperitoneum and are notoriously large.

        b. They are classified as well-differentiated, dedifferentiated, myoxid/round cell and pleomorphic liposarcoma (Figure 15–6).

        c. Prognosis is related to grade and stage.

            (1) Stage 1: Localized low grade, without metastases

(2) Stage 2: Localized small (<5 cm) high-grade tumor

(3) Stage 3: Localized deep and large (>5 cm) high grade

(4) Stage 4: Any tumor with metastases

B. **Fibrous**

1. **Superficial fibromatosis** is a benign nodular proliferation of mature fibroblasts that usually occurs in the palm, foot, and penis.

   a. **Dupuytren contracture** is the name given to the **palmar** variant with nodular thickening of the palmar fascia.

   b. **Peyronie disease** is the name given to **penile** fibromatosis that may cause abnormal curvature of the shaft of the penis.

2. **Deep fibromatoses** (desmoid tumors) are usually large, ill-defined, infiltrative masses similarly composed of fibroblasts.

   a. Desmoid tumors often recur following surgical resection due to their poor circumscription and infiltrative nature.

   b. Intra-abdominal desmoid tumors tend to occur in the mesentery and sometimes are associated with FAP (**Gardner syndrome**).

C. **Fibrohistiocytic**

1. **Dermatofibromas** are common benign skin lesions.

   a. They present as painless, slow-growing, firm, mobile dermal or subcutaneous nodules, typically 1 cm in size.

   b. They are composed of bland spindle cells arranged in a disordered pinwheel-like pattern and may stain for factor 13a.

2. **Dermatofibrosarcomas** are locally aggressive cutaneous tumors.

   a. They are invasive with complex storiform architecture.

   b. Tumor cells immunostain for CD34.

3. **High-grade Pleomorphic Sarcoma** is a malignant undifferentiated neoplasm that usually occurs in the thighs of older adults.

D. **Skeletal Muscle**

1. **Rhabdomyosarcomas** are rare malignant tumors of skeletal muscle.

   a. They usually arise within the head and neck or genitourinary tract of children.

   b. They are classified as embryonal, alveolar, or pleomorphic subtypes.

2. **Embryonal rhabdomyosarcoma** is the most common of the variants and includes sarcoma **botryoides,** a subtype that carries a better prognosis, and characteristically presents as a polypoid, bulky, grape-like mass that protrudes into the vagina of infants.

3. **Alveolar rhabdomyosarcoma** has a worse prognosis and often a characteristic t(2;13) translocation.

4. **Pleomorphic rhabdomyosarcoma** is an aggressive adult sarcoma.

E. **Smooth Muscle**

1. **Leiomyomas** are benign smooth muscle tumors.

   a. They are the most common neoplasm in adult women (usually in the uterine wall, fibroids) but rare in soft tissue.

   b. Leiomyomas are characterized by circumscription, absence of tumor cell necrosis, bland nuclei, and low mitotic index (see Chapter 13).

2. **Leiomyosarcomas** are malignant tumors of smooth muscle and most often occur in adults.

   a. They are characterized by invasion and metastatic potential.

b. They are composed of malignant smooth muscle cells with pleomorphic nuclei, increased mitotic index, and necrosis.

  F. Synovial Sarcomas
    1. Synovial sarcoma is a misnomer; there is no evidence they arise from synovium and are currently categorized as "uncertain origin."
    2. The name arose because they typically arise within deep soft tissues around large joints.
    3. They are usually biphasic with a mixed epithelial:stromal pattern and thin staghorn-like blood vessels.
    4. Diagnosis is supported by identifying the characteristic t(X;18) chromosomal translocation.

CLINICAL PROBLEMS

1. Birbeck granules seen within the cytoplasm of histiocytes by ultrastructural analysis are characteristic of which of the following?

   A. Granulomatous inflammation

   B. Dermatofibroma

   C. Granulocytic sarcoma

   D. Langerhans cell histiocytosis (formerly called histiocytosis X)

   E. Gaucher disease

2. Which of the following features is characteristic of osteoarthritis?

   A. Pannus formation

   B. Heberdon nodes

   C. Baker cyst

   D. Sacroiliitis

   E. Tophi

3. Which of the malignant tumors listed below most commonly presents in children?

   A. Chondrosarcoma

   B. Ewing sarcoma/PNET

   C. Liposarcoma

   D. Leiomyosarcoma

   E. Undifferentiated high-grade pleomorphic sarcoma

4. von Recklinghausen disease of bone is caused by:

   A. Hyperparathyroidism

   B. Hyperuricemia

C. Vitamin D deficiency

D. Fibroblast growth factor receptor 3 (*FGFR3*) gene mutation

E. Increased prostaglandin E production

5. Osteomas of the jaw are associated with which syndrome?

   A. McCune-Albright syndrome

   B. Down syndrome

   C. Lesch-Nyhan syndrome

   D. Neurofibromatosis

   E. Gardner syndrome

6. Which lesion is a palmar variant of fibromatosis characterized by an irregular, nodular thickening of the palmar fascia?

   A. Desmoid fibromatosis

   B. Peyronie disease

   C. Dupuytren contracture

   D. Dermatofibroma

   E. Synovial sarcoma

7. The presence of a bulky, polypoid, grape-like mass protruding from the vagina of a 3-year-old girl should raise concern for which of the following?

   A. Synovial sarcoma

   B. McCune-Albright syndrome

   C. Ewing sarcoma

   D. Embryonal rhabdomyosarcoma

   E. Hand-Schüller-Christian disease

8. An 18-year-old man complains of a subacute onset of knee pain. A radiograph demonstrates an expansile, 10-cm mass arising within the proximal tibia with associated lifting of the periosteum and linear radiating calcifications perpendicular to the bone axis. This mass is concerning for which of the following?

   A. Osteosarcoma

   B. Rheumatoid arthritis

   C. Bone fracture

   D. Osteoid osteoma

   E. Osteomalacia

9. This seronegative spondyloarthropathy is a chronic inflammatory joint disease that typically affects the axial joints (especially the sacroiliac joints) of persons 20-30 years of age, who also test positive for HLA-B27.

   A. Rheumatoid arthritis

   B. Ankylosing spondylitis

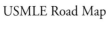

    C. Reiter syndrome

    D. Osteomyelitis

    E. Lyme arthritis

10. Lyme disease is caused by infection with which microorganism?

    A. *Mycobacterium tuberculosis*

    B. *Treponema pallidum*

    C. *Burkholderia cepacia*

    D. *Pseudomonas aeruginosa*

    E. *Borrelia burgdorferi*

ANSWERS

1. The answer is D. Birbeck granules are tennis racket–shaped cytoplasmic structures seen in the Langerhans-like cells of histiocytosis X by electron microscopy.

2. The answer is B. Heberdon nodes are osteophytes at the distal interphalangeal joints of the fingers and are characteristic of osteoarthritis.

3. The answer is B. Ewing sarcoma/PNET is a "small round blue cell" malignant tumor of children that has a characteristic t(11;22) translocation and responds to chemotherapy.

4. The answer is A. von Recklinghausen disease of bone, or osteitis fibrosa cystica, is caused by either primary or secondary hyperparathyroidism and is characterized by widespread osteolytic lesions due to increased osteoclastic activity.

5. The answer is E. Osteomas of the jaw are associated with Gardner syndrome, which also has gastrointestinal polyps and desmoid tumors.

6. The answer is C. Dupuytren contracture is a superficial type of fibromatosis (palmar fibromatosis).

7. The answer is D. This clinical scenario is suggestive of sarcoma botryoides, or embryonal rhabdomyosarcoma, a malignant tumor that typically affects children younger than 5 years of age. This tumor is characterized by a polypoid grape-like mass protruding from the vagina, and carries a better prognosis than other variants of rhabdomyosarcoma.

8. The answer is A. This mass is most concerning for osteosarcoma, which usually arises within the metaphysis of long bones. The peak incidence is between the ages of 10 and 20 years. The classic radiologic appearance is the Codman triangle, caused by lifting of the periosteum by tumor expansion and spiculated sunburst pattern of tumor growth.

9. The answer is B. Ankylosing spondylitis is a chronic inflammatory joint disease that primary affects the axial joints, most commonly the sacroiliac joints. It presents in persons between the ages of 20 and 30 years with symptoms of low back pain and chronic course. The chronic inflammation can lead to rigidity and fixation of the spine resulting from bone fusion (ankylosis). Most patients with this disease test positive for HLA-B27.

10. The answer is E. Lyme disease is most often caused by infection with the spirochete *Borrelia burgdorferi*. This pathogen is transmitted from rodents to humans via the bite of the *Ixodes* deer tick.

CHAPTER 16

CENTRAL NERVOUS SYSTEM, PERIPHERAL NERVES, AND SKELETAL MUSCLE

What a terrible thing to have lost one's mind, or not to have a mind at all.
—Dan Quayle, Vice President of the United States 1988–92

I. Introduction

A. Definitions

1. **Neurons** usually have large nuclei, prominent nucleoli, and abundant basophilic endoplasmic reticulum (Nissl substance).
   a. Lipofuscin is the "garbage" accumulating in aging neurons.
   b. Injury sufficient to cause signs and symptoms of disease are usually associated with neuronal loss and accompanying gliosis (reactive proliferation of glial cells, especially astrocytes).

2. **Glia** are the glue of the central nervous system (CNS).
   a. **Astrocytes** look like "stars" and express glial fibrillary acidic protein (GFAP) and respond rapidly to CNS injury.
   b. **Oligodendroglia** have small dark nuclei; they maintain the myelin sheathing and are therefore abundant in white matter.
   c. **Ependymal** cells are ciliated and line the ventricles.
   d. **Microglial** cells are CNS macrophages.

3. **Meninges** are a fibrous sac encasing the CNS, holding spinal fluid.

B. Developmental Defects

1. **Neural tube** defects are associated with reduced folate levels in the mother.
   a. **Anencephaly** is failed anterior neuropore closure leading to the absence of brain and calvarium.
   b. **Meningomyelocele** is herniation of spinal roots or cord through a posterior neuropore defect.
   c. **Meningocele** is posterior herniation of only meninges.
   d. **Spina bifida** is a failure of posterior vertebral arch fusion and represents the mildest form of neural tube defects.

2. **Holoprosencephaly** is due to a failure of the prosencephalon to cleave into the precursors of the cerebral hemispheres; it is associated with cyclops and is fatal.

3. **Agenesis** of the corpus callosum is often asymptomatic.

C. Trauma

1. **Concussion** is a temporarily altered consciousness.

2. **Contusion** is direct parenchymal injury with hemorrhagic necrosis at the site of trauma (coup injury) and the other side (contra-coup).
3. **Diffuse axonal injury** is caused by shearing stress (eg, shaken baby), and patients are often comatose with poor prognosis.
4. **Cerebral edema** is an increase in the amount of water in the brain due to increased inflow or decreased outflow.
   a. Damage to the **blood-brain barrier** accompanying infections, neoplasms, and stroke is the most common cause of edema.
   b. **Hydrocephalus** is increased cerebrospinal fluid (CSF), which is usually due to obstruction (developmental, neoplasm).
5. **Herniation** results from increased intracranial pressure.
   a. **Uncal herniation** compresses cranial nerve III, leading to ipsilateral pupil dilation and lateral gaze to the side of the lesion.
   b. **Cerebellar tonsillar herniation** through the foramen magnum leads to compression of medullary nuclei and death.

II. Cerebrovascular Disease

A. Global Ischemia
   1. Susceptible areas include **Purkinje cells, hippocampus** pyramidal cells (CA1 sector), and **pyramidal cells** (the third and fifth layers) of the cerebral neocortex.
      a. In the newborn, the susceptible areas to ischemia also include thalamus and pontine nuclei.
      b. Ischemia causes acute cytoplasmic eosinophilic changes (red and dead).
   2. Bilateral border zone (**watershed**) infarcts occur in distal zones of major arterial territories where collateral circulation is poor.
   3. **Respirator brain** refers to the end-stage of global ischemia with widespread necrosis, typically occurring in patients in prolonged mechanical ventilation–dependent comatose state.

B. Focal Ischemia
   1. Cerebral infarct due to ischemic liquefactive necrosis of a defined vascular territory in the brain (eg, middle cerebral artery).
   2. Mechanisms of arterial ischemic infarcts include the following:
      a. In situ atherosclerotic narrowing
      b. **Emboli** from systemic artery (eg, carotid) or heart valve
      c. Systemic disease (eg, **hypertension**)
      d. **Vasculitis** (eg, Behçet syndrome)
      e. Infection (eg, herpes simplex virus [HSV])
      f. **Venous sinus thrombosis,** which can occur in patients with coagulopathy, malignancy, and infection
   3. In the early stages of ischemia, there is diffuse softening of the infarcted territory.
      a. Within days, the dead tissue is discolored and may transform into a hemorrhagic infarct.
      b. Within months to years, there is a progressive cavitation of the infarcted region.
   4. Histologic sections show **red neurons** and neutrophils in acute infarctions with a clear demarcation from the normal adjacent tissue.
      a. This is followed by **macrophage** infiltration and vascular proliferation as well as astrocyte activation.

b. Chronic infarct changes include a meshwork of reactive **astrogliosis** within areas of cystic cavitation.

C. Cerebral Hemorrhage

  1. **Epidural hematoma** is usually from **middle meningeal artery** rupture and is a surgical emergency.

  2. **Subdural hematoma** may be acute or chronic.
     a. Acute cases may be due to trauma or a bleeding disorder.
     b. Chronic cases are due to a past "insignificant" mild trauma, especially in the elderly.

  3. **Subarachnoid hemorrhage** is usually due to congenital berry aneurysms, which occur at the bifurcation of cerebral arteries in the **circle of Willis.**
     a. Sudden death is common after a rupture.
     b. Rebleeding occurs in 50% of cases if not treated.

  4. **Intracerebral hemorrhage** is multifactorial.
     a. Systemic **hypertensive** disease induces Charcot-Bouchard type micro-aneurysms in **basal ganglia,** thalamus, or the brainstem.
     b. Vascular **amyloid** deposits associated with Alzheimer disease leads to superficial intracerebral hematomas.
     c. **Arteriovenous malformations** (AVMs) are common, especially in certain syndromes (eg, **Osler-Weber-Rendu**).
     d. Coagulopathies increase risk of hemorrhage.
     e. Iatrogenic anticoagulation (eg, **warfarin**) increases risk.
     f. Infection (eg, *Aspergillus*) may be angioinvasive.
     g. Metastatic disease (eg, carcinoma, melanoma, choriocarcinoma) leads to hemorrhage.

III. Infections

  A. Meningitis

  1. Acute bacterial infection of the leptomeninges (eg, ***Neisseria gonorrhoeae***) leads to neutrophils in the CSF and may be detected by lumbar puncture, chemistry, culture, and cytology.
     a. The pathogen depends on **patient age** and **immune status.**
     b. Untreated cases lead to involvement of the brain surface with multiple thrombotic infarctions, cerebral edema, diffuse encephalitis, brain abscesses, and death.

  2. **Tuberculosis** may cause caseating **granulomatous** meningitis.
     a. This may lead to hydrocephalus and cranial nerve palsy.
     b. Localized tuberculomas can present as localized mass lesions.

  3. **Neurosyphilis** may be meningovascular (spinal arachnoiditis) and parenchymal (**tabes dorsalis** with general paresis).

  4. **Viral** meningitis is usually self limited and **seasonal**.
     a. Lymphocytes predominate in the CSF by cytology.
     b. It is usually caused by echovirus, coxsackievirus, and mumps.

  5. **Fungal** meningitis may be seen in immunosuppressed patients and is most commonly caused by **cryptococcus.**

  B. Abscess

  1. Bacterial abscesses usually arise from nearby infections, such as sinusitis, otitis media, or thrombi from a **mycotic aneurysm.**

2. Fungi (*Aspergillus, Mucor)* may invade the blood vessel walls (angioinvasive), disseminating into multiple brain abscesses.

3. Toxoplasmosis is usually seen in AIDS patients, presenting as single or multiple intracerebral mass lesions.

C. Encephalitis

1. Viral encephalitis causes chronic inflammation associated with microglial nodules and usually viral inclusion bodies.

   a. HSV encephalitis is the most common cause.

     (1) **HSV-1** causes acute hemorrhagic necrotizing encephalitis with a predilection for the limbic system structures, especially the **temporal lobes**.

     (2) Diagnosis is made by CSF polymerase chain reaction, or brain biopsy revealing **Cowdry A viral inclusions.**

     (3) **HSV-2** or **cytomegalovirus** cause newborn encephalitis.

   b. Eastern equine encephalitis, St. Louis encephalitis, **West Nile**, and others are transmitted via **mosquitoes**, causing diffuse encephalitis without specific viral inclusion bodies.

   c. Primary HIV encephalitis manifests as a chronic progressive dementia with cortical atrophy and myelin rarefaction (pallor).

     (1) HIV is detected in perivascular histiocytes.

     (2) Children may have basal ganglia involvement.

   d. Progressive multifocal leukoencephalopathy from the **JC virus** is multiple demyelinating lesions in immunocompromised patients.

     (1) The JC virus infects the oligodendroglia and induces characteristic intranuclear inclusions.

     (2) Dying oligodendroglial cells lead to demyelination.

   e. Subacute sclerosing panencephalitis is caused by **measles.**

     (1) It leads to a progressive cognitive deterioration in unvaccinated children who have been infected with a replication-defective measles virus.

     (2) Brains show severe involvement of both gray and white matter with neuronal loss, gliosis, and demyelination.

2. Parasites may cause lethal encephalitis and brain injury.

   a. *Naegleria fowleri* is a fresh-water amoeba that may cause primary amebic meningoencephalitis.

   b. *Acanthamoeba* causes a severe acute meningoencephalitis.

   c. Cerebral malaria may lead to hemorrhagic encephalitis.

   d. Cysticercosis (*Taenia solium*) causes cystic lesions.

   e. Echinococcosis may also cause cysts in the liver or lung.

D. Viral Myelitis

1. **Varicella zoster** virus and HSV can involve the spinal ganglia, leading to **painful neuropathy**.

2. **Poliomyelitis** was an epidemic myelitis caused by an enterovirus infecting and killing spinal **motor neurons** in the anterior horn.

3. **HIV** may cause myelitis involving the **thoracic spine**.

E. Prion Disease

1. Insoluble pathologic isoforms of prion protein can be transmitted from diseased individuals, or be inherited as mutant protein, but most occur sporadically.

2. Creutzfeldt-Jakob disease (CJD) involves multiple subsystems of the CNS with **rapidly progressive dementia**, ataxia, and myoclonus.
   a. The disease is usually transmitted from **meat** infected with **bovine spongiform encephalopathy** (mad cow disease).
   b. Sections reveal spongiform change involving the gray matter, reactive gliosis, and neuronal loss.
   c. Since these findings are not entirely specific, definitive diagnosis can be achieved by **immunohistochemical staining** to identify the abnormal prion protein.
  3. Familial forms of prion disease include familial CJD, Gerstmann-Sträussler-Scheinker, and **fatal familial insomnia.**

IV. Demyelinating and Neurodegenerative Diseases

 A. Multiple Sclerosis
  1. Demyelinating diseases lead to loss of salutatory axonal conduction, decreasing or eliminating electrical neuronal signals.
  2. Multiple sclerosis (MS) is the most common demyelinating disorder characterized by **multifocal plaques** that evolve over time.
   a. They are typically adjacent to the **lateral ventricles.**
   b. Active plaques show relative preservation of axons.
  3. Epidemiologic evidence suggests MS may be triggered by exposure to an agent of some kind at a relatively young age; however, there may also be an inherited susceptibility.

 B. Alzheimer Disease
  1. Alzheimer disease is a common dementing illness with **memory loss.**
  2. Definitive diagnosis is made at the time of autopsy.
   a. There is widespread **atrophy** of the cerebrum (Figure 16–1).
   b. Histologic sections show **amyloid plaques,** which are extracellular collections of β-amyloid protein, sometimes with entrapped neuronal processes (neuritic plaques).
  3. All known inherited forms of Alzheimer disease involve mutations involving the amyloid precursor protein, or its processing.
  4. Amyloid plaques are identified by **Congo red stain.**
  5. The distribution and number of neurofibrillary tangles increases with advancing stage of disease.

CLINICAL CORRELATION: "MULTI-INFARCT DEMENTIA"

• *Vascular dementia often progresses in a stepwise fashion and is characterized by cerebral tissue infarction, rather than amyloid.*
• *Over time, this leads to cognitive impairment.*

 C. Pick Disease
  1. Frontotemporal dementia is a clinical syndrome that affects the frontal and temporal lobes preferentially, leading to relatively selective **loss of social inhibitions** and later cognitive loss.
  2. Pick disease is sporadic with characteristic spherical cytoplasmic aggregates (**Pick bodies**).

 D. Parkinson Disease
  1. This movement disorder features reduced facial expression ("masked facies"), stooped posture, rigidity, and tremor.

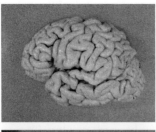
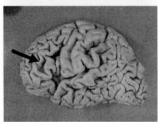
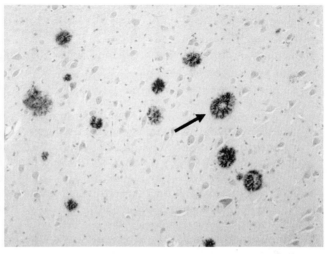

Figure 16–1. Alzheimer disease. The brain on the top left is normal. The one on the bottom is grossly affected by Alzheimer disease with cortical atrophy, shrinkage of the gyri, and enlargement of the sulci (arrow). Histologic sections stained for β-amyloid reveal neuritic plaques.

    2. Symptoms are associated with neuronal loss and gliosis that involves the mid-brain **substantia nigra,** with **Lewy bodies** in surviving pigmented dopamin-ergic neurons.

    3. Rare familial forms are caused by mutations in the *synuclein* gene.

  E. Amyotrophic Lateral Sclerosis

    1. Amyotrophic lateral sclerosis (ALS) affects the upper **motor neurons** of the cerebral cortex and the lower motor neurons of the spinal cord, leading to weakness, muscle atrophy, **fasciculations,** and **spasticity.**

    2. It is usually rapidly progressive and **fatal.**

    3. Most cases are sporadic, but familial syndromes have been linked to muta-tions in the **superoxide dismutase gene.**

    4. There is no treatment to stop progression of the disease.

  F. Trinucleotide Repeat Disorders

    1. These disorders arise from an inherited DNA instability in trinucleotide sequences within a variety of genes.

    2. This leads to a progressive increase in repeat numbers within the inherited allele, which in turn leads to worsening disease in subsequent generations, the so-called "anticipation."

    3. Huntington disease is an **autosomal dominant** disease caused by an expan-sion of polyglutamine sequences in the **huntingtin protein.**

      a. This leads to accumulation of abnormal protein in neuronal nuclei espe-cially in the **caudate nucleus.**

      b. By middle age, this accumulation leads to progressive atrophy and jerky involuntary movements (**chorea**).

    4. Friedreich ataxia is caused by a recessively inherited trinucleotide repeat expan-sion in the gene that encodes **frataxin,** leading to ataxia and sensory neuropathy.

5. **Spinocerebellar ataxia** is an "umbrella" term for a large group of genetically heterogeneous disorders that are characterized clinically by ataxia and additional impairments.

G. **Metabolic Disease**
1. **Leukodystrophies** are dysmyelinating disorders in children.
   a. **Krabbe disease** (autosomal recessive deficiency of galactocerebroside beta-galactosidase) has an early onset and a rapidly progressive course; death occurs within 1 year.
   b. **Metachromatic leukodystrophy** (autosomal recessive deficiency of aryl-sulfatase A) usually manifests within the first 4 years of life with accumulated galacosyl-3-sulfatide in neurons and macrophages, causing brown tissue colorization when stained with cresyl violet ("metachromasia").
   c. **Adrenoleukodystrophy** (X-linked recessive deficiency of peroxisomal enzymes that oxidize long-chain fatty acids) is characterized by variable juvenile and adult onset, central and peripheral demyelination, and adrenal insufficiency.
2. **Mitochondrial encephalomyopathies** are due to defects in mitochondrial function, especially due to abnormalities in mitochondrial proteins.
   a. These can arise due to defects in proteins that are encoded by either nuclear or mitochondrial genes.
   b. Leigh syndrome (**subacute necrotizing encephalopathy**) is characterized by gray matter hemorrhagic necrosis in infants.
   c. Mitochondrial diseases usually have myopathy (see below).

V. Neoplasia

A. **Metastatic Disease**
1. Most malignancies in the brain are metastatic from other sites.
   a. Carcinoma from the lung and breast are most common.
   b. Melanoma and lymphoma/leukemia are also common.

B. **Meningioma**
1. Meningioma arises from the **meningothelial cells** of the craniospinal leptomeninges and arachnoid granulations.
2. Typical sites include olfactory groove, sphenoid wing, parasagittal, tuberculum sella, and foramen magnum.
3. They are slow growing, usually low-grade tumors, in adults.
4. They contrast-enhance by imaging and show a dural tail.
5. Meningioma expresses epithelial membrane antigen (**EMA**).
6. Non-meningothelial tumors can also occur in the meninges, including **hemangiopericytomas,** and skull tumors.
7. Meningiomas are well-circumscribed masses composed of bland epithelioid tumor cells arranged in a **whorling** pattern.
8. Surgery is usually curative.

GRADING PRIMARY CNS NEOPLASMS

- *Grade 1 is slow-growing and curable by surgery (eg, meningioma).*
- *Grade 2 is infiltrative, slow growing, and may transform.*
- *Grade 3 recurs more rapidly, despite therapy.*
- *Grade 4 is very aggressive with multiple recurrences (eg, glioblastoma multiforme).*

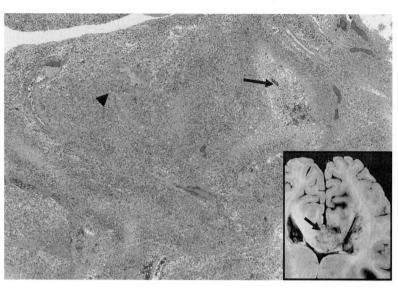

Figure 16–2. Glioblastoma multiforme. The rapidly fatal malignancy involved the corpus callosum (gross inset); it has characteristic palisading of tumor cells around areas of necrosis (arrow) and areas of pronounced angiogenesis (arrowhead).

B. Gliomas
  1. Most adult gliomas are intermediate to high grade and malignant.
     a. They infiltrate the adjacent brain.
     b. Invasive gliomas invariably recur despite chemotherapy and radiotherapy.
  2. **Glioblastoma multiforme** (GBM) is the most common adult glioma.
     a. Patients usually die within 1 year of diagnosis.
     b. GBM may present de novo or progress from an astrocytoma.
     c. Imaging studies reveal a widely invasive malignancy.
     d. Biopsy shows a grade 4 malignancy with conspicuous vascular proliferation (angiogenesis) and characteristic pleomorphic nuclei **pseudopalisading** around areas of necrosis (Figure 16–2).
  3. **Astrocytomas** have features similar to astrocytes (**star-like** cells).
     a. It occurs most commonly in **adults** as a non-enhancing mass with indefinite borders in the white matter.
     b. They are often infiltrative and recur.
     c. Biopsy results show stellate (star-like) tumor cells, sometimes with red cytoplasmic "bellies".
     d. Tumor cells express glial fibrillary acidic protein (**GFAP**) and usually have a p53 mutation in higher-grade lesions.
  4. **Pilocytic astrocytoma** usually occurs in a child's **cerebellum.**
     a. MRI reveals a cyst with a mural nodule.
     b. Surgery is usually curative.
     c. Microscopic features include astrocytes with bipolar piloid (hair-like) processes, and **Rosenthal fibers.**

5. **Oligodendrogliomas** have features similar to oligodendroglial cells.
   a. They constitute only 5–10% of adult gliomas.
   b. They significantly have a **favorable** response to chemotherapy, especially when they have chromosome **1p and 19q deletions.**
   c. They usually present in the frontal or temporal lobes.
   d. They are often calcified.
   e. Histologic sections show characteristic "fried egg" tumor cells with round dark nuclei and abundant clear cytoplasm within a delicate "chickenwire" vascularized stroma.
6. **Ependymomas** have features similar to the ependymal cells lining the ventricles.
   a. It occurs in the fourth ventricle of **children**, and in **lateral ventricles** of adults.
   b. Typical microscopic features are ependymal rosettes and perivascular pseudorosettes.
   c. The extent of surgical resection determines prognosis.
   d. Most recur and some progress to anaplastic ependymoma with seeding metastases into the CSF.

C. Medulloblastoma
   1. Medulloblastoma is a high-grade malignancy, usually located in the **cerebellar vermis** of children.
   2. Biopsy shows a small round blue cell tumor composed of poorly differentiated **neuroectodermal** cells.
   3. The nomenclature changes to primitive neuroectodermal tumor (PNET) if it is supratentorial rather than cerebellar.
   4. Seeding metastasis in the CSF is common and is detected by lumbar puncture and cytology.
   5. Combined chemotherapy and radiotherapy may prolong survival.

D. Germ Cell Tumors
   1. Most are midline and occur in the children and young adults.
   2. Germinoma occurs in the pineal region and is very sensitive to radiotherapy (similar to seminoma in testicle).
   3. Teratoma, yolk sac tumor, and choriocarcinoma are less common.

E. Craniopharyngioma
   1. It is benign, arising from remnants of **Rathke cleft.**
   2. It occurs in the suprasellar region and it is typically calcified.
   3. It may recur if incompletely resected.

F. Pineal Tumors
   1. Pineoblastoma is a PNET of the pineal gland.
   2. Pineocytoma is histologically more mature.

G. Neurocytoma
   1. It presents as a slow-growing calcified mass in the foramen of Monroe or septum pallicidum in the first three decades.
   2. It may recur after surgical treatment.

H. Primary CNS Lymphoma
   1. Primary CNS lymphoma is unusual but may occur in immunosuppressed patients, especially those with AIDS.
   2. Most cases are **diffuse large B cell** lymphomas.

HEREDITARY NEURAL TUMOR SYNDROMES

- *Neurofibromatosis is an autosomal dominant disorder with multiple nerve tissue tumors, cafe au lait spots, and variable expressivity (variable severity).*
- *von Hippel-Lindau syndrome is an autosomal dominant disorder leading to tumors with rich vascular supplies (eg, kidney and cerebellum).*
- *Gorlin syndrome is basal cell carcinoma syndrome that may also develop meningioma or medulloblastoma.*
- *Turcot syndrome is the glioma-polyposis syndrome with adenomatous polyps in the gastrointestinal tract and risk of malignant glioma.*

VI. Nerves

A. Patterns of Nerve Injury
1. **Wallerian degeneration** refers to the degeneration of axons and nerve sheath distal to the point of transaction of a nerve.
2. Regeneration starts from the proximal stump with axonal sprouting and Schwann cell proliferation.
3. Dying-back neuropathy (**distal axonopathy**) starts with a metabolic disturbance in the axon and derangement of axonal transport, which results in degeneration of the distal parts of the axon.
   a. **Metabolic** (diabetes) and **toxic** neuropathies mostly operate as the dying-back mechanism.
   b. There may be recovery, because the distal sheath is intact.

B. Neuropathies
1. Neuropathies are classified according to the size of the nerve, function (motor, sensory, autonomic) and affected element (eg, axon, demyelination), and cause (trauma, entrapment, and so on).
2. **Systemic diseases** may cause neuropathy (eg, diabetes, vasculitis, amyloid, AIDS, Lyme disease, **vitamin B_{12} deficiency**).
3. **Toxins** cause **neuropathy** (eg, lead, cisplatin, arsenic).
4. **Inflammatory demyelinating neuropathy** (eg, **Guillain-Barré**) is a transient neuropathy, rather than chronically progressive.
5. **Paraneoplastic syndrome** and monoclonal gammopathy may cause the so-called immune neuropathy.

C. Peripheral Nerve Biopsy
1. Diagnostic biopsies are usually from the sural nerve for histopathologic evaluation of the presence, etiology, distribution, and severity of polyneuropathy.
2. Disorders such as vasculitis, granulomatous disorders, and amyloidosis may be specifically diagnosed with a nerve biopsy.
3. Primary demyelinating processes may be distinguished from primarily axonal involvement by electron microscopy.
4. Absence of abnormal findings in a sensory nerve may indicate a pure motor neuropathy.

D. Tumors of the Cranial and Peripheral Nerves
1. **Schwannoma** arises from the Schwann cell and forms an encapsulated mass by pushing the axons.
   a. **Acoustic neuroma** is a schwannoma of cranial nerve VIII.

b. Other sites include dorsal nerve roots, and other sensory nerves.
   c. Schwannomas are always benign, and surgery is curative.
2. **Neurofibroma** arises as a neoplastic enlargement of a peripheral nerve, leading to a subcutaneous mass.
   a. Neurofibromas are composed of a mixture of cells, including Schwann cells, perineurial cells, and fibroblasts.
   b. Neurofibromas can occur sporadically, but **plexiform neurofibromas** are pathognomonic for **neurofibromatosis type 1.**
   c. Neurofibromas are benign but can transform into a malignant peripheral nerve sheath tumor, especially in patients with neurofibromatosis type 1.
3. **Malignant peripheral nerve sheath tumor** may occur de novo or may arise in a neurofibroma; it is a high-grade sarcoma with high recurrent and metastatic potential.

VII. Skeletal Muscle Diseases

   A. **Inflammatory Myopathy**
   1. **Dermatomyositis** occurs in children and adults.
      a. Affected patients often have progressive **proximal** symmetric extremity **weakness**, and may have a typical accompanying **rash.**
      b. Older patients with dermatomyositis may have a **malignancy.**
      c. Muscle fiber changes are confined to the periphery of the muscle fascicles (perifascicular atrophy).
      d. Biopsy shows myocyte atrophy and fibrosis (Figure 16–3).
      e. Complement membrane attack complex deposits are seen in capillary walls (see Chapter 1).
   2. **Polymyositis is a necrotizing myopathy** and produces a similar clinical picture to dermatomyositis but does not present with a rash and is more often associated with a connective tissue disorder.
   3. **Inclusion body myositis** is the most common inflammatory myopathy in persons older than age 50.

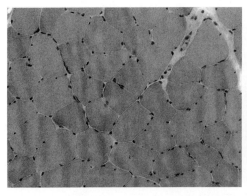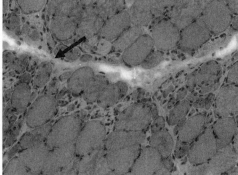

Figure 16–3. Myopathy and muscle biopsies. Compared with normal skeletal muscle (on the left), myopathies show patchy atrophy and fibrosis.

a. It often presents as slowly progressive **combined distal and proximal weakness.**

      b. Biopsy shows typical rimmed vacuoles, amyloid deposits, and inclusion bodies within muscle fibers.

B. Metabolic Myopathy

  1. Pompe disease (glycogenosis type II) is a common recessive disorder of carbohydrate metabolism with a severe infantile and a milder adult form.

      a. The **infantile form** presents as a **hypotonic baby** syndrome with serious cardiac involvement.

      b. Adults show exercise-induced myalgia, fatigue, and weakness.

      c. The defective enzyme is lysosomal alpha-glycosidase.

      d. Muscle biopsy shows glycogen deposits in lysosomal vacuoles.

  2. McArdle disease (myophosphorylase deficiency, type V glycogenosis) is a muscle disorder in adults.

      a. It causes **exercise-induced** cramps and myoglobinuria.

      b. Muscle biopsy shows subsarcolemmal glycogen-filled vacuoles.

  3. Muscle carnitine deficiency induces a slowly progressive limb-girdle myopathy in young adults due to abnormal lipid deposits.

  4. Mitochondrial disorders can be the result of mitochondrial enzyme deficits or mutations in mitochondrial or nuclear DNA.

      a. Manifestations also include ophthalmoplegia and epilepsy.

      b. Syndromes include **Kearns-Sayre syndrome** and **Leigh disease.**

      c. Muscle biopsy shows mitochondrial accumulations in **ragged-red fibers,** absence of cytochrome oxidase by histochemical staining, and abnormal mitochondria by **electron microscopy.**

C. Toxic Myopathy

  1. Statins may cause a range of myopathies, ranging from occasional cramps to necrotizing myopathies and rhabdomyolysis.

  2. Ethanol, amphotericin B, and barbiturates are among agents that can induce rhabdomyolysis.

  3. Zidovudine may cause a secondary mitochondrial myopathy.

D. Muscular Dystrophies

  1. Dystrophies are **genetic myopathies** with a chronic progressive course and variable other systemic findings.

  2. Serum **CK values** are usually **elevated.**

  3. Some dystrophies have a predilection for specific muscle groups.

  4. Most dystrophies are related to mutations of specific genes encoding proteins that are involved in bridging the cytoskeletal function with the extraskeletal matrix.

  5. Duchenne muscular dystrophy is a severe form of **X-linked** muscular dystrophy with early-onset, progressive, symmetric extremity weakness; calf pseudohypertrophy; cardiac involvement; and usually death in the second decade due to respiratory muscle weakness.

      a. Serum CK values are typically very high.

      b. Diagnosis may be made by demonstrating near-total deficiency of **dystrophin** in muscle fiber membranes by immunohistochemical methods, or genetic testing for *dystrophin* gene **mutations.**

      c. Muscle biopsies show progressive loss of myofibers, increased connective tissue, and replacement by adipose tissue.

6. **Becker muscular dystrophy** is an **adult** form with variable clinical course and often partial dystrophin deficiency.
7. **Myotonic dystrophy** type 1 (DM1) is a multisystem disorder with characteristic facies, cardiac and endocrine involvement, **cataracts**, distal extremity atrophy, and myotonia.
   a. Severe neonatal forms occur in children of affected mothers.
   b. The molecular defect is an unstable expansion of a CTG repeat in the untranslated region of a protein kinase.
   c. Muscle biopsy shows a selective atrophy of type 1 fibers.
8. Type 2 myotonic dystrophy affects mostly the type 2 muscle fibers.
9. **Channelopathies** affect subunits of potassium, calcium, and sodium channels and are characterized by episodic and transient weakness.

E. Myasthenia Gravis
   1. An antibody against the **acetylcholine receptor** develops at the postsynaptic membrane of the neuromuscular junction.
   2. It is associated with thymic hyperplasia and **thymoma.**
   3. It presents with episodic weakness, frequent extraocular muscle involvement, **progressive fatigability**, and decremental electromyographic response to repetitive nerve stimulation.
   4. **Lambert-Eaton** myasthenic syndrome is due to an antibody against presynaptic voltage-gated calcium channels in oat cell lung cancer.

CLINICAL PROBLEMS

1. Which of the following would be expected to be an early indication of uncal herniation?
   A. Contralateral hemiplegia
   B. Dilatation of the ipsilateral pupil
   C. Papilledema
   D. Sudden loss of respiratory function
   E. Unilateral loss of hearing

2. Which cells of the CNS are most actively engaged in immune functions?
   A. Neurons
   B. Astrocytes
   C. Microglia
   D. Ependymal cells
   E. Oligodendroglia

3. Which of the following does not reflect a neural tube closing defect?
   A. Anencephaly
   B. Encephalocele
   C. Meningomyelocele

D. Spina bifida

    E. Holoprosencephaly

4. Which of the following areas of the brain is least susceptible to hypoxic/ischemic injury?

    A. Purkinje neurons of the cerebellum

    B. Granular neurons of the cerebellum

    C. The third isocortical layer

    D. CA1 hippocampal neurons

    E. The fifth isocortical layer

5. The most common cause of sporadic viral encephalitis is:

    A. Herpes simplex virus type 1

    B. Herpes simplex virus type 2

    C. West Nile virus

    D Cytomegalovirus

    E. Measles

6. Which of the following statements about Creutzfeldt-Jakob disease is **not** true?

    A. The disease can occur sporadically

    B. The disease can be inherited

    C. The disease is "infectious"

    D. The histologic findings are specific to the disease

    E.　Definitive diagnosis requires immunohistochemistry

7. Which of the following diseases is an example of a tauopathy (neurofibrillary tangles)?

    A. Huntington disease

    B. Creutzfeldt-Jakob disease

    C. Alzheimer disease

    D. Amyotrophic lateral sclerosis (ALS)

    E. Lambert-Eaton syndrome

8. The most common malignancy affecting the CNS is:

    A. Meningioma

    B. Glioblastoma

    C. Oligodendroglioma

    D. Pilocytic astrocytoma

    E. Metastases

9. Which of the following is the most common inflammatory myopathy in patients over the age of 50?

    A. Dermatomyositis

    B. Polymyositis

C. Inclusion body myositis

   D. Toxic myopathy

   E. Muscular dystrophies with inflammation

10. Which of the following statements about muscular dystrophy is false?

   A. They are genetic diseases

   B. Their clinical course is chronic and progressive

   C. Serum CK values tend not to be elevated

   D. Some dystrophies have a predilection for specific muscle groups

   E. Congenital muscular dystrophy causes some hypotonic infant cases

---

ANSWERS

1. The answer is B. Uncal herniation leads to pupil dilation.

2. The answer is C. Microglia are CNS macrophages.

3. The answer is E. Larger neurons are very susceptible to hypoxia, while granular cell neurons are not.

4. The answer is B. Neurons are very susceptible to hypoxia; while granular cells are not.

5. The answer is A. Herpes simplex virus type 1 is the most common cause of viral encephalitis. With global warming and increased mosquito populations, West Nile virus is a growing problem, but not common.

6. The answer is D. Creutzfeldt-Jakob disease can be either inherited or sporadic and may be passed by contact. Immunostaining for the prion protein leads to diagnosis, but histologic features are not specific.

7. The answer is C. Alzheimer disease is the most common tauopathy.

8. The answer is E. Metastatic disease (eg, carcinoma, melanoma, lymphoma) is by far the most common.

9. The answer is C. Inclusion body myositis is more common in the elderly.

10. The answer is C. Serum CK levels are elevated in muscular dystrophy.

CHAPTER 17
LYMPH NODES, BONE MARROW, SPLEEN, AND THYMUS

Conceived of spleen and born of madness...
—William Shakespeare, *As You Like It*

I. Hematopoiesis and Leukopenia

A. Hematopoiesis

1. Prior to birth, the **liver** is the major site of hematopoiesis.
2. By birth, the bone marrow becomes the major site of hematopoiesis.
3. By adulthood, hematopoietic marrow is largely restricted to the vertebrae, ribs, skull, sternum, and pelvis.
   a. In the **bone marrow,** the pluri-potential stem cell gives rise to the common lymphoid and common myeloid progenitors.
   b. Under the influence of granulocyte/monocyte-colony stimulating factor (**GM-CSF**), myeloid progenitors mature to neutrophils in 7–10 days.
4. Every day the bone marrow produces about $50–100 \times 10^9$ neutrophils.
   a. Approximately 5% of neutrophils circulate and 60% are marginated in the spleen and along the blood vessel walls.
   b. Mature neutrophils circulate in the blood for 3–12 hours before migrating into tissues where they live for 2–3 days.
   c. Clinical ranges of absolute neutrophil counts (ANCs) follow:
      (1) Adults normal range: $1.5–7.0 \times 10^3/mm^3$
      (2) Neonates and infants: $2.5–7.0 \times 10^3/mm^3$
      (3) Mild neutropenia: $1.0–1.5 \times 10^3/mm^3$
      (4) Severe neutropenia: $<0.5 \times 10^3/mm^3$

B. Leukopenia

1. **Agranulocytosis** is severe neutropenia.
   a. Causes of neutropenia vary with patient age.
   b. In the neonate, it is usually due to **infection,** maternal drug treatment, or maternal antibody production.
   c. In an infant or child, it is due to infection, drug reactions, and **neoplasms** replacing the bone marrow.
   d. In adults, it is due to drug reaction, infections, neoplasms replacing the bone marrow, and **myeloablative therapies.**

2. **Mechanisms** causing neutropenia are multifactorial.
   a. A **proliferation defect** is a decrease of early myeloid progenitors due to premature destruction caused by toxins, immune destruction, **chemotherapy**, radiation, marrow fibrosis, or a genetic aberration.
   b. A **maturation defect** occurs in **megaloblastic anemias,** such as folate or **vitamin B_{12} deficiency.**
   c. A **survival defect** has normal production and release of neutrophils, but they are rapidly removed from circulation, most often due to **infection.**
   d. A distribution abnormality can occur in **hypersplenism** and in patients with defective release of neutrophils from the marrow.
3. **Lymphocytopenia** means decreased numbers of lymphocytes.
   a. Children have higher lymphocyte counts than adults.
   b. T-cells are the majority of peripheral blood lymphocytes; therefore, most lymphocytopenias are T-cell related.
   c. The causes are multifactorial (Table 17–1).

II. Reactive Proliferation

A. Reactive Lymphoid Hyperplasia

1. Lymphadenopathy is the term to describe enlargement of a single lymph node or group of lymph nodes.
2. In most children and young adults, enlarged lymph nodes are usually a benign reaction to an offending agent (Table 17–2).
3. The frequency of malignant lymph nodes increases in older adults.
   a. Painless firm and mobile lymph nodes suggest lymphoma.
   b. Firm fixed lymphadenopathy suggests metastatic carcinoma.

FINE-NEEDLE ASPIRATION BIOPSY

- *Fine-needle aspiration (FNA) is a minimally invasive means to biopsy enlarged lymph nodes and provide a diagnosis.*
- *Samples may be submitted for culture and molecular testing to evaluate for infection.*
- *Samples may be submitted for flow cytometry to evaluate for lymphoma.*
- *Samples may be stained for antigens to determine origin of carcinoma.*

Table 17–1. Causes of lymphocytopenia.

Severe combined immunodeficiency disease (SCID)	Rheumatoid arthritis
Congenital thymic aplasia (DiGeorge syndrome)	Systemic lupus erythematosus
Wiskott-Aldrich syndrome	Myasthenia gravis
Nutritional deficiencies (eg, protein, zinc)	Systemic diseases
HIV	Sarcoidosis
Influenza	Hodgkin lymphoma
Hepatitis	Renal failure
Tuberculosis	Radiation
Autoimmune disorders	Anti-lymphocyte globulin
	Corticosteroid therapy
	Chemotherapeutic agents

Table 17–2. Common causes of lymphadenopathy.

Anatomic Location	Cause
Occipital	Scalp infections, scalp cancer
Posterior auricular	Rubella
Anterior auricular	Eye infections
Posterior cervical	Cat-scratch disease, malignancy
Anterior cervical	Upper respiratory infections
Submental	Oral infections, malignancy
Supraclavicular	Usually malignant
Mediastinal	Sarcoidosis, malignancy
Axillary	Dermatopathic, malignancy
Retroperitoneal	Usually malignant
Inguinal	Herpes, gonorrhea, malignancy

   4. Surgical excision may be required for definitive diagnosis.
       a. Reactive lymph nodes show the characteristic nodular follicular hyperplasia with prominent germinal centers (Figure 17–1) and conspicuous tingible body macrophages.
       b. If follicular lymphoma is suspected, flow cytometry and immunostaining are used to evaluate for neoplasia.
   B. **Leukocytosis**
       1. It is most commonly due to increased **neutrophils** but can be due to increased levels of other white blood cells.
       2. Leukocytosis is multifactorial.
           a. Most are associated with **bacterial** infections.
           b. **Drugs,** such as corticosteroids, may cause leukocytosis.
           c. Tissue **necrosis** (eg, infarction) causes leukocytosis.
           d. **Metabolic** causes include ketoacidosis and uremia.
           e. **Stress,** exercise, pregnancy, and smoking cause leukocytosis.
       3. Demargination from blood vessels occurs within minutes.
       4. Mobilization from tissues occurs within hours of stimulus.
       5. Increased production requires days of sustained stimulation.
       6. Peripheral blood smears show increased numbers of neutrophils.
           a. There is often a maturation "**left shift,**" which means less mature neutrophil bands, metamyelocytes, and few myelocytes.
           b. The neutrophils may show purple granules and pale blue inclusions (**Dohle bodies**).

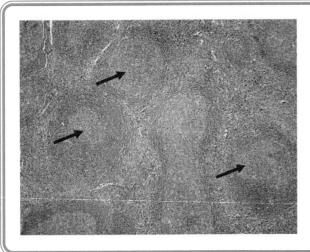

Figure 17–1. Reactive follicular hyperplasia. Prominent germinal centers (arrows) with tingible body macrophages that are rimmed by small lymphocytes characterize a reactive lymph node.

    7. Lymphocytosis is predominantly composed of **T-cells** and fewer numbers of B-cells and NK cells.

      a. Epstein-Barr virus (EBV) is a classic cause of lymphocytosis.

        (1) EBV infects B-cells in the oropharynx, which produce the heterophil antibody (basis of **Monospot test**).

        (2) The infected B-cells disseminate throughout the reticuloendothelial system and provoke an intense T-cell–mediated hyperplasia, including splenomegaly.

      b. Transient stress lymphocytosis is seen in patients with trauma, myocardial infarction, status epilepticus, as well as other acute conditions.

    8. Monocytosis is usually caused by chronic infection or autoimmune disease (eg, collagen vascular disease).

    9. Eosinophilia is usually related to allergic and atopic disorders such as asthma, atopic dermatitis, and allergic rhinitis.

      a. However, it may also be a sign of autoimmune disorders such celiac disease, vasculitides, and inflammatory bowel disease.

      b. Pulmonary disorders such as **Löffler syndrome** and **Churg-Strauss syndrome** are characterized by eosinophilia.

III. Neoplasia

    A. World Health Organization (WHO) Classification of Lymphoid Neoplasms

      1. Lymphoma describes lymphoid neoplasms that form discrete tissue masses without significant peripheral blood or marrow involvement.

      2. Leukemia describes lymphoid neoplasms involving bone marrow AND peripheral blood.

      3. The WHO classification of lymphoid neoplasms distinguishes five categories based on cell of origin.

        a. Precursor B-cell acute lymphoblastic leukemia (ALL) is the most common malignancy in children.

        b. Precursor T-cell ALL is less common (15% of cases)

        c. Peripheral B-cell lymphomas are common and diverse.

Table 17–3. Immunophenotype of mature B-cell lymphomas.

Lymphoma	CD20	CD10	CD5	CD23	BCL6	CD103
Follicular	+	+	−	−	+	−
Large B-cell	+/−	+/−	+/−	−	+	−
Mantle cell	+	−	+	−	−	−
MALT	+	−	−	−	−	−
Burkitt	+	+	−	−	+	−
CLL	+	−	+	+	−	−
Hairy cell	+	−	−	−	−	+

CLL, chronic lymphocytic leukemia; MALT, mucosa-associated lymphoid tissue.

     d. Peripheral T-cell and NK-cell lymphomas are uncommon.
     e. Hodgkin lymphoma has a bimodal distribution (young, old).
  B. Follicular Lymphoma
    1. Follicular lymphoma is common and usually occurs in **older adults** (median age 60 years old).
    2. It presents as **painless lymphadenopathy** (eg, groin, axilla, or neck), but many cases also have bone **marrow involvement** (40%).
    3. The organs (spleen) and peripheral blood are not usually involved.
    4. FNA of a mass lesion with flow cytometry reveals a **CD20** positive B-cell lymphoma with coexpression of the germinal center marker **CD10** and clonal light chain restriction (Table 17–3).
      a. Low-grade lymphoma is predominantly small lymphocytes.
      b. High-grade lymphoma is predominantly large lymphocytes.
      c. It may be difficult to distinguish high-grade follicular lymphoma from diffuse large B-cell lymphoma.
      d. Definitive classification and grading usually involves surgical excision of the lymph node for histologic examination.
    5. Histologic sections reveal a nodular (follicular) pattern similar to reactive lymphoid hyperplasia (Figure 17–1), but the follicular centers lack tingible body macrophages and show poorly formed mantle zones around the germinal centers.
      a. Immunostaining sections for **BCL-2** distinguishes reactive follicular hyperplasia from follicular lymphoma (neoplastic B-cells in the follicular centers are positive for BCL-2; reactive B-cells are negative).
      b. This is because most cases (>90%) have the **(14;18)** **translocation,** which pairs the IgH promoter on chromosome 14 to the **BCL-2 gene** on chromosome 18, leading to **overexpression** of *BCL-2* in neoplastic cells.
    6. Low-grade follicular lymphoma has an indolent course.
      a. Low-grade elements persist and may transform to diffuse large B-cell lymphoma (30–50% of cases).
      b. The median survival is about 10 years from diagnosis.

C. **Diffuse Large B-cell Lymphoma (DLBCL)**
1. DLBCL is **common** (40% of non-Hodgkin lymphomas) and may occur at any age, although most cases arise in older adults.
2. It presents as a rapidly enlarging mass at nodal or extranodal sites, including the gastrointestinal (**GI**) **tract** (most common) and the central nervous system (**CNS**).
3. FNA and flow cytometry reveal a population of large clonal B-cells that may also express CD10 and BCL-6, similar to high-grade follicular lymphoma and Burkitt lymphoma.
4. Surgical excision of the mass lesion shows **diffuse replacement** of normal tissue architecture by large B-cells with **large nuclei** that are $> 3\times$ the size of a normal lymphocyte.
5. 10–20% have the t(14;18) translocation.
6. It is distinguished from follicular lymphoma by the absence of a small cell component and from Burkitt lymphoma by proliferation index and karyotype.

D. **Mantle Cell Lymphoma**
1. Mantle cell lymphoma is uncommon (3–10% of non-Hodgkin lymphoma).
2. The median age is 60 years, and more men are affected than women.
3. It presents as painless lymphadenopathy, often involving the **GI tract,** and may involve **Waldeyer tonsillar ring.**
4. FNA and flow cytometry reveal CD20 positive B-cells that express **CD5** but are negative for CD23 (unlike CLL) and CD10 (unlike follicular lymphoma).
5. Surgical excision of the mass lesion shows architectural effacement by intermediate-sized lymphocytes.
   a. Tumor cells characteristically immunostain for **cyclin-D1.**
   b. This is because they have the **(11;14) translocation,** which couples the heavy chain promoter on chromosome 14 to the cyclin-D1 gene on chromosome 11, leading to overexpression.

E. **Marginal Zone Lymphoma**
1. It may be nodal or extranodal.
   a. Extranodal marginal zone lymphoma usually arises in *mucosa associated lymphoid tissue* (**MALT).**
   b. MALT lymphoma is associated with chronic inflammatory states such as *Helicobacter pylori* **infection** (stomach), **Sjögren syndrome** (salivary or lacrimal glands), and **Hashimoto thyroiditis.**
2. Biopsy reveals small- to medium-sized cells infiltrating around reactive germinal centers in a marginal zone distribution.
3. Flow cytometry reveals a clonal population of CD20 positive B-cells lacking CD5, CD23, and CD10.
4. The lymphoma is **low grade,** indolent, and usually sensitive to therapy (eg, treat the *H pylori* and it may go away).
5. Rare cases may transform to diffuse large B-cell lymphoma.

F. **Burkitt Lymphoma**
1. This high-grade lymphoma has three variants:
   a. **African** (endemic) Burkitt lymphoma occurs in **children** (4 to 7 years old); it often presents as a mass in the **mandible.**
   b. **Sporadic** (nonendemic) Burkitt lymphoma is seen throughout the world and occurs in children and **young adults;** it most often presents as an **abdominal** mass.

c. Burkitt lymphoma associated with **immunodeficiency** has an increased rate in patients with **HIV.**

2. Visible involvement of peripheral blood and bone marrow is uncommon and portends a worse prognosis.

3. Surgical biopsy reveals complete effacement of tissue architecture by sheets of medium-sized lymphoma cells with characteristic baby blue cytoplasm and intermixed macrophages, creating a so-called "**starry sky**" appearance (Figure 17–2).

4. All forms of Burkitt lymphoma are associated with translocations that dysregulate the *MYC* gene on chromosome 8.
    a. The most common translocation is **t(8;14).**
    b. Others are t(8;22) and t(8;2).

5. **EBV infection** is identified in all endemic forms, 25–40% of HIV associated, and 15–20% of sporadic cases.

6. Endemic and sporadic forms are very aggressive but respond well to chemotherapy and are **curable.**

TUMOR LYSIS SYNDROME

- *Treatment and necrosis of high-grade lymphomas may lead to hyperuricemia, hyperkalemia, hyperphosphatemia, lactic acidosis, and hypocalcemia, leading to acute renal failure.*
- *The greater the tumor burden, the higher the risk.*
- *It may be treated with allopurinol (inhibits xanthine oxidase), urinary alkalinization (uric acid solubility), and hydration.*

    G. Chronic Lymphocyte Leukemia (CLL)/Small Lymphocytic Lymphoma (SLL)

1. SLL and CLL are identical, except SLL (a lymphoma) involves lymph nodes and/or spleen and CLL (a leukemia) involves blood and bone marrow.

2. CLL is the **most common leukemia** in the United States and Europe.
    a. Most patients are >50 years old.
    b. Men are affected nearly twice as often as women.

3. Most patients are asymptomatic, but some may have fatigue, infection, splenomegaly, hepatomegaly, or lymphadenopathy.

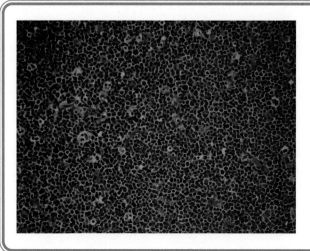

Figure 17–2. Burkitt lymphoma. There are sheets of medium-sized B-cells obliterating normal lymph node architecture. Tumor cells have a very high mitotic index and conspicuous macrophages create a "starry sky."

4. FNA and flow cytometry of an involved lymph node shows small low-grade B-cells with **CD5+/CD23+** coexpression.

5. Surgical biopsy shows diffuse effacement of lymph node architecture by small, monomorphic, lymphocytes with clumped "**soccer ball nuclei**" and occasional larger pro-lymphocytes. CLL cells are fragile and can break apart and smear, forming characteristic **smudge cells.**

6. Most cases (80%) have abnormal cytogenetics by FISH analysis.
   a. **Trisomy 12,** 11q deletions, 17p deletions are most common.
   b. 11q and 17p deletions confer a worse prognosis.

7. The clinical course is indolent and incurable with a median survival of 5–10 years.

8. CLL may transform to DLBCL, so-called **Richter syndrome.**

H. **Hairy Cell Leukemia**
   1. Hairy cell leukemia is **rare** (<2% of non-Hodgkin lymphoma).
      a. Median age is 55 years old.
      b. There is a significant male bias (5:1).
   2. Patients have **splenomegaly,** pancytopenia, recurrent infections, and vasculitis.
   3. Common sites of involvement include the **spleen** and **bone marrow.**
   4. Surgical biopsy reveals medium-sized lymphoid cells with circumferential hairy projections that immunostain for **CD103.**
   5. Disease follows an indolent course with good response to therapy.
   6. Splenectomy may also induce prolonged remission.

I. **Plasma Cell Neoplasms**
   1. Clonal plasma cell proliferations include multiple myeloma, solitary plasma-cytoma, monoclonal gammopathy of undetermined significance (MGUS), and Waldenström macroglobulinemia.
   2. **Multiple myeloma** is the most common and deadly of these diseases.
      a. It is the most common lymphoid malignancy in blacks.
      b. The median age at diagnosis is 70 years.
      c. It usually presents with vertebral pain and infection.
      d. Diagnosis requires multiple clinical features, including **lytic bone lesions,** clonal **M-protein** in the blood (most are IgG), or biopsy proven clonal plasma cell proliferation.
      e. Monoclonal light chains (kappa or lambda) are known as the **Bence Jones protein**, which may be present in the **urine** and are toxic to renal tubular cells culminating in renal failure.
      f. Bone marrow biopsy reveals a clonal proliferation of **CD38/CD138 positive** plasma cells, which comprise greater than **30%** of the overall marrow cellularity.
      g. Plasma cells are mature and contain cytoplasmic inclusions.
         (1) **Mott cell** contains multiple grape-like inclusions.
         (2) **Russell bodies** are Ig cytoplasmic inclusions.
         (3) **Dutcher bodies** are Ig nuclear inclusions.
      h. Multiple myeloma is **not curable** with a median survival of 3 years and less than 10% 10-year survival, despite current drug therapies and bone marrow transplantation.
   3. Solitary **plasmacytoma** is a single mass lesion of clonal plasma cells, lacking the other systemic features of myeloma.

a. A significant percentage of cases progress to myeloma.

b. Some cases are cured by resection and chemotherapy.

4. MGUS is a premalignant and indolent disease that shows serum M-protein and a clonal proliferation of mature plasma cells in the bone marrow (<10% of marrow cells), but does not warrant a diagnosis of multiple myeloma.

a. Smoldering multiple myeloma is an intermediate phenotype.

b. The risk of progression from MGUS to myeloma is 1%/year.

5. Waldenström macroglobulinemia (also called lymphoplasmacytic lymphoma) presents with a serum M-protein composed of **monoclonal IgM,** which can increase the viscosity of the blood.

a. It is rare and indolent with a median age of 63 years old.

b. Hyperviscosity syndrome may be presenting manifestation.

c. It is not curable with a median survival of 5 years.

HYPERVISCOSITY SYNDROME

- *Hyperviscosity syndrome is a consequence of increased blood viscosity due to increased serum proteins.*
- *It can be seen in multiple myeloma but is more often present in association with Waldenström macroglobulinemia.*
- *Symptoms include visual impairment, neurologic problems, bleeding, and cryoglobulinemia.*
- *Treatment for severe cases is plasmapheresis.*

J. T-cell and NK-cell Lymphoma

1. Mature T-cell lymphomas are derived from post-thymic T cells.

2. Because NK-cells have similar immunophenotypic features (similar surface antigen expression) they are grouped with T-cell neoplasms.

3. Characteristic features are summarized in Table 17–4.

4. Mycosis fungoides is a type of T-cell lymphoma that predominantly **involves the skin.**

a. Skin lesions show migration of the lymphoma cells into the epidermis, so-called "**epidermitropism.**"

Table 17–4. Features of T-cell lymphomas.

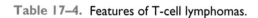

Diagnosis	Clinical Features	Pathology	Prognosis
NK T-cell lymphoma	Destructive mass in nasopharynx	CD3+/CD56+/EBV+	Aggressive Poor
Peripheral T-cell	Lymphadenopathy and skin rash	Eosinophils; clonal T-cell receptor rearrangement.	Aggressive Poor
Anaplastic large cell lymphoma	Lymphadenopathy and "B-symptoms" (eg, high fever)	"Hallmark" cells – large horseshoe shaped nucleus- Rearrangements involving ALK–I.	Favorable in patients with ALK rearrangements.

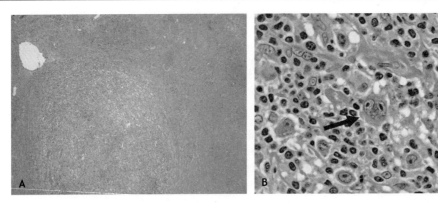

Figure 17–3. Hodgkin lymphoma. A: Low power microscopic view shows a nodular sclerosing pattern, which is the most common variant of Hodgkin lymphoma. **B:** Characteristic Reed-Sternberg cell (arrow) in a background of mixed inflammatory cells, including neutrophils and eosinophils.

      b. **Pautrier abscesses** are characteristic aggregrates of lymphoma cells with irregular "cerebriform" nuclei that occur in the epidermis.

      c. There is also usually a band-like lymphoma infiltrate in the superficial dermis.

    5. Sézary syndrome is the **leukemic** form of mycosis fungoides.

      a. Tumor cells are present in blood.

      b. It is indolent with median survival of 10 years.

  K. Classical Hodgkin Lymphoma

    1. Hodgkin lymphoma has characteristic **Reed-Sternberg cells.**

      a. Reed-Sternberg cells are derived from germinal center B-cells and are characterized by 2 nuclear lobes with large red nucleoli and abundant cytoplasm (Figure 17–3).

      b. Reed-Sternberg cells are typically positive for CD30 and negative for CD45.

    2. There is a **bimodal age** distribution with peaks at 15–35 years and after the age of 50.

    3. Clinical features include lymphadenopathy, "**B symptoms**" (fever, night sweats, weight loss), and rarely involvement of organs (usually spleen) or bone marrow.

    4. FNA and flow cytometry are not informative unless Reed-Sternberg cells are identified in the smears, warranting excisional biopsy of the suspicious lesion.

    5. Histologic sections of the mass lesion reveal characteristic Reed-Sternberg cells in a mixed inflammatory background.

    6. Nodular sclerosing type is most common (70%) and shows characteristic thick bands of fibrosis (Figure 17–3).

  L. Hodgkin Lymphoma, Lymphocyte Predominant Type

    1. This type is less common (5% of cases).

    2. It may lack Reed-Sternberg cells

    3. Instead, this type has mononuclear 'popcorn cells' that may express CD20 (B-cell marker).

Table 17–5. Clinical staging of Hodgkin and non-Hodgkin lymphomas.

Stage	Definition
I	Involvement of a single lymphoid tissue (eg, lymph node, spleen, thymus, Waldeyer tonsillar ring)
II	Involvement of multiple lymphoid tissues on the same side of the diaphragm
III	Involvement on both sides of the diaphragm
IV	Disseminated involvement

4. Hodgkin lymphoma is usually **curable** with radiation and chemotherapy (>90% of stage 2 disease is cured; 70% of stage 4).
5. **Stage** is related to lymphoma distribution (Table 17–5).

M. **Acute Lymphoblastic Leukemia**
1. 75% of cases occur in **children** <6 years old.
2. Clinical features include bone marrow failure with thrombocytopenia (**bleeding**), neutropenia (**infection**), and **anemia.**
3. Biopsy shows small to medium blasts with scant cytoplasm, condensed to dispersed chromatin, and indistinct nucleoli.
4. Flow cytometry of bone marrow biopsy reveals blasts that frequently express **TdT (expressed only in pre-B and pre-T lymphoblasts),** CD19 (since most are B-cell), and CD10.
   a. Precursor **T-cell ALL** (CD3+) is less common (15% of cases) and usually arises in the thymus of **adolescent males.**
   b. Recall the four **terrible Ts** of the anterior mediastinum (**T-cell leukemia, thymic** carcinoma, **teratoma,** and **thyroid**).
5. Cytogenetics often reveals a high association of pre-B ALL in infancy with translocations involving *MLL* **gene** on **chromosome 11.**
6. Most cases (80%) are cured in the pediatric population.
   a. Poor prognostic factors include age <2 years or >10 years.
   b. **Philadelphia chromosome t(9;22)** involving *BCR-ABL* **genes** is seen in some cases.

N. **Myelodysplastic Syndromes**
1. Myelodysplastic syndromes (MDS) are a group of clonal hematopoietic bone marrow diseases characterized by **dysplasia** (ringed sideroblasts, bilobed Pelger-Huet neutrophils, mononuclear megakaryocytes) and **ineffective hematopoiesis.**
2. Myeloblasts may be present but account for **<20% blasts.**
3. Typically, patients have peripheral blood cytopenias and hypercellular bone marrows for their age.
4. Prevalence increases with age, about 1/50,000 in 70-year-olds.
5. Prognosis is generally poor with median survival of 3 years.

> a. Some patients suffer from sequelae of bone marrow failure.
> b. Patients often get multiple red cell transfusions.
> c. About 30% of patients progress to **acute leukemia.**

REFRACTORY ANEMIA WITH EXCESS BLASTS

CLINICAL CORRELATION

- *Patients commonly have fatigue, macrocytic anemia, and neutropenia.*
- *Bone marrow biopsy is hypercellular for age.*
- *Erythroid and myeloid precursors are dysplastic with 10% blasts.*
- *Cytogenetics may show part of chromosome 7 deleted.*

> **N. Chronic Myeloproliferative Diseases (CMD)**
>   1. Chronic myeloproliferative diseases (CMD) are a group of clonal hematopoietic bone marrow diseases characterized by proliferation in the bone marrow of one or more myeloid cell lines.
>   a. CMD typically shows hypercellular bone marrow, but, unlike MDS, the peripheral blood in CMD has increased hematopoietic cells.
>   b. For example, in **chronic myelogenous leukemia (CML),** which is a type of CMD, the peripheral blood has increased neutrophils and there may be **extramedullary hematopoiesis** in the **liver** and **spleen** causing hepatosplenomegaly.
>   c. Myeloblasts may be present, but similar to CMD, blasts are less than the 20% required for a diagnosis of acute leukemia.
>   2. CMD is most common in middle aged and older adults; patients have fatigue, weight loss, night sweats, and splenomegaly.
>   3. Other than CML, other subtypes of CMD include **essential thrombocythemia,** which presents with high platelet counts and atypical megakaryocytes; **chronic idiopathic myelofibrosis,** which is a proliferation of megakaryocytic and granulocytic cells in the marrow and evolves to marrow fibrosis; **polycythemia vera,** which is characterized by uncontrolled production of red cells.
>   4. **JAK2** is a cytoplasmic tyrosine kinase that is abnormal in most cases of polycythemia vera and occasionally in other CMD cases; it provides a potential targeted therapy for these diseases.

CLINICAL CORRELATION "CHRONIC MYELOGENOUS LEUKEMIA AND GLEEVEC"

CLINICAL CORRELATION

- *CML provides a model for new targeted therapies that rely on understanding molecular pathways.*
- *The Philadelphia Chromosome t(9;22) results in the BCR gene on chromosome 22 to be fused to the ABL on chromosome 9, creating an abnormal tyrosine kinase, which is the target for new and effective targeted therapies such as STI571, or Gleevec.*

> **O. Acute Myelogenous Leukemia (AML)**
>   1. The differences between acute and chronic myeloid malignancies is an **aggressive** clinical course and **>20% blasts.**
>   2. Acute myelogenous leukemia usually presents in adults as anemia or thrombocytopenia, or both.
>   a. It is rare (3/100,000).
>   b. The median age of onset is 60 years old.
>   c. **Radiation** (Hiroshima) and **cytotoxic therapy** (alkylating agents for chemotherapy) increase the risk of AML.

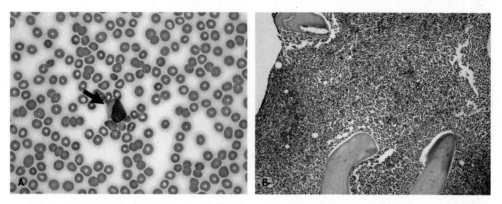

Figure 17–4. Leukemia. A: A blood smear from a patient with leukemia shows a blast (arrow) with an Auer rod. **B:** A bone marrow biopsy reveals a hypercellular marrow filled with blasts.

3. **Granulocytic sarcoma,** or chloroma (green tumor), is a mass lesion of myeloid blasts that may be a presenting feature of AML; they may be solitary or multi-focal and usually arise beneath the periosteum of the skull, spine, and ribs.

4. Diagnosis is made by **biopsy, flow cytometry,** and **cytogenetics.**

   a. AML may be classified by blast morphology (Figure 17–4).

   b. Immunophenotype, which can be ascertained by flow cytometry and im-munostains on tissue biopsies, helps classify AML.

   c. Increasingly important are assays that identify genetic abnormalities; bal-anced chromosomal translocations have a more favorable prognosis (eg, t(8;21)(q22;q22);(*AML1/ETO*)).

   d. AML with inversion or **inv(16)**(p13q22) generally has a favorable prog-nosis and is associated with granulocytic differentiation and abnormal looking **eosinophils.**

   e. Acute promyelocytic leukemia (**APL**) typically has prominent and numer-ous **Auer rods**; patients may already have disseminated intravascular coag-ulation (**DIC**) by the time they seek medical attention, but respond well to all-trans **retinoic-acid** due to the **t(15;17) RAR-PML fusion.**

   f. AML with multi-lineage dysplasia usually occurs in elderly patients and has an unfavorable prognosis.

5. Most patients achieve **remission** with chemotherapy, but <25% remain free of disease.

P. Langerhans Cell Histiocytosis

   1. Langerhans cell histiocytosis is a neoplastic proliferation of immature **den-dritic cells,** which express **CD1a** and **S-100.**

   2. **Birbeck granules** (tennis-rackets) are seen by electron microscopy.

   3. **Letterer-Siwe disease** is multifocal histiocytosis.

      a. It occurs in infants.

      b. Presents as skin lesions resembling seborrheic dermatitis.

      c. Untreated disease is fatal.

      d. With chemotherapy, survival is 50%.

4. **Eosinophilic granuloma** is a mass lesion of Langerhans tumor cells within the medullary cavity of bones (eg, **skull,** ribs, femur).
   a. Tumor cells are intermixed with numerous eosinophils (hence the name), plasma cells, and neutrophils.
   b. It is a relatively **benign lesion** that usually occurs in **children** and young adults.
   c. It may **spontaneously resolve** within 1–2 years of diagnosis.
   d. Otherwise, curettage to relieve mass effects is curative.
5. **Hand-Schüller-Christian** disease is the combination of skull lesions causing mass effects, including **exophthalmos** and compression of the posterior pituitary stalk leading to **diabetes insipidus.**
   a. Most cases **spontaneously regress.**
   b. If needed, chemotherapy ameliorates mass effects.

IV. Spleen

A. Splenomegaly
1. The spleen filters blood, removing senescent or abnormal cells.
2. Normally, the spleen weighs approximately 150 g.
3. The cut surface reveals pale specks representing the white pulp in histologic sections.
   a. **Red pulp** represents the sinuses filled with blood.
   b. **White pulp** represents lymphoid centers.
4. An accessory spleen associated with the pancreas is a very common congenital anomaly.
5. The spleen enlarges in response to congestion (**cirrhosis),** infection (eg, **mononucleosis),** portal or splenic vein **obstruction,** myeloid malignancies (eg, **CML or polycythemia vera),** autoimmune disease (eg, systemic lupus erythematosus), and storage diseases (eg, Gaucher disease).
6. A large spleen in turn may sequester blood elements leading to multiple **cytopenias,** which may be treated by splenectomy.

B. Splenic Infarction
1. Infarction occurs when the splenic artery becomes occluded, usually from emboli originating from **thrombi** in the heart.
2. Emboli may also be from tumors or infection.

C. Splenic Rupture
1. The most common cause is blunt force **trauma.**
2. Spontaneous rupture may present in patients with splenomegaly associated with infection (mononucleosis, **malaria),** and malignancy.
3. Splenic rupture results in massive blood loss and **shock** requiring immediate splenectomy to stop the bleeding.

D. Neoplasia
1. The spleen is rarely the site of primary malignancy.
2. Benign tumors include fibromas and hemangiomas (cavernous type).

V. Thymus

A. Development
1. The thymus is the site of **T-cell maturation.**
2. It is located in the anterior mediastinum.

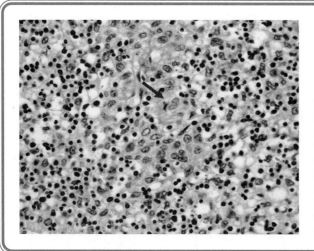

Figure 17–5. Thymoma. Benign thymoma resembles normal thymic tissue, or thymic hyperplasia, but is encapsulated; as it enlarges, it causes mass effects on surrounding mediastinal structures. They are often associated with myasthenia gravis.

3. At birth, it weighs 30 g and continues to grow until adulthood, reaching a maximum weight of 50 g; thereafter, it **involutes.**
4. Histologic sections show cytologically bland thymic epithelial cells in a background of small round lymphocytes.

B. **Developmental Disorders**
1. **Thymic hypoplasia** or aplasia is associated with **DiGeorge syndrome.**
2. Thymic cysts are common and are usually incidental.
3. **Thymic hyperplasia** describes an enlarged gland for age with hyperplastic lymphoid follicles; it is often associated with **myasthenia gravis.**

C. **Neoplasia**
1. Benign thymoma may be cortical or medullary.
   a. **Cortical thymoma** resembles thymic hyperplasia (Figure 17–5).
   b. **Medullary thymoma** resembles a spindle cell neoplasm.
2. **Invasive thymoma** resembles cortical thymoma, but penetrates the capsule of the gland and infiltrates surrounding tissues (eg, lung).
3. **Thymic carcinoma** has a malignant epithelial component, resembling squamous cell carcinoma, or lymphoepithelial carcinoma.
4. All thymic neoplasms are tumors of adults.
   a. Most present because of mass effects.
   b. About 33% of cases are associated with **myasthenia gravis.**

CLINICAL PROBLEMS

1. A 40-year-old female smoker has an elevated lymphocyte count on a routine complete blood count. What are the likely findings by flow cytometry?

A. A clonal B-cell population is present

B. CD4 T cells are reduced

C. CD4 T cells are increased

D. NK cells are elevated

E. There is a proportional increase in B-cells, which are polyclonal

2. A 13-year-old girl presents with sore throat, fatigue, and cervical adenopathy. Which of the following findings do you NOT expect?

A. Complete blood count shows a lymphocytosis

B. Peripheral smear review shows atypical (reactive) lymphocytes

C. Liver function tests are elevated

D. A heterophil antibody is detected

E. The patient reports recent exposure to a neighbor's cat

3. A 65-year-old man has a leukocytosis. Which of the findings would argue against a reactive neutrophilia?

A. Peripheral smear review shows toxic granulation

B. Neutrophils have Dohle bodies

C. Peripheral smear review shows neutrophil bands and metamyelocytes

D. The absolute neutrophil count is $120.0 \times 10^3/mm^3$

E. The patient has a fever and a productive cough

4. Which of the following is *incorrect* about AML:

A. In adults, AML is more common than ALL

B. Some AML blasts have inv(16) associated with eosinophilia

C. WHO includes "AML with recurrent genetic abnormalities"

D. Diagnosis of AML generally requires at least 30% blasts

E. APL is closely associated with t(15;17) and many Auer rods

5. A 65-year-old man complains of increasing fatigue. Complete blood counts show that he has had a macrocytic anemia for the past 8 months, but his white blood cell count and differential and platelet count are normal. Some neutrophils on his peripheral blood smear are Pelgeroid. He takes no prescription medications. Cytogenetic studies on his bone marrow show 10% of cells have a part of chromosome 7 deleted. Which of the following is the best answer?

A. He likely has a JAK2 positive chronic myeloproliferative disease

B. His marrow is hypercellular and he has AML

C. His marrow is hypercellular and he has MDS

D. His marrow is hypocellular and he has AML

E. His marrow is hypocellular and he has MDS

6. A 50-year-old woman is found to have a white blood cell count of 150,000 cells/mcL consisting mostly of mature neutrophils, as well as a basophilia and a mild thrombocytosis. Red cells and platelets are unremarkable. Which of the following is the best answer?

A. The patient has AML with inv(16)

B. The patient has acute promyelocytic leukemia with DIC

C. The patient has CML with t(15;17)

D. The patient has CML with t(9;22)

E. The patient has a JAK2 positive chronic myeloproliferative disease

7. All of the following are associated with a poor prognosis in pre-B acute lymphoblastic leukemia EXCEPT which of the following?

A. Age less than 2 years old

B. t(9:22) (Philadelphia chromosome)

C. Presentation in adolescence

D. Hyperdiploidy

E. Elevated blast count in peripheral blood

8. A 68-year-old African American man complains of low back pain. Radiographs show multiple lytic lesions in the lumbar vertebra. Laboratory studies demonstrate anemia as well as a serum M-protein. What additional clinical feature is characteristic of this disease?

A. Serum monoclonal IgM

B. Free light chains in urine

C. Splenomegaly

D. Hyperviscosity syndrome

E. Lymphadenopathy

9. A 48-year-old woman shows lymphocytosis on complete blood cell count. Review of the peripheral smear showed numerous small, mature appearing, monomorphic lymphocytes and smudge cells. She does not have anemia, and her platelet count is normal. What is the most likely diagnosis?

A. Mantle cell lymphoma

B. Chronic lymphocytic leukemia (CLL)

C. Acute lymphoblastic leukemia

D. Follicular lymphoma

E. Marginal zone lymphoma

10. An 18-year-old man complains of shortness of breath. Radiograph demonstrates a large mediastinal mass. Biopsy of the mass shows a mixed inflammatory infiltrate with occasional larger cells having two nuclear lobes and prominent eosinophilic nucleoli. What is the diagnosis?

A. Precursor T-cell acute lymphoblastic leukemia/lymphoma (pre-T ALL)

B. Nodular lymphocyte predominant Hodgkin lymphoma

C. Classic Hodgkin lymphoma

D. Thymoma

E. Diffuse large B-cell lymphoma

ANSWERS

1. The answer is E. This is a case of persistent polyclonal B-cell lymphocytosis. Flow cytometry is a diagnostic modality that permits the evaluation of antigens on individual cells using specific monoclonal antibodies conjugated to fluorochromes. A polyclonal B-cell population will have both kappa and lambda light chains.

2. The answer is E. This history is a classic presentation of infectious mononucleosis. The laboratory findings include an atypical lymphocytosis, positive Monospot, and mild hepatitis (elevated liver function tests).

3. The answer is D. Neutrophilias in excess of $100 \times 10^3/mm^3$ are often neoplastic. The other choices are associated with reactive neutrophilias.

4. The answer is D. The diagnosis of AML generally requires 20% blasts in marrow or blood according to the World Health Organization. The requirement under the older FAB classification scheme was 30% blasts. There are some special cases, like the presence of t(8;21) or inv(16), a diagnosis of AML might be made with less than 20% blasts.

5. The answer is C. There is no evidence that the patient has AML. The clinical history of a refractory anemia, the evidence of dysplasia (Pelgeroid neutrophils) and the deletion of part of chromosome 7 are good evidence of MDS. Most MDS marrows are hypercellular. Even if the patient has 20% of marrow cells with a deletion of part of chromosome 7 it does not mean that there are 20% blasts because in MDS non-blast cells have cytogenetic abnormalities.

6. The answer is D. The patient likely has leukemia. It is most likely CML, which has the t(9:22) involving the *BCR/ABL* fusion gene (known as the Philadelphia chromosome). CML is typically accompanied by a basophilia and a mild thrombocytosis. There are no increased numbers of blasts, precluding a diagnosis of AML. There is no evidence of DIC, and the WBC of 150,000 cells/mcL is mostly mature neutrophils and not promyelocytes. There is no mention of abundant Auer rods as seen in APL with its typical t(15;17). Although CML is a chronic myeloproliferative disease (MPD), it is not associated with JAK2 mutations as are polycythemia vera, essential thrombocythemia, and idiopathic myelofibrosis.

7. The answer is D. Hyperdiploidy, age between 2 and 10, low white count, and early pre-B phenotype are associated with a favorable prognosis. Age less than 2 and greater than 10, the presence of specific cytogenetic abnormalities including the Philadelphia chromosome, and a high blast count at presentation confer a worse prognosis.

8. The answer is B. This patient has multiple myeloma. Free light chains in the urine are seen in approximately 75% of multiple myeloma patients called Bence Jones proteinuria. A serum monoclonal IgM is commonly associated with Waldenström macroglobulinemia and only rarely seen in multiple myeloma. Splenomegaly and lymphadenopathy are not characteristic.

9. The answer is B. Neoplastic lymphocytes in chronic lymphocytic leukemia (CLL) have a tendency to break apart and form characteristic smudge cells. Whereas other lymphomas can involve the blood, it is less likely than CLL, which is the most common cause of a neoplastic lymphocytosis. The lymphocytes are mature, while ALL would look immature.

10. The answer is C. The large cells with two nuclear lobes and prominent eosinophilic nucleoli are Reed-Sternberg cells characteristic of classic Hodgkin lymphoma. These would stain with CD15 and C30, but not CD45. Nodular lymphocyte predominant Hodgkin lymphoma has L&H cells, a variant of the Reed-Sternberg cells that would be CD20 positive and negative for CD15 and likely negative for CD30. The other entities listed do not demonstrate the histologic features described.

CHAPTER 18
BLEEDING DISORDERS AND TRANSFUSION MEDICINE

All bleeding stops eventually . . .
—aphorism

I. Red Cells

A. Anemia

1. The World Health Organization defines anemia as a serum hemoglobin level less than **13 g/dL** for men and less than **12 g/dL** for women.
    a. Approximately 2.5% of the population is anemic.
    b. This proportion is higher among preterm infants, menstruating women, and the elderly.

2. The severity of symptoms, range from fatigue and dyspnea to intermittent claudication and angina.

3. **Claudication** is cramp-like pain, particularly in the calf or thighs, that intensifies with exertion and resolves with rest.

4. Physical findings include **pallor,** tachycardia, and murmurs.

5. Compensation includes increased cardiac output, redistribution of blood flow, and lowered hemoglobin oxygen affinity.
    a. Slowly evolving anemia allows sufficient time for these physiologic adjustments and may mask the presence of hemolysis or hemorrhage.
    b. Rapid large-volume loss increases the risk of low blood pressure, oliguria, and multi-organ system failure.

6. Anemia is further classified by specific red cell indices as summarized in Table 18–1 with associated diagnoses.
    a. **Mean corpuscular hemoglobin concentration (MCHC)** is obtained by dividing the hemoglobin concentration by the hematocrit; the usual reference range is 32–36 g/dL.
    b. **Mean corpuscular volume (MCV)** is an average red cell volume.
        (1) 80–100 femtoliters (fL) is considered normal.
        (2) Because MCV is an average, it may not identify a mixed population of undersized and excessively large cells.

7. The more common etiologies of anemia may be grouped as either blood loss, impaired production, or enhanced destruction (hemolysis).

Table 18–1. Classification of anemia by red cell morphology.

Microcytic Anemia (MCV < 80 fL)	Normocytic Anemia (Normal)	Macrocytic Anemia (MCV > 100 fL)
Iron deficiency	Chronic disease	Vitamin B$_{12}$ Deficiency
Thalassemia	Hemolytic anemia	Folate deficiency

  B. **Blood Loss**
  1. As its name implies, **acute posthemorrhagic anemia** is due to blood loss over a short period of time (minutes to hours).
  2. The subsequent shift of third space fluid into the vascular compartment leads to a **normocytic anemia.**
  3. Otherwise healthy individuals may tolerate acute blood losses of 10–15% of total blood volume (500–700 mL in adults).
     a. Acute losses in excess of 20% of blood volume cause postural hypotension, and patients are frequently symptomatic.
     b. Symptoms and signs of hemorrhagic shock occur when short-term blood losses reach 30–40% of blood volume; under these circumstances, red blood cell (RBC) transfusion is warranted.

ESTIMATING BLOOD LOSS

- *A drop in hematocrit of three points is equivalent to 500 mL of blood.*
- *Hematocrit does not fall instantaneously after an acute bleed.*
- *Normal or only mildly abnormal results immediately following hemorrhage can be misleading and may delay appropriate therapy.*

  C. **Impaired Production**
  1. **Iron deficiency** is the most common cause of anemia; it is seen in 20% of women of childbearing age and in 2% of men.
     a. The lack of available iron, whether due to insufficient intake, **menstrual losses,** or **chronic gastrointestinal bleed,** limits hemoglobin synthesis.
     b. Iron requirements increase during pregnancy and lactation.
     c. Disorders with reduced intracellular hemoglobin, such iron deficiency and thalassemia, tend to be **microcytic anemia.**
     d. Aside from microcytosis noted on a complete blood cell (CBC) count, other clues to iron deficiency anemia include decreased serum iron, serum **ferritin,** and transferrin saturation, while total iron-binding capacity **(TIBC) is increased.**
  2. Anemia of **chronic disease** also involves impaired iron use.
     a. It is observed with chronic infections, rheumatologic diseases, neoplasms, and other debilitating chronic illnesses associated with inflammation.

b. The inflammatory cytokines hobble iron metabolism and promote resistance to erythropoietin.

c. While anemia of chronic disease may share some features of iron deficiency (**microcytosis** in half of cases, low serum iron, decreased percentage saturation, and increased free RBC protoporphyrin), the **TIBC is decreased.**

3. **Megaloblastic anemia** results from **vitamin B$_{12}$** or **folate** deficiency.

a. These cofactors are required for DNA synthesis, and when they are deficient, nuclear maturation is defective.

b. Immature cells are destroyed before leaving the bone marrow.

c. **Autoimmune gastric atrophy** leads to decreased production of intrinsic factor that, in turn, hampers vitamin B$_{12}$ absorption, causing **pernicious anemia.**

   (1) Intrinsic factor is measured by the **Schilling test.**

   (2) Inadequate dietary intake is noted among the **elderly.**

   (3) It is also observed among chronic **alcoholics** with poor nutrition or during pregnancy.

d. It is characterized by **macrocytic anemia** with a reduced reticulocyte index, an abnormal Schilling test (if pernicious anemia), and low serum vitamin B$_{12}$ or folate levels.

SCHILLING TEST

- *The Schilling test involves the use of radiolabeled vitamin B$_{12}$ to trace the gastrointestinal absorption and renal excretion.*
- *Diminished urinary excretion (less than 7% over 24 hours) may be due to either pernicious anemia or malabsorption.*
- *Increased excretion of the labeled vitamin B$_{12}$ with intrinsic factor is diagnostic of pernicious anemia.*

4. **Bone marrow failure** leads to severe normocytic anemia, which requires a bone marrow biopsy for definitive diagnosis.

a. **Diamond-Blackfan anemia** is a congenital chronic pure RBC aplasia presenting in infancy.

b. **Aplastic anemia,** by contrast, results from a failure of all three hematopoietic cell lines.

   (1) Constitutional forms of aplastic anemia include **Fanconi anemia,** and Shwachman-Diamond syndrome.

   (2) Acquired aplastic anemia may be idiopathic or secondary to medications (chemotherapy), toxins, and infections.

c. **Neoplastic infiltrates** displace normal hematopoietic tissue.

D. Hemolysis

1. **Hemolytic anemia** results from RBC destruction.

a. Regardless of the location, the initial response to hemolysis is increased RBC production (reticulocytosis); however, when RBC loss exceeds capacity, anemia results.

b. **Intravascular hemolysis** is marked by **hemoglobinemia,** hemoglobinuria, hemosiderinuria, and low haptoglobin.

c. **Extravascular hemolysis** elevates levels of **serum bilirubin** and lactate dehydrogenase (LDH).

Table 18–2. Differential diagnosis associated with red blood cell shape.

Disease	RBC Shape
Hereditary spherocytosis	Spherocytes
Megaloblastic anemias and myelofibrosis	Ovalocytes
Fibrin deposition disorders	Schistocytes
Iron deficiency, liver disease, thalassemic syndromes, and hemoglobinopathie	Target cells
Myelofibrosis; severe iron deficiency	Dacrocytes (teardrops)

2. **Hereditary spherocytosis** is an autosomal dominant defect of the erythrocyte membrane protein **spectrin** that limits RBC deformability, leading to splenic mediated hemolysis (Table 18–2).
   a. It is the most common RBC membrane disorder (1:5000).
   b. Laboratory findings include spherocytes, elevated MCHC, and **increased osmotic fragility.**
3. **Hereditary elliptocytosis** is an autosomal dominant defect of cytoskeletal structural proteins that results in large numbers of elliptical RBC with less resistance to shear forces.
   a. Nearly all of these patients (90–95%) are asymptomatic.
   b. The increased prevalence of this condition among patients with **African** and **Mediterranean** ancestry is a legacy of malaria.
   c. At least 25% of the RBCs are normochromic elliptocytes on a peripheral blood smear, but unlike hereditary spherocytosis, the osmotic fragility is normal.
4. **Glucose-6-phosphate dehydrogenase (G6PD) deficiency** is an X-linked defect in oxidative phosphorylation.
   a. The enzyme catalyzes the oxidation of glucose-6-phosphate to 6-phosphogluconate while simultaneously reducing the oxidized form of nicotinamide adenine dinucleotide phosphate ($NADP^+$) to nicotinamide adenine dinucleotide phosphate (NADPH).
   b. NADPH is required for multiple biosynthetic reactions, especially maintaining **glutathione** in its reduced form.
   c. An inability to reduce $NADP^+$ to NADPH upstream of glutathione conversion predisposes cells to oxidative damage.
   d. Exposure to **fava beans, sulfa antibiotics,** and **nitrofurantoin** increases oxidative stress and may precipitate hemolytic crises.
   e. As with hereditary elliptocytosis, this condition is also more common among those of Mediterranean ancestry in whom shortened RBC lifespan once conferred a relative advantage against malarial parasites.
   f. "**Bite cells**" and RBCs with **Heinz bodies** (clumps of denatured hemoglobin) are present on a peripheral smear.

5. **Pyruvate kinase deficiency** is a common autosomal recessive disorder affecting an enzyme critical for glycolysis and adenosine triphosphate production in RBCs.
   a. Because of their dependence on anaerobic metabolism, any impairment of the glycolytic pathway shortens the RBC lifespan (normally around 120 days).
   b. Severity varies from an asymptomatic chronic anemia to severe hemolytic anemia requiring transfusions in childhood.
6. **Autoimmune hemolytic anemia** occurs with immunoglobulin-mediated destruction of host RBCs by host antibodies.
   a. **Warm autoimmune hemolytic anemia** is mediated by **IgG** antibodies directed against universal **Rh antigens** causing hemolysis and transfusion-dependent chronic anemia.
      (1) It is associated with **lupus,** chronic lymphocytic leukemia, **Evans syndrome,** and medications (methyldopa).
      (2) Laboratory findings include spherocytes on peripheral smear and a positive direct antibody test (DAT).
   b. **Cold autoimmune hemolytic anemia** is mediated by **IgM** antibodies that react at cold temperatures and can result in **ABO** typing discrepancies.
      (1) These antibodies may cause cold agglutinin syndrome or paroxysmal cold hemoglobinuria (PCH).
      (2) There are spherocytes and a positive DAT.
7. **Microangiopathic hemolytic anemia** stems from intravascular hemolysis as RBCs are shredded by fibrin strands attached to injured endothelial beds.
   a. **Aortic stenosis** is the most common association.
   b. It may also be associated with hemolytic uremic syndrome (HUS), **thrombotic thrombocytopenic purpura** (TTP), disseminated intravascular coagulation (DIC), HELLP (*h*emolysis, *e*levated *l*iver enzymes, and *l*ow *p*latelet count)syndrome, eclampsia, heparin-induced thrombocytopenia, and sepsis.
   c. **Schistocytes** and nucleated RBCs are present in blood.
8. **Paroxysmal nocturnal hemoglobinuria** results from a rare acquired hematopoietic stem cell mutation of **phosphatidylinositolglycan A (*PIG-A*)** gene on the X chromosome.
   a. A decrease in this anchoring protein limits the expression of both decay-accelerating factor **(DAF** or **CD55)** and membrane inhibitor of reactive lysis **(MIRL** or **CD59).**
   b. Ordinarily, these proteins inhibit complement-mediated intravascular hemolysis.
   c. A decline in these protective factors leaves affected RBCs vulnerable to premature rupture leading to **red urine.**
   d. The diagnosis was once based on increased RBC lysis in acidified serum **(Ham test)**; however, **flow cytometry** is now used to identify the absence of DAF (CD55) and MIRL (CD59).
9. **Drug-induced hemolysis** is an under diagnosed yet medically significant cause of hemolysis and anemia.
   a. RBC destruction may be immune- or nonimmune-mediated.
   b. In **immune-mediated hemolysis,** the drug usually binds the RBC, acts as a **hapten,** and stimulates antibodies that target the drug-RBC combination.

(1) Occasionally, immune complexes of drugs and antibodies nonspecifically bind to the RBC and lead to "innocent bystander" hemolysis.

(2) It is associated with the use of **penicillins** and **cephalosporins.**

   c. In **nonimmune-mediated hemolysis,** the drug has a direct toxic effect on RBCs; underlying genetic variations, such as G6PD deficiency, predispose patients to this type of hemolysis.

10. In **infection-induced hemolysis,** the mechanism of RBC destruction varies with specific actions of the pathogen.

   a. These include physical rupture from accumulation of intracytoplasmic parasites, RBC breakdown by bacterial hemolysins, and host-mediated immune RBC destruction directed against bacterially modified RBC antigens.

   b. Several pathogens and infections cause hemolysis.

     (1) **Malaria** is a massive public health issue, and hemolysis and anemia are features of infection.

     (2) Hemolysis also occurs in **babesiosis** and occasionally complicates infections with *Clostridium perfringens, Streptococcus pneumoniae* and *Haemophilus influenzae.*

     (3) Three members of the herpesviridae (varicella-zoster virus, cytomegalovirus, and Epstein-Barr virus) are also sometimes associated with hemolytic anemia.

   c. The routine work-up consists of CBC with smear evaluation, LDH, bilirubin, urinalysis, and microbial culture (to varying degrees based on suspected agent).

E. **Hemoglobinopathies**

1. Normal hemoglobin is a tetramer composed of four globin chains each of which is linked to an iron-chelating porphyrin (heme).

   a. The genes encoding the various types of globin are located on chromosomes 11 and 16, and the relative expression of these genes varies with age.

   b. **Embryonic hemoglobin** is two zeta and two epsilon chains.

   c. **Fetal hemoglobin** (hemoglobin F or HbF) is composed of two alpha chains and two gamma chains.

   d. After birth, the relative proportion of HbF declines as normal **adult hemoglobin** (HbA), made of two alpha and two beta chains, rises (Table 18–3).

   e. **Variant hemoglobin,** HbA_2, has a delta chain rather than beta.

   f. Over 900 hemoglobin variants are known, and they all may cause anemia by one of several mechanisms.

     (1) The hemoglobin molecule may be structurally abnormal as in hemoglobin S (HbS) or hemoglobin C (HbC).

     (2) Subunit production may be impaired (eg, thalassemia).

2. **Hemoglobin S** is a point mutation within the β-globin gene that limits RBC deformability and causes hemolytic anemia.

   a. The mutation is more common in persons of African ancestry.

   b. Heterozygotes (S trait) are mostly asymptomatic with reduced susceptibility to malaria.

   c. Homozygotes (SS) experience clinically variable ischemia, organ damage, and pain.

   d. HbS aggregates under lower oxygen tension and creates the characteristic **sickle cell** erythrocyte.

Table 18–3. Hemoglobin variants.

Type	Composition or Alteration	Relative Abundance
Normal		
A	$\alpha_2\beta_2$	95–98%
A_2	$\alpha_2\delta_2$	2–3.5%
F (fetal)	$\alpha_2\gamma_2$	<0.5%
Abnormal		
β chain		
S	*Valine at codon 6 of β chain (β^S)*	1:625 / African, eastern Mediterranean, Middle Eastern
C	Lysine at codon 6 of β chain (β^C)	1:5900 / West African
E	Lysine at codon 26 of β chain (β^E)	Southeast Asian: Thai and Khmer most affected

   e. The impaired cellular plasticity limits microcirculation and leads to tissue damage in areas served by affected vasculature.
   f. Through its effects on circulation, sickle cell disease has several potential clinical manifestations.
      (1) Vascular occlusion **crises** include cerebral infarcts, angina, renal papillary necrosis, priapism, avascular necrosis of the femoral head and other bones.
      (2) Severe anemia is caused by RBC destruction.
      (3) Infection, particularly by encapsulated organisms (*H influenzae* and *S pneumoniae*), is common among patients with functional **asplenia** secondary to ischemic splenic damage.
   g. Screening involves the sickle solubility test and confirmation with hemoglobin electrophoresis.
3. **Hemoglobin C** (HbC) shares many similarities with HbS; it is also the result of a point mutation that reduces RBC deformability and causes normocytic anemia.
   a. Hemoglobin C trait is a relatively benign disorder found in persons of **West African** descent.
   b. Hemolysis dominates the clinical picture in homozygotes but is not as severe as with SS disease.
   c. When C trait combines with S trait (hemoglobin SC), retinal vascular lesions are worse.
   d. Laboratory evaluation includes both a CBC and hemoglobin electrophoresis.

Table 18–4. Clinical presentation of α-thalassemia.

Type	Genotype	Laboratory	Clinical
Silent carrier	−α/αα	RBC indices usually normal	Normal
α Trait	−α/−α or −−/αα	Microcytic, increased RBC	Usually normal
Hb H disease	−−/−α	Microcytic, increased RBC, inclusion bodies	Mid anemia, splenomegaly, icterus
α-Hydrops fetalis	−−/−−	Anisocytosis, poikilocytosis	Intrauterine or neonatal death

RBC, red blood cell.

4. **Hemoglobin E** (HbE) disease stems from a relatively common β-globin mutation among **Southeast Asians** (prevalence can reach 30–40%).
   a. The mutation reduces synthesis of the abnormal β-globin, and when paired with a normal hemoglobin allele, the imbalance mimics the clinical features of β-thalassemia.
   b. HbE results in a heterogeneous group of disorders whose phenotype range from asymptomatic to severe.
5. **α-Thalassemia** is due to a **deletion** of one or more α-globin genes that decreases α-globin production (Table 18–4).
   a. The excess unpaired beta and gamma chains form the nonfunctional, unstable tetramers **hemoglobin H** and **hemoglobin Bart's,** respectively.
   b. Clinical impact worsens with the number of affected genes.
   c. Bone marrow hyperplasia leads to skeletal deformities.
   d. The mutation is most common in the Mediterranean and Asia.
   e. CBC may show microcytosis and hypochromasia.
6. **β-Thalassemia** refers to a group of disorders that result from a variable genetic deficiency in β-globin synthesis.
   a. It is also more common in the Mediterranean and Asia.
   b. Clinical presentation is summarized in Table 18–5.
   c. In contrast to α-thalassemia, most forms of β-thalassemia are point mutations rather than complete gene deletions; suppression of β-globin expression varies from no expression ($\beta 0$) to variable deficiency ($\beta +$).
   d. The laboratory findings are similar to α-thalassemia.
      (1) Patients have an increased hemoglobin A_2 (>2.5%) and a decreased fraction of hemoglobin A (<97.5%).
      (2) In 30% of cases, fetal hemoglobin is elevated.

II. Platelets

A. Normal
   1. Platelets are an essential element of primary hemostasis.
   2. They arrest initial bleeding by forming a plug and induce clotting to stabilize the plug (thrombin burst).

Table 18–5. Clinical presentation of β-thalassemia.

Type	Genotype	Laboratory Features	Clinical
β–Thalassemia minor (Trait)	β/β0; β/β+	Microcytic, increased RBC, target cells, elevated HbA_2, HbF	Usually normal, but mild anemia can occur
β–Thalassemia Intermedia	β+/β+	Same as with trait	Non-transfusion dependent anemia
β–Thalassemia major (Cooley anemia)	β+/β+ β0/β+ β0/β0	Microcytosis, schistocytes, nucleated RBCs	Transfusion-dependent anemia, splenomegaly, bone deformities,

RBCs, red blood cells.

    3. Normal platelet count is 150,000 to 400,000/mcL.
      a. Counts less than 10,000/mcL are associated with spontaneous hemorrhage.
      b. Counts less than 50,000/mcL are associated with excessive bleeding.
    4. Defects may be quantitative or qualitative (Table 18–6).
    5. Medications may inhibit platelet function to prevent thrombosis (eg, aspirin suppresses the production of prostaglandins and thromboxanes, decreasing platelet aggregation).
  B. Thrombocytopenia
    1. It often presents as an abrupt drop in platelet count.

Table 18–6. Clinical disorders of platelets.

Quantitative Platelet Disorders	Qualitative Platelet Disorders
Drug-induced thrombocytopenia	Uremia
Bone marrow failure	von Willebrand disease
Hypersplenism	Bernard-Soulier syndrome
Disseminated intravascular coagulation	Glanzmann thrombasthenia
Idiopathic thrombocytopenic purpura	Myeloproliferative disorders
Thrombotic thrombocytopenic purpura	Drugs and dietary supplements
Hemolytic uremic syndrome	Postcardiac bypass platelet dysfunction
Viral infections	

2. Signs and symptoms include petechial hemorrhages and ecchymoses following unexplained fever, nausea, lightheadedness, and vomiting.
3. There are two main mechanisms leading to thrombocytopenia.
    a. **Medications** (eg, methotrexate) may **impair marrow function.**
    b. **Peripheral destruction** may be accelerated with drugs, including heparin, valproic acid, and vancomycin.
4. Platelet count is the cornerstone of diagnosis.
    a. Platelet factor 4 enzyme-linked immunosorbent assay (ELISA) is used to rule out **heparin-induced thrombocytopenia.**
    b. A complex of heparin and platelet factor 4 incites an antibody response to platelets.
5. If the causative agent is identified and discontinued, symptoms often resolve within a few days, and the platelet count returns to normal within a week.
6. **Idiopathic thrombocytopenic purpura** is a diagnosis of exclusion.
    a. Also known as immune thrombocytopenic purpura, many cases are attributed to IgG antibodies directed against platelet membrane **glycoproteins IIb-IIIa or Ib-9.**
    b. Antibody coating facilitates subsequent **opsonophagocytosis** by splenic macrophages.
    c. Despite this activity, there is no splenic enlargement.
    d. Bleeding may range from bruising to cerebral hemorrhage.
    e. Treatment aims to boost the platelet count(corticosteroids or intravenous immunoglobulin) and limit consumption (splenectomy).
    f. Immunosuppression (azathioprine, mycophenolate mofetil, rituximab, or vincristine) is increasingly being used.
    g. Platelet transfusion is not indicated except in cases of profuse, potentially life-threatening hemorrhage.
7. **Thrombotic thrombocytopenic purpura** is a rare life-threatening multisystemic disorder characterized by **disseminated microthrombi.**
    a. In most cases, a deficiency or inhibition of **ADAMTS13** permits the accumulation of multimeric **von Willebrand factor.**
    b. These long strands admixed with snared platelets cause shear stress in the microcirculation and cause hemolysis.
    c. This condition may be congenital (defect within the ADAMTS13 gene) or acquired (ADAMTS13 autoantibodies, pregnancy, or HIV).
    d. The classic pentad of TTP consists of fever, anemia (microangiopathic hemolytic), thrombocytopenia, renal failure, and neurologic symptoms (altered mental status and seizures).
    e. If untreated, the mortality rate approaches 95%.
    f. The mainstay of therapy is **plasmapheresis,** replacing the patient's plasma and eliminating the offending antibody.
    g. While no single parameter (platelet count, extent of schistocytosis, ADAMTS13 level, or LDH level) is, by itself, diagnostic, both improving trends and gradually resolving symptoms indicate therapy has been successful.
    h. Patients with an inherited ADAMTS13 deficiency (**Upshaw-Schulman syndrome**) undergo periodic prophylactic exchange to maintain sufficient levels of ADAMTS13.
    i. Platelet transfusions must be avoided because the additional platelets promote further thrombosis.

C. **von Willebrand Disease**
       1. This is a group of bleeding disorders related to quantitative (type I) or qualitative (type II) von Willebrand factor (vWF) abnormalities resulting in poor platelet adhesion and decreased stabilization of **factor VIII.**
          a. vWF is constitutively produced by endothelium and stored within **Weibel-Palade bodies.**
          b. In the absence of bound vWF, factor VIII is rapidly degraded.
       2. **Type 1** has less vWF, but vWF and factor VIII function normally.
       3. **Type 2** has qualitative vWF functional defects.
       4. **Type 3** is the most severe form with deficiencies of both vWF and factor VIII resulting in profound hemorrhage.

III. Coagulation and Fibrinolysis

    A. **Coagulation**
       1. The **coagulation cascade** may be activated by the intrinsic or extrinsic reaction pathways to produce a fibrin clot (Figure 18–1).
          a. The intrinsic and extrinsic coagulation cascades may be individually assessed by **partial thromboplastin time** (PTT) and **prothrombin time** (PT)/international normalized ratio (INR).
          b. The PTT may be lengthened with deficiencies of factors within the **intrinsic pathway**—factors XII, XI, IX, or VIII.
          c. The PT is often reported as an INR, a mathematical conversion to standardize the variability of laboratory reagents, and may be prolonged by

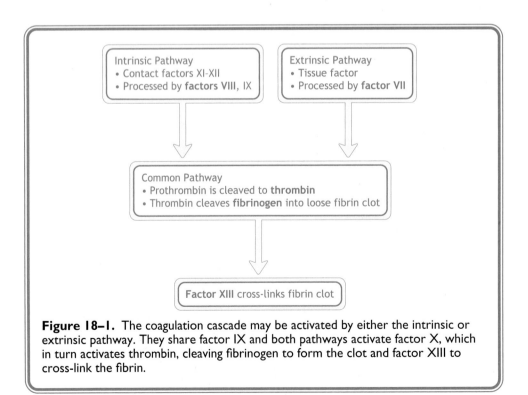

Figure 18–1. The coagulation cascade may be activated by either the intrinsic or extrinsic pathway. They share factor IX and both pathways activate factor X, which in turn activates thrombin, cleaving fibrinogen to form the clot and factor XIII to cross-link the fibrin.

abnormalities within the **extrinsic and common pathways**—factors VII, X, V, or II.

    (1) Factor VII has the shortest half-life.

    (2) Factor VII is vitamin K–dependent.

    (3) A decline in factor VII may be due to warfarin therapy or an early sign of vitamin K deficiency or liver disease.

  d. Clotting factors from both pathways (eg, II, VII, IX, and X) are dependent on vitamin K; therefore, vitamin K deficiencies secondary to malabsorption, poor diet, or warfarin toxicity can lengthen both PTT and PT/INR.

VITAMIN K, WARFARIN, AND FACTOR VII

- *Vitamin K is synthesized by bacteria in the gut and is essential for liver synthesis of vitamin K–dependent clotting factors (II, VII, IX, and X) in addition to protein C and protein S.*
- *Warfarin inhibits vitamin K function.*
- *Recombinant factor VIIa is the most rapid means for emergency reversal of anticoagulation from excess warfarin.*

  2. Coagulation factors are maintained at about three times the concentrations needed to maintain normal function.

    a. Congenital and acquired conditions that lower clotting factor concentrations below 30% of normal predispose patients to bleeding.

    b. Conversely, conditions that lower the concentrations of antithrombotic factors (protein C, protein S, and antithrombin) result in hypercoagulable states (thrombophilia).

      (1) Protein C is a serine protease that, in concert with protein S, inhibits both factors Va and VIIIa.

      (2) Protein S is a cofactor for protein C.

    c. The enzymatic linchpin of the coagulation system is thrombin.

      (1) It circulates as the inactive precursor prothrombin.

      (2) Once prothrombin is cleaved by factor X, thrombin acts as a serine protease, cleaving multiple targets, including fibrinogen into fibrin.

      (3) Thrombin activates factors V, VIII, and IX.

      (4) It binds to thrombomodulin to induce protein C to inactivate factors Va and VIIIa as negative feedback.

      (5) Factors favoring thrombin generation include inflammation, infection, low blood flow, endothelial damage, and platelet activation.

    d. **Antithrombin,** formerly known as antithrombin 3 or AT3, is a non–vitamin K–dependent factor that is a potent inhibitor of thrombin, and its activity is potentiated by **heparin.**

  B. Fibrinolysis

    1. There is a stoichiometric balance between clotting and fibrinolysis.

    2. The web of cross-linked fibrin polymers during clotting also ensnares the inactive proenzyme **plasminogen** from the circulation, which is then converted into **plasmin** by plasminogen activator released by endothelial cells.

      a. Activation is also promoted by thrombin and urokinase.

      b. Recombinant tissue plasminogen activator (t-PA) is used therapeutically to promote fibrinolytic activity and remove newly formed clots following thrombosis.

(1) If given early enough, t-PA helps reestablish circulation and prevents irreversible ischemic damage.

    (2) But, it increases the risk of secondary hemorrhage.

  3. Plasmin lyses cross-linked fibrin and individual fibrin monomers into **D-dimers** and **fibrin split products.**

    a. D-dimers are specifically derived from the fibrin mesh that was previously stabilized by factor XIII.

    b. D-dimers may indicate disseminated intravascular coagulation (**DIC**), deep venous thrombosis (**DVT**), or pulmonary embolism (**PE**).

  4. Like thrombin, the action of plasmin is tightly regulated by both α_2-antiplasmin and α_2-macroglobulin.

  5. Antifibrinolytics are used to treat excessive bleeding.

C. Coagulopathies

  1. Pathology is divided into increased bleeding and clotting.

  2. Excess hemorrhage is a clinical feature shared by von Willebrand disease, the hemophilias (A, B, and C), liver failure, dilutional coagulopathies, and DIC.

  3. Hemophilia is a group of hereditary coagulopathies defined in part by a decrease of a specific component of the coagulation cascade.

    a. Hemophilia A (classic hemophilia) is the most common form and results from a deficiency of **factor VIII.**

    b. Hemophilia B (**Christmas disease**) is the second most common and is a deficiency of **factor IX.**

    c. Hemophilia C, a deficiency of factor XI, differs from the other two forms of hemophilia both in severity (relatively mild) and inheritance (autosomal recessive).

  4. The **liver** synthesizes all but one of the clotting factors; therefore, any process that impairs liver function (infectious disease, toxins, metabolic dysfunction, or ischemia) may manifest as a coagulopathy.

    a. Infectious causes include hepatitis A, B, and C; Epstein-Barr virus, cytomegalovirus (CMV), herpes, and parvovirus.

    b. Hepatotoxins include **acetaminophen,** salicylates, methanol, and isoniazid.

    c. A long list of metabolic disorders (eg, hemochromotosis, Wilson disease) may also contribute to liver failure.

  5. Dilutional coagulopathy occurs when platelets and clotting factors are essentially washed out by aggressive fluid resuscitation or multiple RBC transfusions without plasma replenishment.

  6. DIC is an extremely dangerous hemorrhagic condition with simultaneous activation of thrombin and plasmin.

    a. It may arise in many settings, including the following:

      (1) Infections (bacterial, viral, fungal, parasitic)

      (2) Pregnancy (eg, preeclampsia, amnionic fluid embolism)

      (3) Malignancy (eg, lung cancer)

      (4) Acute liver failure

      (5) Inflammation (eg, sarcoidosis, ulcerative colitis)

    b. Clotting factors are consumed in a vicious cycle of uncontrolled thrombosis and fibrinolysis.

    c. Laboratory findings include low platelets, low fibrinogen, prolonged PT/INR, activated PTT, and positive D-dimer.

7. **Thrombophilias** may be primary (factor V Leiden, antithrombin deficiency, protein C or protein S deficiency) or acquired (DIC and antiphospholipid syndrome).

    a. **Factor V Leiden** is a common hereditary thrombophilia resulting from a single point mutation that alters the inactivation site used by protein C.

        (1) The subsequent resistance to inactivation permits ongoing conversion of prothrombin to thrombin.

        (2) These patients are prone to repeated thromboembolic events and may require prophylactic anticoagulation.

    b. **Antithrombin (AT) deficiency,** whether congenital or acquired through sepsis, leads to prolonged circulation of activated coagulation factors.

        (1) These patients are at increased risk for thromboembolic events, particularly in unusual sites (eg, mesentery).

        (2) AT deficiency leaves patients relatively resistant to the therapeutic effects of heparin.

    c. **Protein C deficiency** is clinically associated with warfarin-induced skin necrosis by exacerbating the hypercoagulable state.

    d. **Protein S deficiency** is also worsened or acquired de novo through warfarin administration.

    e. **Antiphospholipid syndrome** antibodies are directed against membrane phospholipids (eg, anticardiolipin antibody).

        (1) It is associated with recurrent arterial or venous thrombosis and recurrent fetal loss (recurrent abortion).

        (2) Terminology is potentially misleading as the antibody is sometimes called the **lupus anticoagulant** despite the fact that it is thrombotic and not specifically associated with systemic lupus erythematosus.

IV. Transfusion Medicine

A. Blood Products

1. Blood products are available to treat volume depletion, ischemia, coagulation, and immune deficiency.

2. Several basic blood products are derived from whole blood donations; these may be used individually or in combination as part of component therapy.

3. **Component therapy** administers only the fraction required to correct the patient's immediate deficiency (eg, RBCs for anemia; platelets for thrombocytopenia; plasma for coagulopathies; granulocytes for immunosuppression.)

4. RBCs are available as leukoreduced RBCs, packed RBCs, or whole blood for symptomatic patients with deficient oxygen capacity.

    a. Hemoglobin <**6 g/dL** usually requires **transfusion.**

    b. Hematocrit can be misleading, especially in the setting of acute blood loss; the decision to transfuse should weigh all pertinent clinical findings and not rely solely on a single hemoglobin measurement.

    c. Each unit is approximately 300 mL.

    d. The standard dose is 2 units for adults or **10 mL/kg** in pediatric patients.

    e. The expected response to each unit is an increase of 1 g/dL hemoglobin and three points of hematocrit.

5. **Platelets** are available as either platelet units (drawn from a single donor), or platelet concentrates (pooled from whole blood).

    a. Counts less than 10,000/mcL require prophylactic transfusion.

b. Greater than 50,000/mcL is required for surgery.

c. A platelet target of 100,000/mcL is appropriate for neurosurgery and during massive transfusion.

d. Platelets are frequently **ineffective** in patients with **idiopathic thrombocytopenic purpura** and are **contraindicated** in patients with **TTP.**

e. The standard adult dose is 1 unit or **10 mL/kg** in pediatric patients, and the expected response is a platelet count increase of 30,000–60,000/mcL.

6. **Plasma** is available as fresh frozen plasma (FFP) or thawed plasma.

   a. Plasma products should be administered to increase the level of clotting factors in patients with a demonstrated deficiency.

      (1) If the PT and PTT are less than 1.5 times normal, FFP is rarely needed.

      (2) Compared with FFP, thawed plasma has reduced concentrations of labile plasma factors such as factors VII and VIII, but the two products are used interchangeably.

   b. Plasma should not be used for volume expansion or when virally inactivated factors concentrates are available to treat specific factor deficiencies.

   c. The standard dose is 2–3 units in adults or 15 mL/kg in pediatric patients; however, a dose of 4–6 units or **20 mL/kg** is often required for full correction.

7. **Cryoprecipitate** is a concentrated solution of factor VII (the antihemophilic factor), fibrinogen, and fibronectin produced from plasma frozen to −70 °C then thawed to 4 °C.

   a. These products are used to correct hypofibrinogenemia.

   b. Therapy with cryoprecipitate is most effective when the serum fibrinogen level is less than 80 mg/dL.

   c. The standard dose is 10 units for adults or 1 unit/10 kg in pediatric patients.

   d. The expected response is an increase in fibrinogen of about 50 mg for every 10 units.

8. **Factor concentrates** are derived from fractionation of human or animal plasma and recombinant factor concentrates.

   a. **Factor VIII** concentrate has replaced cryoprecipitate as the treatment of choice for **hemophilia A,** but neutralizing antibodies develop in some patients rendering them refractory.

   b. **Recombinant factor VIIa** is licensed for use in hemophilia A patients resistant to factor VIII concentrates, and it is also used for emergent reversal of warfarin-induced hemorrhage.

   c. **Factor IX** concentrates may be used to treat hemophilia B and severe von Willebrand disease.

9. **Granulocyte concentrates** are collected by apheresis in about 200-300 mL containing an average of 5×10^9 granulocytes.

   a. The product must be infused within 24 hours of collection.

   b. Granulocytes cannot be leuko-reduced. To make them CMV-virus safe, the unit must be from a donor who is CMV negative.

   c. These products are indicated for short-term support of **leukopenic patients** with life-threatening fungal or bacterial infections that have not responded to antibiotics.

B. Compatibility Testing

   1. **Pretransfusion processing** is used to ensure the safety and compatibility of blood products.

a. Potential donors are excluded on the basis of risk factors, including infectious disease status (HIV, hepatitis, or malaria), history of injection drug use, or recent transfusion.

    b. The risk of malaria and Creutzfeldt-Jakob disease is considered with the travel history.

    c. Each unit of donated whole blood for allogeneic transfusion is screened for the following:

        (1) Hepatitis B core antibody (anti-HBc)

        (2) Hepatitis B surface antigen (HBsAg)

        (3) Hepatitis C virus antibody (anti-HCV)

        (4) HIV-1 and HIV-2 nucleic acid and antibodies

        (5) Human T-cell virus (HTLV-1 and HTLV-2) antibodies

        (6) West Nile virus

        (7) Infection with *Treponema pallidum*

2. Leukoreduction is the filtration of white blood cells to decrease the quantity of white cells by 99.9%.

    a. It reduces the risk that the recipient will raise antibodies to the donated blood, a process known as alloimmunization, and this makes febrile transfusion reactions less likely.

    b. The process also reduces the potential for CMV transmission, since CMV infects only white cells.

    c. **Irradiation** lowers the mitotic index of donor T-lymphocytes and is considered for patients who are either immunocompromised (secondary to hereditary conditions, HIV, chemotherapy, or stem cell transplantation) or enrolled in directed-donation program.

    d. Despite these procedures, small but quantifiable risks of disease transmission remain (Table 18–7).

3. Compatibility testing helps ensure both transfusion safety and maximal survival of transfused cells.

    a. Safety begins with the patient blood sample in the correct type tube (usually purple) and properly labeled with the patient's name and medical record number; blood samples that do not meet these criteria must be rejected and recollected.

    b. Pretransfusion testing involves determining the recipient's blood type and the presence of any recipient antibodies that may cause hemolysis.

    c. Typing includes ABO and Rh expression.

    d. The process takes approximately 1 hour.

TYPE, SCREEN, AND CROSSMATCH

CLINICAL CORRELATION

- *Transfusion compatibility testing is based on agglutination.*
- *The direct antibody (or Coombs) test assesses the presence of immunoglobulin or complement bound to RBCs.*
- *The indirect antibody test uses a multistep process to screen for a specific antigen, alloantibody, or crossmatch reaction.*
- *Antibody identification involves a complex procedure where 11 or more reagent cells are tested against patient plasma.*
- *A crossmatch order asks the laboratory to reserve a particular RBC unit for a particular patient.*

Table 18–7. Risks of transfusion-transmitted infection.

Disease	Estimated Risk
HIV	I in 2 million
Hepatitis C	I in 2 million
Hepatitis B	I in 500,000
Bacterial infection (platelets)	I in 75,000, if culture negative
West Nile virus	Extremely rare

C. Blood Groups
  1. More than 630 distinct antigens are expressed on the surface of RBCs; however, only a few cause significant problems.
  2. **ABO** antigens were among the earliest characterized and are the most familiar to healthcare professionals.
     a. The A and B codominant genes code for glycoproteins, the A and B antigens, which are added to an H precursor.
     b. Patients homozygous for the O gene produce neither the A nor the B antigen, only the H precursor.
     c. Anti-A or anti-B antibodies are produced to the ABO antigen not expressed by the host.
     d. When blood products are required emergently, type O RBCs and type AB plasma may be given with the least concern for transfusion reaction (Table 18–8).
  3. The **Rh (Rhesus) antigens** are a large class of more than 50 related antigens, including D, C, c, E, and e.
     a. Rh-positive individuals produce the D antigen.

Table 18–8. Summary of ABO antigens and compatibilities.

Recipient Phenotype	Genotype (alleles)	ABO Antigens	Antibodies	Compatibility
O	OO	None	Anti-A and B	Universal donor
A	AA or AO	A	Anti-B	A or AB plasma
B	BB or BO	B	Anti-A	B or AB plasma
AB	AB	A and B	None	Universal recipient

Table 18–9. Red blood cell antigens and antibodies.

Antigen	Antibody	Frequency and Significance
D	Anti-D	Extremely common Most frequent cause of hemolytic disease of newborn
Kell	Anti-K	Common; 10% of blood incompatible May cause newborn hemolytic disease
Kidd	Anti-Jka or Anti- Jkb	Dangerous ("killer Kidd") Causes acute hemolytic transfusion reaction
Duffy	Anti-Fya or Anti-Fyb	Anti-Fya most common

    b. Rh-negative individuals do not produce the antigen and do not produce antibodies to D unless exposed to it through pregnancy or another form of transfusion.

    c. These Rh antibodies may induce hemolytic reactions.

  4. In addition to the Rh system, other clinically significant antigens include Kell, Kidd, and Duffy and are listed with their associated antibodies in Table 18–9.

 D. Complications

  1. Reactions to transfused products must be recognized.

  2. Potential complications may be characterized by **timing** (acute or chronic) and **temperature** (febrile or afebrile).

  3. Adverse transfusion reactions are common.

    a. Fever (increase of 1 °C) occurs in 1:200 transfusions.

    b. Allergic reaction occurs in 1:300 transfusions.

    c. Fatal hemolytic reaction is rare (1:250,000)

    d. Recipients must understand risks and benefits to give informed consent prior to transfusion.

    e. When there are signs or symptoms of a transfusion reaction, the transfusion must be stopped immediately.

  4. In addition to obtaining vital signs and performing a brief physical examination, a posttransfusion blood specimen is evaluated for **hemoglobinemia,** antibody coating, and confirmatory typing.

  5. Febrile nonhemolytic reactions are the most common complication of either platelet or RBC transfusion, and are caused by recipient antibodies against donor leukocytes.

    a. Fever, chills (rigors), and dyspnea occur 1–6 hours after transfusion, and these are usually self-limited.

    b. Patients may be premedicated with acetaminophen.

    c. The use of **leukoreduced** cellular products also reduces the incidence of this type of reaction.

    d. No hemolysis is detected during routine workup.

6. **Transfusion-related acute lung injury** is currently the most common cause of fatal transfusion reactions.

    a. It is due to donor anti-HLA or anti-neutrophil antibodies that incite host neutrophil activation and subsequent adherence to pulmonary epithelium.

    b. Similar to acute respiratory distress syndrome, symptoms include **fever and shortness of breath** with signs of oxygen desaturation and noncardiogenic pulmonary edema pattern on chest radiograph, all arising within 1–6 hours after infusion.

7. **Acute hemolytic transfusion reactions** may be fatal.

    a. These usually involve a type O patient receiving a non-O RBC unit due to an **administrative error** (patient misidentification, mislabeled specimens, etc).

    b. Early-onset fever, hypotension, wheezing, burning, or impending sense of doom are part of the clinical picture, and subsequent DIC may lead to later bleeding.

    c. The transfusion must be stopped immediately.

    d. Prevention requires meticulous attention to patient identification during phlebotomy (sampling for pretransfusion testing) and infusion.

8. **Allergic reactions** to various donor proteins are the second most common type of adverse event overall.

    a. A range of allergic reactions is possible from mild urticaria and pruritus to severe anaphylaxis with respiratory difficulty.

    b. The symptoms of **mild allergic reactions** usually begin at the very onset of transfusion.

    c. **Anaphylactic reactions** are potentially life-threatening.

    d. The cause may lie with either the donor or the recipient.

        (1) Donor anaphylatoxins (such as C3a and C5a) or IgE antibodies can respond to recipient antigens.

        (2) Conversely, recipient antibodies may arise against donor plasma antigens, especially among recipients with an underlying selective **IgA deficiency.**

    e. In mild cases, an antihistamine is helpful both in the immediate management and prophylaxis of future episodes; severe anaphylaxis, however, mandates more extensive supportive care and avoidance of plasma-containing products.

9. **Transfusion-associated circulatory overload** (TACO) results from poorly compensated volume expansion by transfused products.

    a. It is more prevalent among infants, the elderly, and patients with impaired cardiac function (eg, congestive heart failure); therefore, these patients are less tolerant of volume status changes and may experience dyspnea, orthopnea, and edema.

    b. Signs and symptoms include shortness of breath, wheezing, and oxygen desaturation.

        (1) These occur after significant volume has been infused.

        (2) Cardiogenic pulmonary edema is seen on chest radiograph.

    c. Treatment includes stopping the transfusion and placing the patient in an upright position as well as administering oxygen, diuretics, and cardiac medication.

d. TACO may be prevented with a combination of slower infusion rate (1 mL/kg/h), volume-reduced products, and diuretics before, during, or after infusion.
10. **Chronic (or delayed) reactions** may occur long after transfusion, between 24 hours and 3 months later.
    a. Delayed hemolytic transfusion reactions may not be reliably associated with fever; however, they are distinguished from acute hemolytic reactions by the location of hemolysis.
      (1) Acute hemolytic reactions occur intravascularly, producing gross hemoglobinemia and hemoglobinuria.
      (2) Delayed hemolytic reactions are a form of extravascular **hemolysis** resulting in decreased circulating erythrocytes with increased bilirubin.
    b. They are most often caused by IgG antibodies that are raised in response to a previous transfusion or pregnancy.
      (1) These antibodies may then fall to such low levels as to be undetected on subsequent antibody screens.
      (2) Another dose of a blood product containing the originally offending antigen induces an **anamnestic response** that marks the donor RBCs for engulfment by macrophages (extravascular hemolysis).
    c. Many common antigens have been implicated, including members of the Rh, Kell, Kidd, Duffy, and MNSs systems.
11. **Transfusion-associated graft-versus-host disease** (TA-GVHD) results from **donor T-lymphocytes** engrafting within an immunocompromised recipient and attacking host tissue.
    a. These patients have rash, diarrhea, liver abnormalities, and pancytopenia.
    b. The **prognosis is grim;** most cases are fatal.
    c. TA-GVHD does not respond to drugs used to control GVHD in transplant recipients.
    d. This complication, however, may be prevented with the use of irradiated (not simply leukodepleted) blood products as described above.

CLINICAL PROBLEMS

1. Why are hemoglobinemia, hemoglobinuria, and hemosiderinuria not seen in hereditary spherocytosis (HS)?
   A. Hemolysis in HS is predominantly intravascular
   B. Hemolysis in HS is predominantly extravascular
   C. The anemia of HS is due to ineffective erythropoiesis
   D. The anemia of HS is due to defective hemoglobin synthesis
   E. Increased spectrin associated with HS scavenges free hemoglobin

2. Which disorder is rarely, if ever, associated with microcytic-hypochromic anemia?
   A. Iron deficiency anemia
   B. Thalassemia minor

C. Anemia of chronic disease

D. Sickle cell anemia

E. Anemia secondary to chronic gastrointestinal bleeding

3. Which of the following findings would favor a diagnosis of thalassemia minor over iron deficiency?

   A. Mean corpuscular volume (MCV)75 fL, low serum iron, low red blood cell (RBC) count

   B. MCV 75 fL, high serum iron, low RBC count

   C. MCV 75 fL, high RBC count, hemoglobin $A_2 > 2.5\%$

   D. MCV 75 fL, low RBC count, hemoglobin $A_2 < 1\%$

   E. MCV 105 fL, normal RBC count, hemoglobin A_2 2%

4. Which laboratory profile is most characteristic of anemia of chronic disease?

   A. Normal serum iron, normal total iron-binding capacity (TIBC), normal ferritin

   B. Low serum iron, normal TIBC, normal ferritin

   C. Low serum iron, high TIBC, low ferritin

   D. Low serum iron, high TIBC, high ferritin

   E. High serum iron, high TIBC, high ferritin

5. Thrombotic thrombocytopenic purpura is characterized by which of the following?

   A. Thrombocytopenia, schistocytes, elevated lactate dehydrogenase

   B. Thrombocytopenia, spherocytes, and elevated LDH

   C. Thrombocytopenia, schistocytes, and normal LDH

   D. Thrombocytosis, spherocytes, and elevated LDH

   E. Isolated thrombocytopenia with no identifiable cause

6. Severe microvascular bleeding and oxygen desaturation develop in a patient undergoing emergency cesarean section for amniotic fluid embolism. Which of the following is the presumptive cause of bleeding?

   A. Thrombocytopenia

   B. von Willebrand disease

   C. Hemolytic uremic syndrome

   D. Hypofibrinogenemia

   E. Uterine rupture

7. A 68-year-old woman with chronic anemia and a dangerously low hematocrit is given 4 units of RBCs over 1 hour; severe orthopnea, rales, and infiltrates on chest radiograph develop. About how much transfused volume did she receive?

   A. 250 mL

   B. 500 mL

   C. 1200 mL

D. 1800 mL

E. 4 L

8. A patient's cells show 4+ agglutination with anti-A and anti-B. Patient plasma does not agglutinate A or B cells. What statement is true about the patient's ABO group?

A. Least common ABO type

B. Second most common ABO type

C. Most common ABO type

D. ABO discrepancy prevents determination of type without testing

E. Patient should receive RhoGAM if given Rh-positive platelets

9. Which of the following blood transfusions would result in an immediate hemolytic transfusion reaction?

A. Group O recipient with a group A donor

B. Group A recipient with a group O donor

C. Group B recipient with a group O donor

D. Group AB recipient with a group A donor

E. Group AB recipient with a group O donor

10. A 70-kg man with a platelet count of 35/mcL is going for major surgery and the surgeon wants the platelet count above 50/mcL. What is the correct number of platelets to order?

A. 12 random donor units

B. 2 random donor units

C. 6 pheresis units

D. 3 pheresis units

E. 1 pheresis unit

ANSWERS

1. The answer is B. Hereditary spherocytosis is characterized by extravascular hemolysis. Spherocytes are poorly deformable, are retained within the spleen, and lysed. Disease improves with splenectomy.

2. The answer is D. In addition to the obvious crescent-shaped cells, a peripheral blood smear from a patient with sickle cell disease may display a range of morphologic abnormalities such as nucleated RBCs and ovalocytes. The cytoplasm of non-sickled cells is generally normochromic.

3. The answer is C. Iron deficiency anemia is usually associated with decreases in RBC count, hemoglobin concentration, mean corpuscular volume, and reticulocyte count. The laboratory indices with thalassemia are more variable, but typically the RBC count is higher and proportion of hemoglobin A_2 is elevated.

4. The answer is B. Anemia of chronic disease is a disorder of iron use marked by reduced reticulocyte response despite adequate iron stores. The serum iron level is decreased while the TIBC is decreased or normal.

5. The answer is A. Schistocytes are RBC fragments with two or more points that may be observed in several conditions, such as microangiopathic anemia, uremia, DIC, hemolytic uremic syndrome, and TTP. An elevated lactate dehydrogenase (LDH) is similarly nonspecific but is often considered an indicator of hemolysis. The presence of hemolysis (evidenced by RBC fragments and elevated serum LDH) and thrombocytopenia is highly suspicious for TTP.

6. The answer is D. Debris in amniotic fluid is a potent activator of the coagulation cascade leading to heavy consumption of fibrinogen.

7. The answer is C. The average unit of RBCs is approximately 300 mL in volume (roughly 200 mL of red cells, 50 mL of plasma, and a variable amount of additive solution).

8. The answer is A. Both the forward type (patient cells with known antisera) and the reverse type (patient plasma with known red cells) indicate that this patient has AB blood. This is the least common phenotype within the ABO system.

9. The answer is A. Type O is the universal donor and type AB is the universal recipient.

10. The answer is E. The expected increase (or "bump") with a single pheresis unit is between 30,000 and 60,000 platelets/mcL.

CHAPTER 19
PEDIATRIC PATHOLOGY AND CONGENITAL SYNDROMES

Children are not little adults.
—aphorism

I. Perinatal Morbidity

A. Intrauterine Growth Retardation (IUGR)

1. IUGR is a syndrome of restricted growth, rather than immaturity, defined by birth weight less than the tenth percentile for age.
2. Most cases are detected by prenatal ultrasound based on biparietal diameter (BPD) and foot length.
3. **Fetal** causes include congenital infections, anatomic anomalies, multiple gestations, and chromosomal abnormalities.
4. **Placental** causes include uteroplacental insufficiency, placental abruption, infarction, and chronic umbilical cord obstruction.
5. **Maternal** causes include conditions pertaining to the mother's health or habits that interfere directly (eg, teratogens) or indirectly (eg, uteroplacental insufficiency) with fetal growth.
6. IUGR may be symmetric or asymmetric.
   a. **Symmetric IUGR** is the proportionate undergrowth of all organ systems, usually resulting from fetal factors.
   b. **Asymmetric IUGR** is the disproportionate undergrowth of organ systems, usually resulting from uteroplacental insufficiency.

B. Respiratory Distress Syndrome (RDS)

1. RDS is caused by a lack of **surfactant** in premature lungs; production of type II pneumocytes does not start until after 35 weeks' gestational age.
2. Increased surface tension within the alveoli causes collapse and severely labored breathing within 30 minutes of birth.
3. It is characterized microscopically by alveolar **hyaline membranes.**
4. Mechanical ventilation and increased oxygen requirement may lead to bronchopulmonary dysplasia, retinal damage, necrotizing enterocolitis, and intraventricular hemorrhage.

C. Necrotizing Enterocolitis

1. This is the most common severe gastrointestinal disorder in neonates, characterized by acute necrotizing inflammation of the gut.

2. It usually involves the terminal ileum and ascending colon.

3. Onset coincides with first oral feeding.

4. It is thought to result from failure of the immature intestinal immune system to cope with bacterial colonization of the gut.

5. It is characterized by edema, hemorrhage, necrosis, bacterial overgrowth, and gas in the intestinal wall.

6. Affected areas appear grossly gangrenous.

7. Bowel perforation and septic shock may occur.

8. Surgical intervention is usually required.

D. Erythroblastosis Fetalis (Hemolytic Disease of the Newborn)

    1. It results from incompatibility between fetal and maternal blood groups, most commonly involving the **Rh system** (D antigen).

    2. Sensitization of the mother is required.

        a. Blood from Rh-positive fetus passes into the circulation of Rh-negative mother (>1 mL required).

        b. Passage is usually transplacental during labor.

        c. This leads to the formation of maternal anti-Rh IgM antibodies, which cannot cross the placenta.

        d. The maternal immune response matures and IgG antibodies are formed, which can cross the placenta in subsequent pregnancies.

        e. The resulting hemolysis varies in degree but may be detected in amniotic fluid samples.

    3. Mild cases show increased fetal red blood cell production sufficient to maintain the fetal circulation.

        a. **Extramedullary hematopoiesis** is seen in the liver and spleen.

        b. The child is born pale and variably anemic.

        c. Hepatosplenomegaly may be present.

    4. Severe cases present with severe anemia and hypoxia leading to fetal organ failure.

        a. Fluid moves into the extravascular spaces, resulting in massive, generalized edema (**hydrops fetalis**).

        b. Unconjugated hyperbilirubinemia (**jaundice**) develops.

        c. Bilirubin also deposits in the brain, primarily in the basal ganglia (**kernicterus**).

    5. Treatment includes exchange transfusion and **phototherapy,** which oxidizes bilirubin into nontoxic, water-soluble molecules.

    6. The most effective treatment is **prevention.**

        a. Rh-negative mothers carrying Rh-positive fetuses are treated prenatally (~28 weeks) and shortly after delivery (<72 hours) with **anti-D Rhesus immune globulin (RhoGAM).**

        b. RhoGAM prevents sensitization by binding to fetal red cells in the maternal circulation, rendering them non-antigenic.

    7. A similar process, though less severe, can be seen in **ABO** incompatibilities and **glucose-6-phosphate-dehydrogenase (G6PD) deficiency.**

E. Sudden Infant Death Syndrome (SIDS)

    1. SIDS is a sudden unexpected death of an infant within the first year of life that is unexplained despite comprehensive investigation, including autopsy, review of the clinical history, adequate testing for known causes of sudden death, and forensic investigation of the scene and circumstances of death.

2. SIDS is attributed to 2000 deaths annually in the United States.
   a. It is the third leading cause of death (~8% of total deaths) in infants less than 1 year old.
   b. Most cases (85%) occur between 2 and 4 months of age.
   c. Race bias is blacks > whites > Hispanics > Asians.
3. Risk factors appear to be multifactorial.
   a. Maternal factors are age less than 20 years old, cigarette smoking, drug abuse, multiple gestation, family history, and low socioeconomic status.
   b. Infant risks are prematurity, male gender, low birth weight, and sleeping in the **prone** position.
4. The cause is unknown, but current leading hypotheses include:
   a. Heart conduction anomalies may lead to cardiac arrhythmia.
   b. Prolonged apneic episodes (lasting greater than 20 seconds) may be implicated since infants appear to be chronically hypoxemic prior to death.

SUDDEN INFANT DEATH SYNDROME

- *There is no evidence of trauma or toxins by autopsy.*
- *The manner of death appears natural, but the cause is unknown.*
- *Because sleeping in the prone position may be a risk factor, "back to sleep" is the current recommendation to reduce the risk of SIDS.*

II. Congenital Anomalies

A. Syndromes and Sequences
1. Morphologic abnormalities are present at the time of birth.
2. Causes may be genetic, environmental, or multifactorial.
   a. **Malformation** is a primary anomaly related to defective organ or organ system development (eg, transposition of the great vessels, spina bifida, esophageal atresia).
   b. **Deformation** is an anomaly related to global mechanical forces (eg, oligohydramnios) that restrict or otherwise impede normal growth (eg, club feet).
   c. **Disruption** is a secondary anomaly resulting from local destruction of normally developing tissue (eg, limb and amniotic bands).
   d. **Sequence** is a group of anomalies that occur secondary to an original insult (eg, autosomal recessive polycystic kidneys or renal dysplasia, leading to reduced amnion production, which causes pulmonary hypoplasia, flattened facies, and club feet in Potter sequence).
   e. **Syndrome** is a cluster of anomalies that has been clinically observed and described without an anatomic or embryologic relationship (eg, DiGeorge syndrome, which comprises parathyroid and thymic gland hypoplasia and outflow tract defects in the heart; the cause is usually 22q11 deletion).

B. Aneuploidy
1. Most chromosomal anomalies are lethal, accounting for most miscarriages (spontaneous abortions), especially in the first trimester of pregnancy.
2. The most common chromosomal anomalies detected by karyotype are:
   a. **Trisomy,** which is a gain of one autosomal or sex chromosome.
   b. **Monosomy,** which is a loss of one autosomal or sex chromosome.
   c. **Triploidy,** which is three copies of the genome (eg, 69XXY).

3. Trisomy 21 is Down syndrome, 47XX+21 or 47XY+21.
    a. It is the most common aneuploidy in live births (1/700).
    b. It usually results from maternal meiotic non-disjunction.
    c. Incidence increases with maternal age (1/25 live births in mothers >45 years).
    d. The classic phenotype is:
        (1) **Mental retardation**
        (2) **Epicanthal folds**
        (3) **Single palmar crease**
        (4) Congenital **heart defects**
        (5) Increased risk of acute **leukemia**
        (6) **Neurodegenerative disease** in adulthood
4. Trisomy 18 is Edwards syndrome, 47XX+18, or 47XY+18.
    a. It is also caused by maternal meiotic non-disjunction.
    b. The classic phenotype is:
        (1) **Intrauterine fetal demise**
        (2) **Micrognathia** (small jaws)
        (3) **Rocker bottom feet**
        (4) Severe mental retardation
        (5) Prominent occiput
        (6) Low set ears
        (7) Congenital heart defects
        (8) Horseshoe kidney
5. Trisomy 13 is Patau syndrome, 47XX+13 or 47XY+13.
    a. It is also cased by maternal meiotic non-disjunction.
    b. The classic phenotype is:
        (1) **Intrauterine fetal demise**
        (2) **Microphthalmia** (small eyes)
        (3) **Cleft lip and palate**
        (4) Microcephaly
        (5) Severe mental retardation
        (6) **Polydactyly**
        (7) Cardiac and renal anomalies
        (8) Rocker bottom feet
C. Sex Chromosomal Anomalies
  1. Monosomy X is **Turner Syndrome,** 45XO.
    a. Loss of the X chromosome occurs during spermatogenesis.
    b. It occurs in 1/3000 live female births (98% fatal).
    c. In stillborn infants, fetal hydrops with nuchal (neck) **cystic hygroma** is classically seen.
    d. The classic phenotype (usually genetic **mosaic**) is:
        (1) Broad, shield-like chest
        (2) Webbed neck
        (3) **Aortic coarctation**
        (4) Gonadal dysgenesis (**streak ovaries**)
        (5) Infertility
        (6) Renal defects (**horseshoe kidney**)
        (7) Short stature

2. Trisomy XXY is **Klinefelter syndrome,** 47XXY in 80% of cases.
   a. It results from the presence of two or more X chromosomes in conjunction with one or more Y chromosomes.
   b. It occurs in 1/850 live male births.
   c. The classic phenotype is:
      (1) **Long legs**
      (2) **Gynecomastia**
      (3) Hypogonadism (small atrophic testes)
      (4) Delayed or absent puberty
      (5) Infertility
3. Trisomy **XYY syndrome** results from an extra Y chromosome.
   a. It occurs in approximately 1 in 1000 live male births.
   b. Patients are usually not dysmorphic, but tend to be tall and have mildly decreased intelligence.
4. **True hermaphroditism** requires the presence of both ovarian and testicular tissue, separately or together as an **ovotestis.**
   a. It is extremely rare with a broad spectrum of phenotypes.
   b. It is usually 46XX, but may be 46XY, or mosaic.
5. **Pseudohermaphroditism** is a discordance between gonadal sex and phenotype (eg, "testicular feminization").

PENIS AT 12

- *In rare cases, "females" may develop a penis at puberty.*
- *Genetic studies may reveal a 46XY genotype in these girls.*
- *Additional studies reveal a mutation in the androgen receptor, which masked their male development until androgen levels rose at puberty.*

III. Classic Single Gene Disorders in Children

A. Autosomal Dominant Disorders

1. **Achondroplasia** is a prominent cause of **dwarfism** characterized by early, abnormal ossification of the epiphyseal plates.
   a. It results from a point mutation in the fibroblast growth factor receptor 3 (*FGFR3*) gene.
   b. There is no association with mental retardation, early death, or infertility.
   c. However, it may be lethal in utero if homozygous.
2. **Osteogenesis imperfecta** is characterized by deranged type I **collagen** synthesis and extremely **brittle bones.**

B. Autosomal Recessive Disorders

1. **Cystic fibrosis** is caused by a mutation in the transmembrane regulator *CFTR* gene.
   a. 1/20 Northern Europeans have a mutation, but it is silent in heterozygotes (only symptomatic if homozygous for mutation).
   b. There is a 1/400 chance of having a baby with cystic fibrosis in these populations.
   c. Mutations in the *CFTR* gene lead to **chloride channel** deficit.
   d. Loss of chloride channel in epithelial cells leads to an inability to reabsorb chloride.

e. In sweat gland ducts, this produces the increased **sweat** chloride levels measured in diagnostic testing.

f. In the epithelia of the intestine, pancreas, and bronchi, the situation is reversed; loss of the chloride channel prevents adequate secretion of chloride, causing thick viscous mucous, culminating in **obstruction.**

g. Signs of intestinal malabsorption appear due to blockage and fibrosis of the pancreas.

h. Similar effects are seen in the vas deferens of male patients, resulting in infertility.

i. The most severe complications arise in the **lungs** where secretions become trapped in the airways leading to persistent lung infections (eg, caused by *Pseudomonas* sp.), and chronic obstructive pulmonary disease (COPD).

j. Therapy addresses malabsorption with replacement of pancreatic enzymes and supplementation of the fat-soluble vitamins (A, D, E, and K) as well as ensuring adequate caloric intake and periodic antibiotics to control infection.

2. **Infantile polycystic kidney disease** is characterized by diffuse bilateral cystic dilation of the renal collecting ducts.

   a. Most of the renal cortex is also destroyed.

   b. The absence of urine production leads to oligohydramnios, which in turn fails to promote fetal lung development (via fetal breathing of amnionic fluid), culminating in pulmonary hypoplasia, respiratory distress and death (Potter sequence).

3. **Oculocutaneous albinism** is the reduced or absent production of melanin with loss of skin, hair, and eye pigmentation, leading to poor vision and increased sensitivity to ultraviolet light.

   a. Subtypes exist, which vary in severity and underlying genetic defect (all autosomal recessive).

   b. Absence of tyrosinase results in the most severe phenotype.

C. **X-Linked Recessive Disorders**

1. **Duchenne muscular dystrophy** is an X-linked recessive disease caused by mutations in the **dystrophin** gene on Xp21.

   a. It is characterized by progressive onset of weakness, primarily involving **proximal muscle** groups (Gower sign).

   b. Males appear normal at birth.

   c. There is an onset of weakness by age 4.

   d. The calf muscles are enlarged (pseudohypertrophy).

   e. Patients can no longer walk by 10 years of age.

   f. Adolescents die of cardiac or respiratory failure.

2. **Becker muscular dystrophy** is a variant of Duchenne muscular dystrophy with later onset and milder phenotype, also involving Xp21.

3. **Color blindness** is usually caused by defects in the photopigment genes on the q-arm of the X chromosome.

   a. It is usually a red-green color blindness in males.

   b. Approximately 5% of men and 0.5% of women are affected.

IV. **Metabolic Disorders**

A. **Storage Diseases**

1. **Lysosomal storage diseases** are related disorders caused by enzyme deficiencies leading to lysosomal accumulation of the substrate.

a. There are over 400 variants with an incidence of 1/8000.
b. Accumulating substrates include lipid, sphingolipid, polysaccharides, mucopolysaccharides, and proteins.

2. **Hurler syndrome (mucopolysaccharidosis I)** is the prototypic mucopolysaccharidosis characterized by deficient degradation of long-chain carbohydrates.
   a. Deficiency of the enzyme **α-L-iduronidase** leads to accumulation of heparan and dermatan sulfates in cells throughout the body.
   b. Clinical features include:
      (1) Prominent **supraorbital ridges**
      (2) **Dwarfism**
      (3) Hepatosplenomegaly
      (4) Mental **retardation**
   c. The diagnosis is made by detecting urinary mucopolysaccharides and visualizing abnormal lysosomes by electron microscopy.
   d. Treatment is enzyme replacement and bone marrow transplant.
   e. Death usually occurs in childhood from cardiac disease.

3. **Gaucher disease** is an autosomal recessive disease that is more common in the Jewish population.
   a. **β-Glucocerebrosidase deficiency** leads to accumulation of glucocerebroside in the cells of the reticuloendothelial (phagocytic) system.
   b. **Macrophages** become distended by the accumulated lipid, identified light microscopically by the '**crumpled tissue paper**' appearance of the cytoplasm (Gaucher cells).
   c. Type 1 (non-neuronopathic) occurs in early adolescence and has a chronic course with normal life expectancy.
   d. Type 2 (infantile, acute neuronopathic) occurs early (3–6 months of age) with neuronal effects and demise within a year.

B. **Disorders of Amino Acid Metabolism**
   1. These disorders are defined by a deficiency of enzymes critical to amino acid metabolism.
   2. **Phenylketonuria** (PKU) is caused by phenylalanine hydroxylase deficiency leading to failed conversion of phenylalanine to tyrosine.
      a. Without treatment, marked hyperphenylalaninemia develops causing the following classic symptoms:
         (1) Severe mental **retardation** by 6 months
         (2) Sweat and urine smell **musty** (due to excretion of the shunt pathway metabolite phenylacetic acid)
         (3) Abnormal hair pigmentation
         (4) Focal demyelination, abnormal gyri, and white matter gliosis associated with seizures
      b. Treatment involves dietary restriction of phenylalanine; if started early this allows normal brain development.
   3. **Alkaptonuria** is a deficiency of homogentisic acid oxidase, which causes connective tissue deposition of homogentisic acid.
      a. When exposed to light, homogentisic acid polymerizes to form **blue-black pigment** in the ear, cartilage, sclera, and joints.
      b. Excretion of homogentisic acid produces the **black urine.**
      c. After 10 years of age patients present with arthritis and atherosclerosis.

C. **Disorders of Purine Metabolism**
1. **Adenosine deaminase deficiency** (ADA) is an inherited disorder (recessive) that leads to impaired DNA synthesis affecting mostly lymphocytes (T and B cells).
   a. This results in severe combined immunodeficiency (**SCIDS**).
   b. The condition is diagnosed in the first 6 months of age.
   c. It is very rare (1/million births), but children are prone to repeated and persistent infections that may cause death.
2. **Lesch-Nyhan syndrome** is characterized by **hyperuricemia** due to deficiency of hypoxanthine guanine phosphoribosyltransferase leading to neonatal crystalluria.
   a. **Megaloblastic anemia** may be present.
   b. In childhood, patients exhibit choreoathetosis, spasticity, and a propensity for **self-mutilation.**

V. **Benign Childhood Tumors**

A. **Hemangioma**
1. This is the most common neoplasm in children.
2. They usually arise in the skin but may involve solid organs.
3. Grossly, they are reddish blue and can be elevated ("strawberry hemangiomas") or flat (Port-wine stains).
4. Elevated lesions commonly regress prior to school age.
5. Malignant transformation is very rare.

B. **Lymphangioma**
1. Lesions are composed of a proliferation of lymphatic vessels.
2. They tend to enlarge with time and do not usually regress.
3. Deleterious effects are due to obstruction.
4. **Cystic hygromas** are large lymphangiomas of the neck.

C. **Teratoma**
1. Benign teratomas are primarily cystic lesions containing mature, **well-differentiated,** elements of various embryologic origins, including skin, bowel, brain, cartilage, bone, and teeth.
2. They are usually in the **sacral** region, **ovary,** thorax, and **brain.**
3. In the head and neck, they can be large and disfiguring.
4. Approximately 10% are malignant, with **immature elements,** usually neural, or extra-embryonic components (eg, yolk sac tumor).
5. Immature elements are not malignant in congenital teratomas.

VI. **Childhood Malignancies**

A. **Leukemia and Lymphoma**
1. The most common malignant childhood neoplasms arise from the **lymphoid** lineage (eg, acute lymphoblastic leukemia [ALL]) rather than from myeloid lineage (AML), which is more common in adults.
2. **Leukemia** accounts for more cancer **deaths** in children than all of the other childhood malignancies combined.
3. Burkitt lymphoma, lymphoblastic lymphoma, and Hodgkin disease are the most commonly seen lymphomas in children.
4. Symptoms include fever, weight loss, anemia, bruising, and pain.
5. Survival has greatly improved with chemotherapy, which is often started immediately after the diagnosis.
6. Bone marrow transplantation is required for some cases.

B. **Soft Tissue and Bone Tumors**
  1. The most common soft tissue tumor in children is **rhabdomyosarcoma.**
  2. **Alveolar rhabdomyosarcoma** has the characteristic t(2;13) translocation and is more aggressive than **embryonal** type (eg, botryoid rhabdomyosarcoma arising from the vagina).
     a. Rhabdomyosarcoma usually arises in the head and neck.
     b. It is a small round blue cell tumor with striated muscle-like features and immunostains for muscle antigens (eg, **myogenin**).
  3. The most common childhood bone malignancies are **osteosarcoma** and **Ewing sarcoma** (see Chapter 15 for details).

C. **Neuroblastoma**
  1. Neuroblastoma is the most common malignant neoplasm affecting infants less than 1 year of age (Figure 19–1).

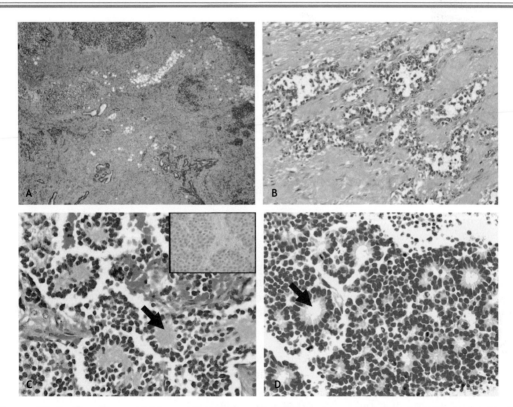

Figure 19–1. Small round blue cell tumors. A: Wilms tumor with triphasic pattern of epithelial glandular cells, primitive blastema, and fibrous stroma. **B:** Alveolar rhabdomyosarcoma appears as loosely cohesive tumor cells lining alveolar-like spaces. **C:** Neuroblastoma is arranged in Homer Wright rosettes with no lumens (similar to Ewing/PNET), but immunostains for the neuroendocrine marker chromogranin (inset). **D:** In contrast, retinoblastoma is arranged in Flexner-Wintersteiner rosettes, which do have a lumen (like neural ependymoma).

2. Neuroblastoma arises from the neural crest and is most commonly found in the adrenal medulla; although it may arise anywhere along the sympathetic chain, including the neck.
3. Abdominal mass and fever are presenting signs.
    a. Some are incidentally found by prenatal ultrasound.
    b. Diffusely metastatic tumors to liver, bone marrow, and skin produce the so-called '**blueberry muffin**' clinical appearance.
4. Neuroblastomas secrete catecholamines (vanillylmandelic acid [VMA] and homovanillic acid [HVA]); urine testing for these compounds can confirm the diagnosis and monitor for recurrence.
5. Microscopically, these tumors are arranged in sheets and pseudorosettes of small round blue cells.
    a. Tumor cells immunostain for neuroendocrine markers, such as **chromogranin.**
    b. In time, or after treatment, these tumors may mature revealing ganglion cells and mature neural tissue.
6. Genetic aberrations include deletion of 1p, **N-myc** gene amplification, and hyperdiploidy.
    a. *N-myc* amplification is associated with aggressive behavior.
    b. Hyperdiploidy is associated with a better prognosis.
D. **Wilms Tumor (Nephroblastoma)**
    1. Wilms tumor is the most common primary **renal tumor** in children; most cases are diagnosed after the first year of life.
    2. Wilms tumor arises from nephrogenic blastemal cells; malignant cells are primitive small round blue cells, but may differentiate into a variety of distinct cell types.
    3. Classically, Wilms tumor is triphasic, with blastemal, stromal, and epithelial elements (Figure 19–1).
        a. Blastemal cells are primitive cells with high nuclear:cytoplasmic (N:C) ratios.
        b. Stromal cells form fibromyxoid areas.
        c. The epithelial component often shows some basic recapitulation of renal tubular elements.
        d. The presence of marked nuclear atypia is referred to as **anaplasia** and is associated with an unfavorable outcome.
    4. Mutations may be found in the *WT-1* gene (a zinc-finger transcription factor involved in renal and gonadal development).
        a. Aberrations of *WT-2*, a protein of unknown function, is also seen in Beckwith-Wiedemann syndrome.
        b. Sporadic nephroblastomas often fail to reveal mutations.
    5. Treatment is surgery and adjuvant chemotherapy.
    6. Prognosis is generally good (>90% long-term survival).
    7. Wilms tumor may present as part of a syndrome.
        a. **Beckwith-Wiedemann syndrome** is characterized by **macroglossia,** hypoglycemia, organomegaly, renal cysts, and Wilms tumor.
        b. **WAGR syndrome** is characterized by *W*ilms tumor, *a*niridia, *g*enital abnormalities, and mental *r*etardation.
        c. **Denys-Drash syndrome** is characterized by **gonadal dysgenesis,** renal failure, and Wilms tumor.

E. **Medulloblastoma**

1. Medulloblastoma is a primitive neural tumor that occurs in the cerebellum, predominantly in children (see Chapter 16).
2. Metastatic disease into the cerebrospinal fluid is evaluated by lumbar puncture and cytology.

SMALL ROUND BLUE CELL TUMORS

- *Most malignant childhood tumors present as small round blue cell tumors, which means they are immature or rapidly dividing, leading to high nuclear:cytoplasmic ratios with little cytoplasm or evidence of differentiation.*
- *Small round blue cell tumors are distinguished by location, morphology, immunohistochemistry (eg, WT-1 in Wilms tumor), and cytogenetics (eg, t(11;22) for Ewing sarcoma; t(2:13) for alveolar rhabdomyosarcoma; N-myc amplification (2p24) in neuroblastoma).*
- *The mnemonic for these childhood malignancies is LERN: leukemia/lymphoma, Ewing, rhabdomyosarcoma, and neuroblastoma.*

CLINICAL PROBLEMS

1. Which of the following is a direct consequence of respiratory distress syndrome?
   A. Intraventricular hemorrhage
   B. Hyaline membrane formation
   C. Necrotizing enterocolitis
   D. Retinal damage
   E. None of the above

2. An Rh-negative primigravida woman is pregnant with an Rh-positive fetus. Which of the following is the best course of action?
   A. Do nothing, there is no threat to the fetus
   B. Give anti-D rhesus immune globulin before the next pregnancy
   C. Perform maternal plasmapheresis
   D. Give RhoGAM at 28 weeks gestation and within 3 days of delivery
   E. Answers B and C are correct

3. Which of the following is **true** regarding sudden infant death syndrome (SIDS)?
   A. SIDS is a diagnosis of exclusion
   B. SIDS is more common in children who sleep in the supine position
   C. SIDS is most common in Asians
   D. SIDS is more common in singleton births
   E. None of the above

4. Which is **NOT** usually associated with mental retardation?

   A. Trisomy 21

   B. Trisomy 18

   C. Trisomy 13

   D. Monosomy X

   E. All the above are usually associated with mental retardation

5. Which of the following is a feature of Duchenne muscular dystrophy?

   A. Late onset with indolent course

   B. Death in the first decade of life

   C. Sparing of cardiopulmonary function

   D. Gower sign

   E. None of the above

6. Which of the following is a lysosomal storage disease?

   A. Phenylketonuria

   B. Lesch-Nyhan syndrome

   C. Gaucher disease

   D. Adenosine deaminase deficiency

   E. All the above

7. Which of the following is a characteristic of cystic fibrosis?

   A. Vitamin B deficiency

   B. Patients have decreased sweat chloride levels

   C. The underlying genetic defect involves chromosome 7

   D. Secretory diarrhea

   E. All the above

8. Which of the following is **true** regarding benign tumors of childhood?

   A. Flat hemangiomas will spontaneously regress

   B. Cystic hygroma is common in Klinefelter syndrome

   C. Malignant transformation is sometimes seen in teratomas

   D. Teratomas are most common in the head and neck

   E. None of the above

9. Which of the following is **false** regarding common malignancies of childhood?

   A. Neuroblastoma is a small round blue cell tumor

   B. Follicular lymphoma is common in children

   C. Alveolar rhabdomyosarcoma shows a t(2;13) translocation

   D. Osteosarcoma is the most common childhood bone tumor

   E. None of the above are false

10. Which of the following is **true** regarding Wilms tumor?

    A. Predominance of stromal elements portends a worse prognosis

    B. Mutations in the *WT-2* gene are seen in WAGR syndrome

    C. Wilms tumor most commonly arises in the lung

    D. Prognosis is generally good (> 90% long-term survival)

    E. All the above

ANSWERS

1. The answer is B. Hyaline membranes form when direct damage to alveolar lining cells allows protein rich exudative fluid to enter the alveolus. The remaining choices represent complications of mechanical ventilation and oxygen toxicity.

2. The answer is D. Anti-D rhesus immune globulin must be given at 28 weeks gestation and again following delivery to prevent sensitization of the mother. There is no threat to the current pregnancy (it is the mother's first), but the objective is to prevent complications in subsequent pregnancies.

3. The answer is A. Sudden infant death syndrome (SIDS) is diagnosed only when all other possible causes of death are ruled out. Studies have demonstrated that sleeping in the supine position reduces the incidence of SIDS. This finding was the impetus behind the "back to sleep" program instituted by pediatricians.

4. The answer is D. Turner syndrome (Monosomy X) is usually associated with normal intelligence. The other choices are associated with moderate to severe mental retardation.

5. The answer is D. As proximal muscle weakness worsens, children with Duchenne muscular dystrophy will often use their arms to aid in standing by placing their hands on the knees and pushing up (Gower sign). Onset is usually evident by 4 years of age, and death usually results from cardiopulmonary compromise.

6. The answer is C. Gaucher disease is a lysosomal storage disease. The other choices represent other metabolic disorders.

7. The answer is C. The *CFTR* gene is on chromosome 7. Vitamin deficiencies are restricted to the fat-soluble vitamins (A, D, E, K). Secretions are viscid, leading to ileus. Sweat chloride levels are increased.

8. The answer is C. Malignant transformation occurs in teratomas, represented by histologically immature cells (eg, yolk sac). Teratomas are most common in the sacrococcygeal region. Cystic hygromas are seen in Turner syndrome. Elevated hemangiomas tend to regress; flat (macular) hemangiomas do not.

9. The answer is B. Follicular lymphoma is extremely uncommon in children. Burkitt and Hodgkin lymphoma are the common childhood malignancies.

10. The answer is D. Prognosis is generally good with combination surgery, chemotherapy, and radiation. *WT-2* gene defects are seen in Beckwith-Wiedemann syndrome. Preponderance of blastemal elements indicates a worse prognosis. Wilms tumor (nephroblastoma) arises in the kidney.

CHAPTER 20

IMMUNE SYSTEM MEDIATED DISEASE

*And though all streams flow from a single course to cleanse
the blood from polluted hand, they hasten on their course in vain.*
—Aeschylus

I. Congenital Disorders of Hypoimmunity

A. Humoral Immunodeficiency

1. **Common variable immune deficiency** is a group of diseases characterized by marked reductions in serum IgG and IgA levels.
   a. It occurs in males and females with equal frequency.
   b. There are normal numbers of circulating B lymphocytes, but there are defects in terminal B-cell maturation leading to reductions in immunoglobulin.
   c. These patients are susceptible to bacterial infections, especially respiratory and gastrointestinal infections.
   d. There is an increased risk of gastric carcinoma, lymphomas, and amyloidosis.

2. **Bruton** (also called **X-linked**) **agammaglobulinemia** is a disorder of B-cells where a mutation in a cytoplasmic Bruton tyrosine kinase (**BTK**) causes maturation arrest in B-cells.
   a. Infant boys are normal until 4–6 months of age as maternal antibody protection wanes.
   b. Patients suffer from recurrent bacterial infections, especially pneumonia, meningitis, otitis, with **encapsulated pyogenic bacteria** (*Streptococcus pneumoniae*, *Haemophilus influenzae*, group A streptococcus).
   c. While lymphoid precursors can be identified in bone marrow, lymph node tissue will be markedly hypoplastic with essentially absent germinal center formation and decreased plasma cells.
   d. Replacement with immune globulin is the cornerstone of treatment along with prompt antibiotic use.

3. **IgA deficiency** is the most common primary immune deficiency.
   a. It has a prevalence of 1 in 350 individuals.
   b. The hallmark of this disorder is a very low, often undetectable, serum IgA level.
   c. It predisposes to respiratory and gastrointestinal tract infections.
   d. IgA deficiency is also associated with celiac disease, as well as autoimmune and lupus-like syndromes.

e. IgA-deficient patients are prone to **anaphylaxis** if they receive blood products from non–IgA-deficient patients.

    f. Treatment centers around antibiotics and avoiding sensitization to IgA-containing blood products.

  4. Selective immunoglobulin class and subclass deficiencies typically involve the IgG class of immunoglobulins.

    a. Patients can be asymptomatic or have recurrent infections.

    b. The total immunoglobulin level of the serum can be normal or decreased, depending on the IgG subclass involved.

    c. About one-fifth of IgA-deficient patients will have a concomitant IgG subclass deficiency.

B. Cellular Immunodeficiency

  1. DiGeorge syndrome is a defect in neural crest development of the third and fourth pharyngeal pouches leading to thymic hypoplasia.

    a. Defective T-cell mediated immunity leaves patients prone to viral, fungal, and protozoal infections.

    b. Patients also have other manifestations of **third and fourth pharyngeal pouch developmental problems,** including parathyroid gland abnormalities, cardiac anomalies, facial defects, great vessel anomalies, and esophageal atresia.

    c. About 90% of cases involve a **mutation or deletion of chromosome 22q11.**

C. Combined Immunodeficiency Disorders

  1. Severe combined immunodeficiency (SCID) is characterized by a nearly complete absence of humoral and cellular immune function.

    a. Affected patients nearly always die within a short time unless they can be isolated from the environment and receive a bone marrow transplant.

    b. There are several types of SCID, most of which are autosomal recessive and X-linked in inheritance.

    c. SCID presents within the first few months of life, with episodes of respiratory and cutaneous bacterial infections, viral infections (such as cytomegalovirus [CMV]), candidal infections, and opportunistic infections (such as pneumocystis pneumonia).

  2. Adenosine deaminase (ADA) deficiency is an autosomal recessively inherited decrease in **purine metabolism** with excess accumulation of metabolites particularly toxic to developing lymphocytes.

    a. ADA deficiency manifests just like SCID, but **skeletal abnormalities** may also be present.

      (1) Radiographic findings include flared ribs (similar in appearance to rickets) and abnormalities of the vertebral transverse processes.

      (2) The **thymic shadow is absent** from chest films.

    b. Another enzyme involved in purine metabolism called purine nucleoside phosphorylase (PNP) can result in a SCID-like state.

  3. Hyper-IgM syndrome is caused by a mutation in the **CD40 ligand,** which is responsible for antibody class switching.

    a. Most cases are X-linked, but some are autosomal recessive.

    b. There are decreased serum levels of **IgG, IgA,** and **IgE.**

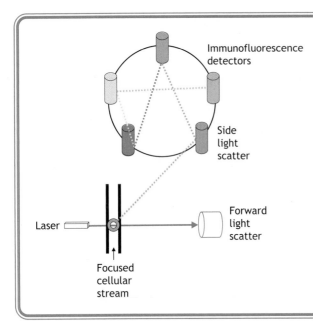

Figure 20–1. Flow cytometry. Light beams from lasers strike the cells as they flow through a focused stream. Laser light scattered in a forward direction is proportional to **cell diameter.** Laser light reflected at an angle (side scatter) is proportional to cellular granularity. Fluoresced light from labeled antigens is also collected at an angle. Laboratories use from one to ten fluorescent probes to dissect the complex mixture of cells found in blood, bone marrow, and lymphoid tissue.

   c. Lymph nodes are abnormal and lack germinal centers.
   d. Patients suffer from recurrent infections.

  D. **Flow Cytometry**
    1. Flow cytometry is the characterization of cell populations by patterns of light scatter and fluorescence detected from individual cells as they stream past an excitation light source, typically a laser (Figure 20–1).
    2. Forward scatter is a measure of cellular size, while side scatter is dependent on cytoplasmic granularity (Figure 20–2A).
    3. With the addition of fluorescent-tagged antibodies to specific surface antigens, sets of cells may be identified, and even sorted, by these characteristics.
    4. More specific than a complete blood count, flow cytometry quantifies the proportion of cell subsets, such as the CD4 to CD8 ratio, and thus, it provides additional data for the diagnosis of immune deficiency, as with DiGeorge syndrome or AIDS (Figure 20–2).
    5. Aberrant expression of antigens from normally distinct cell populations, such as CD3 (T-cells) and CD20 (B-cells), is characteristic of malignancy (Table 20–1).
    6. Potential specimen sources include peripheral blood, and bone marrow aspirate as well as normally paucicellular specimens, such as cerebrospinal fluid and bronchoalveolar lavage.

  E. **Complement Deficiency**
    1. **Complement deficiencies** are rare disorders accounting for less than 1% of all immune deficiency states.
    2. Complement deficiency may result in recurrent infection, but also **systemic lupus erythematosus** (SLE) and other lupus-like conditions.
     a. **Deficiency of C1q** is almost always associated with SLE and recurrent bacterial infections.

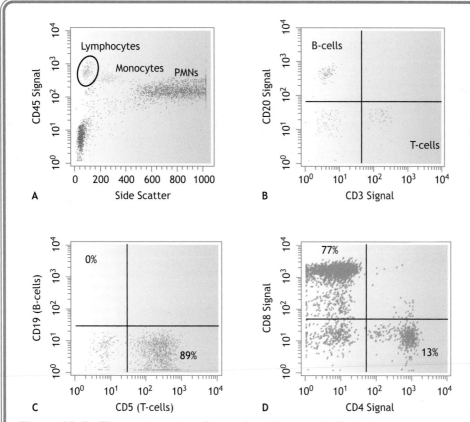

Figure 20–2. Flow cytometry diagnosing disease. A: Typical two parameter dot plot of CD45 versus side scatter. Each dot represents a cell with the correlated values of both parameters. Three colored clusters show lymphocytes, monocytes, and granulocytes. Dots near lower left corner are debris. **B:** Patients with DiGeorge syndrome may have a normal, reduced, or absent T-cell population. In this case, the percentage of T-cells is reduced (normal > 55%). **C:** Only lymphocytes are displayed with CD19 to label B-cells and CD5 to label T-cells. No CD19+ B-cells are present in a male patient with X-linked agammaglobulinemia. **D:** Only lymphocytes are displayed with CD4 versus CD8 from a case of HIV infection. CD4+ T lymphocytes are greatly decreased. In healthy individuals, there are more CD4+ than CD8+ T lymphocytes. PMNs, polymorphonuclear neutrophils.

    b. **Deficiency of C1 esterase inhibitor** results in inappropriate activation of C1 and generation of C2 kinin.
        (1) The latter increases vascular permeability and is thought to mediate **angioedema** among patients with C1 esterase inhibitor deficiency.
        (2) The subsequent edema involves subcutaneous tissue as well as the respiratory and gastrointestinal tracts.
    c. Patients with **homozygous C2 deficiency** have a 50% risk of developing lupus or recurrent infections.

Table 20–1. CD antigens and cellular expression.

Antigen	Cellular Expression
CD3	Pan T cell
CD4	Helper T cell
CD8	Cytotoxic T cell
CD19 and CD20	Pan B cell
CD13 and CD33	Myeloid cells
CD14 and CD68	Macrophages and monocytes
CD56	Natural killer (NK) cells
CD34	Hematopoietic stem cells
CD45	Leukocyte common antigen
CD55 and CD59	Decay-accelerating factor (DAF) and membrane inhibitor of reactive lysis (MIRL)
CD117 (c-kit)	Hematopoietic stem cells

    d. **C3 deficiency** leads to reduced opsonization of bacteria.
      (1) Patients with C3 deficiency are at increased risk for infections with encapsulated bacteria (*S pneumoniae*).
      (2) Patients with C3 deficiency may be clinically similar to those who have undergone splenectomy.
    e. Patients with heterozygous deficiencies of early proteins, **C2, C3, and C4,** also have an increased prevalence of autoimmune disorders.
    f. Deficiencies of the late components, **C5, C6, C7, and C8,** lead to susceptibility to neisserial infections (ie, meningitis).

  F. **Phagocytic Function Deficiency**
    1. **Chronic granulomatous disease** is a group of disorders with impaired respiratory burst of phagocytic cells.
      a. The impaired ability of phagocytic cells to generate oxidants results in susceptibility to recurrent infections by **catalase-positive organisms** (staphylococci, *Pseudomonas, Campylobacter, Neisseria gonorrhoeae,* and *Moraxella catarrhalis*).
      b. Mutations involving the genes that encode for components of the reduced form of nicotinamide adenine dinucleotide phosphate **(NADPH) oxidase system** results in the inability of phagocytic cells to generate reactive oxygen species.
      c. Severe forms of glucose-6-phosphate dehydrogenase (G6PD)-deficiency can result in a chronic granulomatous disease-like picture, since this enzyme is also involved in NADPH regeneration.

d. The **nitroblue tetrazolium (NBT) slide test** was a previous test of oxidative function in which neutrophils take up colorless NBT and form a deep blue cytoplasmic precipitate in the presence of adequate oxidant formation; there is no color change among patients with chronic granulomatous disease.

      e. Newer tests include flow cytometry, which detects oxidation of certain molecules within the cytoplasm.

  2. Leukocyte adhesion deficiency, as its name implies, is the relative absence of several molecules belonging to the β_2 or leukocyte integrin family.

      a. The integrins are a superfamily of adhesion molecules.

      b. This is a heterogeneous group of disorders that results in various decreases of leukocyte adhesion and, therefore, variable severity of immune deficiency.

      c. Patients suffer from recurrent bacterial infections, especially of the soft tissues (*S aureus* and *Pseudomonas).*

      d. There is often a classic history of delayed loss of the umbilical cord stump.

      e. Laboratory findings include markedly elevated leukocyte counts in the peripheral blood.

      f. Diagnosis is made by demonstrating lack of normal adhesion molecules, either by leukocyte aggregation studies (older technology) or by flow cytometry (newer).

  3. Chédiak-Higashi syndrome is caused by an autosomal recessive mutation of the *CHS1* gene involved with cytoplasmic organelles.

      a. The mutation causes several clinical features including **oculocutaneous albinism,** neuropathy, **enlarged neutrophil granules,** and abnormal platelets.

      b. The lack of pigmentation is caused by abnormal melanosomes.

      c. Leukocyte counts are decreased (leukopenia), especially the fraction of neutrophils (neutropenia).

      d. Multiple lines of white cells are affected with **abnormally functioning lysosomes** rendering the patient vulnerable to recurrent fungal and bacterial infections of the skin and lungs.

      e. The primary and secondary granules of neutrophils fuse into large granules that do not function properly in phagocytosis.

      f. The patients also possess a true platelet defect with decreased levels of adenosine diphosphate and serotonin resulting in abnormal aggregation.

G. Miscellaneous Disorders

  1. Wiskott-Aldrich syndrome is an immunodeficiency state with associated **eczema** and **thrombocytopenia.**

      a. It is an X-linked recessive disorder mapped to Xp11.23 which encodes the Wiskott-Aldrich syndrome protein (WASP) involved with cytoskeleton structure and cell membrane signaling.

      b. Patients have a defective antibody response to polysaccharide and protein antigens.

      c. They have **decreased** levels of **IgM,** normal IgG levels, and **increased** IgE and **IgA** levels.

      d. There is a decrease in the number of circulating T-cells with progressive loss of T-cell zones in the thymus.

  2. Hyper-IgE syndrome (Job syndrome) presents with an odd assortment of symptoms, including pruritic, **eczematous skin lesions** with intermittent staphylococcal **"cold" abscesses** without the usual pain, erythema, and warmth of a typical abscess.

   a. Mucocutaneous candidiasis and onychomycosis are seen.

   b. There is also a predisposition to bone fractures.

   c. There are no confirmatory or diagnostic tests available; the disorder is recognized by its clinical manifestations and markedly **elevated IgE** levels.

   d. Patients have a phenotype similar to chronic granulomatous disease, but neutrophil function is normal.

3. Chronic mucocutaneous candidiasis is characterized by chronic *Candida* infections of the skin and mucous membranes.

   a. This disorder is not fatal.

   b. The exact immune deficiency mechanism is unknown.

   c. Testing of the immune system can be normal.

   d. Affected patients can have associated endocrine disorders.

   e. Treatment includes antifungal agents.

4. Ataxia-telangiectasia is one of the autosomal recessive ataxias with associated immune system dysfunction.

   a. The gene for ataxia-telangiectasia is on chromosome 11 (the *ATM* gene) and is involved in regulation of the cell cycle.

   b. There is both **thymic hypoplasia** and **immunoglobulin deficiencies** (especially IgG and IgA).

   c. Symptoms and signs present in the first decade with ataxia due to **cerebellar dysfunction, telangiectasia,** and immune dysfunction.

      (1) Patients are prone to recurrent infections.

      (2) There is an **increased risk of cancer,** especially lymphoma (non-Hodgkin and Hodgkin) and T-cell acute lymphoblastic leukemia.

      (3) These patients are also at increased risk for **diabetes mellitus** and other endocrine disorders.

II. HIV/AIDS

  A. Epidemiology

    1. HIV is an **RNA retrovirus** with a high affinity for CD4 T-lymphocytes and monocytes.

      a. There are two strains of HIV, designated type 1 and type 2.

      b. **HIV-1** is found throughout the world and is responsible for most of the cases of AIDS worldwide.

      c. **HIV-2** is predominantly in West Africa and follows a **more indolent** course compared to HIV-1.

    2. Transmission is primarily through sexual contact or inoculation.

      a. **Parenteral transmission** has occurred in several groups at risk, including injection drug users, persons with hemophilia, and recipients of infected blood.

      b. Transmission from mother to infant occurs through direct **transplacental spread,** trauma occurring in the birth canal, and through breastfeeding.

      c. HIV is not passed through casual contact.

  B. Diagnosis and Monitoring

    1. HIV screening most often involves enzyme-linked immunosorbent assay (**ELISA**) for anti-HIV antibodies within the peripheral blood.

      a. This technique has high sensitivity and specificity.

b. Despite this, false-positive results are possible, especially among low-risk populations or during pregnancy.

         (1) Antibodies against **similar pathogens** may cause false-positive results.

         (2) SLE and other autoimmune diseases are another source of false-positive results.

      c. Positive ELISA results are confirmed by **Western blot.**

         (1) In a Western blot (protein immunoblot), proteins are separated by gel electrophoresis, transferred to nitrocellulose paper, then bound to an antibody specific to the protein of interest.

         (2) Patients with both a positive ELISA screening test and negative Western blot are usually monitored with repeat tests but are usually not truly infected.

  2. In cases of suspected acute HIV infection with negative antibody results, there are other methods to make a diagnosis.

      a. Assays that detect the **p24 antigen** of the virus can be used.

      b. Viral culture from peripheral blood mononuclear cells is also possible but may take several weeks.

      c. The presence of viral nucleic acids may be detected in peripheral blood by **real-time polymerase chain reaction (PCR).**

         (1) Of all the methods for detecting acute HIV, reverse transcription (RT)-PCR is probably the best.

         (2) The addition of **nucleic acid testing** to the screening panel for blood donations has significantly decreased the time from infection to detection.

  3. The **CD4+ lymphocyte count** is used to monitor patients with confirmed HIV infection and is considered the best marker of disease progression (Figure 20–2D).

      a. Normal CD4 counts in adults are 500–1500 cells/mcL.

      b. HIV-positive individuals with counts under 200 cells/mcL are considered to have AIDS regardless of symptomatology.

      c. The count helps determine the risk of particular opportunistic infections.

         (1) When counts fall **below 200 cells/mcL,** patients are at increased risk for **opportunistic infections.**

         (2) Counts less than 50 cells/mcL strongly indicate risk of **CMV infections,** especially retinitis.

      d. A single CD4 count should not be used for initial diagnosis of HIV infection because there are many conditions associated with a low CD4 count.

         (1) Systemic steroid therapy may decrease the count, while acute viral illnesses (influenza and herpes simplex infection) may raise the CD8 count.

         (2) CD4 counts also exhibit a diurnal variation with a relative decline in the morning.

C. Pathophysiology of HIV

  1. HIV infection follows a typical clinical course.

      a. Acute infection is characterized by the **HIV syndrome** in which the virus spreads throughout susceptible tissues over weeks.

      b. A period of latency, lasting from weeks to many years, follows during which HIV is actively replicating without causing any symptoms or leading to opportunistic infection.

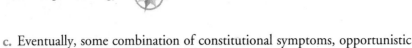

    c. Eventually, some combination of constitutional symptoms, opportunistic infection, or neoplasia leads to a diagnosis of AIDS.

  2. Aside from a diminished CD4 count, AIDS is defined clinically by the presence of one or more opportunistic infections and neoplasms.

    a. **Fungal infections** include candidiasis of the upper aerodigestive tract, cryptococcal infection of the central nervous system (CNS), pneumocystis pneumonia as well as disseminated histoplasmosis and coccidioidomycosis.

    b. **Protozoal infections** include cryptosporidiosis and other gastrointestinal infections along with CNS toxoplasmosis.

    c. **Bacterial infections** typically involve atypical *Mycobacteria.*

    d. **Viral infections** with CMV and disseminated infections with herpes simplex virus and varicella zoster virus are observed.

    e. **Kaposi sarcoma,** B-cell lymphomas (especially involving the CNS), and invasive cervical carcinoma are associated with AIDS.

III. Systemic Rheumatic Diseases

  A. Systemic Lupus Erythematosus

    1. SLE is the prototypical systemic autoimmune disease that is most prevalent in women of childbearing age, but can occur in anyone.

    2. The etiology is unknown.

    3. The diagnostic criteria for SLE, as promulgated by the American College of Rheumatology, include the following:

      a. **Malar rash**

      b. Photosensitivity

      c. Oral ulcers

      d. **Discoid rash**

      e. Nonerosive arthritis

      f. Pleuritis or pericarditis

      g. Nephropathy

      h. Hemolytic anemia, leukopenia, lymphopenia, or thrombocytopenia

      i. Positive antinuclear antibody (ANA) study

      j. **Specific autoantibodies** to ds-DNA, Sm nuclear antigen, or antiphospholipid antibodies

    4. To be diagnosed, a patient must exhibit at least four of the above, either all at once or sequentially over any time period.

    5. The hallmark of this disease is the presence of **circulating autoantibodies to DNA** with tissue injury caused by circulating immune complexes composed of native DNA and anti-DNA antibodies.

    6. Most patients with SLE have a broad spectrum of polyclonal autoantibodies.

    7. Several of the autoantibodies have certain diagnostic characteristics and associations.

      a. **Anti ds-DNA** is the most specific marker for SLE and often follows disease activity—elevated in active SLE (Table 20–2).

      b. **Anti-SM and anti-RNP,** the Smith antigen, is also considered specific for SLE, and it may be predictive of renal disease and CNS manifestations.

      c. **Anti-SS-A/Ro and SS-B/La** are associated with SLE and Sjögren syndrome; they may be linked to nephritis, vasculitis, leukopenia, and photosensitivity.

Table 20–2. Markers of autoimmune disease.

Marker (Anti-)	Condition
Acetylcholine	Myasthenia gravis
GBM	Goodpasture syndrome
Centromere	CREST syndrome
Histone (alone)	Drug-induced lupus (hydralazine, isoniazid, and procainamide)
IgG (Fc part)	Rheumatoid arthritis
Microsomal	Chronic autoimmune thyroiditis
Double stranded DNA	SLE
Single stranded DNA	SLE and others
Smith	SLE (pathognomic) (30% of cases)
Antinuclear antibody	SLE (95% of cases), Sjögren syndrome
SSA (Ro)	Sjögren syndrome
SSB (La)	Sjögren syndrome
RNP	Sjögren syndrome, arthritis, and mixed connective tissue disease
Scl-70	Diffuse scleroderma
Topoisomerase	Diffuse scleroderma
c-ANCA	Wegener granulomatosis, Churg-Strauss
p-ANCA	Polyarteritis nodosa, colitis

GBM, glomerular basement membrane; c-ANCA, cytoplasmic antineutrophil cytoplasmic antibody; CREST, calcinosis cutis, Raynaud phenomenon, esophageal dysmotility, sclerodactyly, and telangectasia; p-ANCA, perinuclear antineutrophil cytoplasmic antibody; SLE, systemic lupus erythematosus.

   d. **Anti-phospholipid antibodies** are found in up to two-thirds of SLE patients and are associated with thrombosis (arterial and venous), thrombocytopenia, hemolytic anemia, and miscarriage.
8. In SLE, there is defective clearance of apoptotic cellular debris resulting in the characteristic **LE cell,** a phagocyte (neutrophil or macrophage) visibly loaded with engulfed apoptotic cells.
9. **Renal involvement** is especially prominent in SLE, and it remains a major cause of morbidity in the lupus patient.

a. The World Health Organization (WHO) has developed a classification system for lupus renal disease.
       (1) Class I (no detectable renal lesion on biopsy)
       (2) Class II (mesangial lupus glomerulonephritis)
       (3) Class III (focal proliferative glomerulonephritis)
       (4) Class IV (diffuse proliferative glomerulonephritis)
       (5) Class V (membranous glomerulonephritis)
   b. None of the renal lesions are specific for SLE.
10. **Drug-induced lupus** typically spares the kidney and is associated with the presence of **anti-histone antibodies.**
    a. Drugs known to incite drug-induced lupus include hydralazine, procainamide, and isoniazid, but these are now rarely used in medical practice.
    b. In drug-induced lupus, there are other antibodies present, including **anti-ss-DNA** and **anti-chromatin antibodies.**
11. **Chronic discoid lupus** is a benign cutaneous form of lupus without the associated systemic disease.

B. Sjögren Syndrome
   1. This is an autoimmune disease characterized by progressive chronic inflammation of the lacrimal glands and salivary glands.
   2. These patients have the **sicca complex,** xerostomia and xerophthalmia (dryness of the mouth and eyes, respectively).
   3. Females are typically affected more than males; there is an association with rheumatoid arthritis, SLE, dermatomyositis, and mixed connective tissue disease.
   4. Sjögren syndrome can also manifest as cutaneous vasculitis, interstitial pneumonitis, and lymphadenopathy.
   5. Biopsies of the salivary glands are often used to make the diagnosis, with the predominant finding a lymphocytic infiltration of the glands with gland atrophy and destruction.
   6. Sjögren syndrome can develop into a **B-cell lymphoma.**
   7. The autoantibodies associated with Sjögren syndrome are **anti-SS-A/Ro and anti-SS-B/La.**
   8. The sensitivity of these autoantibodies is low, between 30% and 60%, but the presence of both together in a patient is specific for primary Sjögren syndrome.

C. Rheumatoid Arthritis
   1. This is a systemic rheumatic disease characterized by a chronic, **symmetrically destructive** arthritis.
   2. Joints most commonly involved are the metacarpal-phalangeal joints, proximal interphalangeal joints, wrists, knees, feet; the axial skeleton is typically spared with the exception of the atlanto-occipital joint, which can become subluxed with trauma.
   3. **Rheumatoid nodules** arise on the extensor surfaces of joint, typically the upper extremities, and have a characteristic histologic pattern of necrotic granulomas.
   4. Extra-articular manifestations include rheumatoid nodules, cutaneous vasculitis, interstitial lung disease, and effusions.
   5. **Felty syndrome** is a combination with chronic neutropenia.

6. Several common laboratory tests help diagnose arthritis.
   a. **Rheumatoid factor** is an antibody directed against the Fc portion of the antibody molecule.
   b. Anti-citrullinated peptides are antibodies measured by ELISA that are about 60–70% sensitive, and 90% specific.

D. **Scleroderma (Progressive Systemic Sclerosis)**
1. This is a multisystem disorder of unknown cause, although some cases have been associated with environmental and ingested toxins.
2. Clinically, there is subcutaneous and soft tissue fibrosis with associated vasculopathy.
3. The **CREST syndrome,** a variant of scleroderma, is less aggressive, and consists of the following:
   a. **C**alcinosis cutis
   b. **R**aynaud phenomenon
   c. **E**sophageal dysmotility
   d. **S**clerodactyly
   e. **T**elangectasia
4. Vascular lesions are particularly common in the kidney that may lead to malignant hypertension.
5. The vascular lesions can also lead to pulmonary hypertension.
6. There are several autoantibodies associated with scleroderma and the CREST syndrome.
   a. **Autoantibodies** to **centromere antigens** are seen in CREST syndrome and less aggressive forms of scleroderma (typically with less pulmonary fibrosis).
   b. Autoantibodies to **Scl-70** are seen in scleroderma that follows a more aggressive clinical course, with increased pulmonary complications and increased mortality.
   c. Autoantibodies to RNA polymerases are specific for scleroderma, especially of the diffuse type of scleroderma (as opposed to the CREST syndrome).

IV. Allergic Diseases

A. **Allergic Rhinitis**
1. This is one of the most prevalent medical conditions, with over 20% of individuals having allergies by **positive skin testing** results.
2. Allergic rhinitis is characterized by IgE-mediated nasal congestion, sneezing, lacrimation, and increased mucus production.
3. This is an example of a **type I hypersensitivity** response, mediated by airborne allergens, animal dander, pollens, and dust mites.
4. Checking nasal mucus for the presence of **eosinophils** has been used in the past to distinguish allergic rhinitis.
5. Allergic rhinitis can become complicated by otitis media and maxillary sinusitis.

B. **Asthma**
1. Asthma is hyperactive airway disease with chronic inflammation.
2. Not all asthma is driven by an allergy, and it is estimated that only about one-fifth of asthmatics have an allergic component.
3. **Extrinsic asthma** refers to type I hypersensitivity, while **intrinsic asthma** is due to nonimmune causes, such as aspirin, viral infections, stress, or exercise.

4. Type 2 helper T-cells are thought to be the major player in the chronic inflammation associated with asthma.

5. In allergen-triggered asthma, there are two responses—an immediate phase followed by a late phase.

    a. The **immediate phase** is mediated by **IgE** bound to IgE receptors on mast cells in the airways and lasts for minutes.

    b. Release of mediators by inflammatory cells already in the airways leads to influx of inflammatory cells which leads to development of the **late phase.**

6. There are several pathologic findings in acute asthma, usually observed in patients suffering from status asthmaticus.

    a. There is increased thick mucus occluding airways.

    b. Because of the mucous plugging, there is over-distention of the lungs, with foci of atelectasis.

    c. There can be **pneumothorax.**

    d. On microscopic sections, there can be mucosal edema, infiltration by eosinophils and mast cells, hypertrophy of the submucosa, hypertrophy of the bronchial smooth muscle, and eosinophil by-products (**Charcot-Leyden crystals**).

7. The relationship of asthma with allergic rhinitis and eczema is known as atopy.

C. Urticaria and Angioedema

    1. Urticaria can be acute (less than 6 weeks) or chronic.

    2. In most cases of urticaria, the exact etiology cannot be pinpointed; however, most cases of acute urticaria are considered to be secondary to infection (viral infections, streptococcal pharyngitis, early hepatitis B, and infectious mononucleosis).

    3. Only some cases of urticaria are mediated by **IgE,** while others can be triggered by nonspecific stimuli such as **cold** weather or a **physical stimulus.**

    4. The pathophysiology of angioedema is similar to urticaria, but it involves deeper tissues.

    5. Many patients have both urticaria and angioedema.

    6. Mast cell disorders, such as systemic mastocytosis and urticaria pigmentosa, can manifest as urticaria.

    7. Hereditary angioedema usually presents in the second decade of life and results from a deficiency of the **C1 esterase inhibitor.**

        a. It is rare and presents with oral and facial angioedema.

        b. The lack of C1 esterase inhibitor allows for unchecked activation of the complement system.

        c. Patients can have a quantitative loss of the C1 esterase inhibitor (majority), or a qualitative impairment of function (about 15%).

        d. The best screen is to test a C4 level, which will be low due to unchecked complement activation.

D. Anaphylaxis

    1. Anaphylaxis is a severe systemic manifestation of a **type I (immediate) hypersensitivity** response (mediated by IgE).

    2. The hallmark findings are vascular collapse and shock due to marked vasodilation and capillary leak, bronchospasm and laryngeal edema with airway obstruction, urticaria, and angioedema.

    3. Individuals must be sensitized to the antigen.

        a. Any substance may act as an antigen.

b. Milk, eggs, peanuts, and **wheat** are common food antigens in **children.**

      c. **Peanuts** and **shellfish** are common food antigens in **adults.**

  4. The severity of response depends on the level of sensitization.

  5. Anaphylaxis may still occur in patients who have demonstrated previous tolerance to an antigen.

  6. Treatment includes removing offending antigen and administration of epinephrine, intravenous fluids, corticosteroids, and antihistamines.

CLINICAL PROBLEMS

1. The risk of celiac disease is increased in patients with which condition?

  A. Rheumatoid arthritis

  B. Ankylosing spondylitis

  C. IgA deficiency

  D. Scleroderma

  E. Chronic granulomatous disease

2. Because of the increased risk of anaphylaxis, plasma-containing blood products should **NOT** be given to patients who have which of the following conditions?

  A. Complement deficiency

  B. Hereditary angioedema

  C. Systemic lupus erythematosus

  D. IgA deficiency

  E. Combined variable immune deficiency

3. A 37-year-old patient arrives at the emergency department with a several-week history of increasing dyspnea, cough, and chest tightness. A complete blood count demonstrates an elevated eosinophil count. A serum IgE level performed after admission is markedly elevated. Cultures are negative. Which is correct?

  A. The infiltrate may be related to community-acquired pneumonia

  B. The infiltrate may be related to mucous plugging and atelectasis

  C. The patient could potentially have bronchopulmonary aspergillosis

  D. Corticosteroids should be considered as part of the treatment plan

  E. All of the above are correct

4. A 45-year-old woman complains of fatigue, muscle aches, and pains in her joints, specifically her hands and wrists. On physical examination, she does have some swelling of her wrists and metacarpal-phalangeal joints. Which tests may be useful in her evaluation?

  A. Complete blood count

  B. Antinuclear antibody screen

C. Erythrocyte sedimentation rate

D. Urinalysis

E. All of the above

5. 25-year-old man complains of having fever, malaise, headache, and a rash on his chest and abdomen. He has a history of injection drug use. Which of the following tests would **not** be a useful first test?

A. Serum markers for hepatitis B

B. Quantitative CD4+ determination

C. Enzyme-linked immunosorbent assay for HIV

D. Antibodies to hepatitis C virus

E. Polymerase chain reaction for HIV

Questions 6–15: Match the finding with the condition.

6. HLA-B27

7. Anti-U1nRNP

8. Parathyroid hypoplasia

9. Recurrent infections from *Neisseria* sp.

10. Antibodies to the Fc region of immunoglobulin

11. Anti-SS-A/Ro

12. Giant neutrophil granules

13. Dermatitis and thrombocytopenia

14. Mutation in the CD40 ligand

15. Bruton tyrosine kinase (BTK) mutation

    A. Rheumatoid arthritis

    B. Ankylosing spondylitis

    C. Sjögren syndrome

    D. DiGeorge syndrome

    E. Scleroderma

    F. Hyper-IgM syndrome

    G. Complement deficiency

    H. Chédiak-Higashi syndrome

    I. X-linked agammaglobulinemia

    J. Wiskott-Aldrich syndrome

ANSWERS

1. The answer is C. Patients with IgA deficiency also have an increased risk of celiac disease.

2. The answer is D. Patients with IgA deficiency are at risk for anaphylaxis if given blood products from normal donors, which contain IgA in plasma. These patients often need blood products from IgA deficient patients or washed products to remove the offending plasma.

3. The answer is E. In a patient with asthma and worsening symptoms, it is important to look for an underlying cause. In extrinsic asthma, there can be a peripheral eosinophilia and elevated IgE. This can also be seen in allergic bronchopulmonary aspergillosis, which is also associated with marked sputum eosinophilia, thick mucus with plugging and atelectasis. The infiltrate may also be indicative of a community-acquired pneumonia.

4. The answer is E. In evaluating a patient with a possible systemic rheumatologic disorder, it is important to consider the diagnostic criteria for systemic lupus erythematosus (SLE) as well as the other rheumatic disorders.

5. The answer is B. Remember that a low CD4+ is nonspecific and does not indicate HIV infection. In the presence of HIV infection, the CD4+ count is useful in determining disease severity.

6. The answer is B. Ankylosing spondylitis is associated with HLA-B27.

7. The answer is E. Scleroderma is associated with autoantibodies to U1nRNP.

8. The answer is D. DiGeorge syndrome is associated with branchial pouch developmental anomalies, including parathyroid hypoplasia. Postoperative hypocalcemia is a concern in these patients who often have associated cardiac defects that require surgical treatment.

9. The answer is G. Complement deficiency, especially the late complement components, is associated with recurrent neisserial infections.

10. The answer is A. Rheumatoid arthritis is associated with the rheumatoid factor, an autoantibody against the antibody Fc region.

11. The answer is C. This autoantibody is associated with Sjögren syndrome and systemic lupus erythematosus.

12. The answer is H. The mutation in Chédiak-Higashi syndrome causes problems in intracytoplasmic organelle physiology, leading to formation of giant cytoplasmic granules in neutrophils.

13. The answer is J. Dermatitis and thrombocytopenia are seen in Wiskott-Aldrich syndrome.

14. The answer is F. The CD40 ligand is responsible for antibody class switching in the mature B-cell. If this ligand is defective, then no switch occurs, and IgM persists, leading to elevated IgM levels and defective humoral immunity.

15. The answer is I. The BTK mutation prevents normal B-cell maturation, leading to severe humoral immune deficiency.

RAPID REVIEW GLOSSARY

"The question is," said Alice, "whether you can make words mean so many different things."
—Lewis Carroll, *Alice in Wonderland*

I. COMMON TERMS

Abscess "Pocket" of contained liquefactive necrosis with prominent inflammatory cell infiltrate

Acinar Cells arranged around a central lumen; seen in exocrine tissue, such as sebaceous, mammary, and pancreatic glands

Adenocarcinoma Malignant neoplasm arising from glandular tissue, most commonly in the breast, lung, colon, and prostate

ADAMTS-13 Protease that cleaves von Willebrand factor; reduced in cases of thrombotic thrombocytopenic purpura (TTP)

Adenomatoid Resembling a glandular structure, or related to a set of rare benign, possibly mesothelial-derived, neoplasms that may arise within the genital tract

Adenomyosis Presence of ectopic endometrial tissue within the myometrium

Adenosis Increased number of acinar units within a lobule

Adenosquamous Mixed glandular and squamous features

Agenesis Absence or developmental failure

Aggressive Having high recurrence, invasive or metastatic potential

Allograft Organ or tissue transplant from a member of the same species with a different genotype

Alopecia Absence or loss of hair

Amphophilic Staining with either acidic or basic dyes

Anamnestic Property of lymphocyte-mediated immune memory that produces an increased number of antibodies more rapidly with subsequent exposure to an antigen

Anaplasia Loss of cellular differentiation, or dedifferentiation, observed within many types of neoplastic tissue

Aneuploidy Any number of chromosomes that is not a multiple of 23

Anergy Inability to mount an antigen-specific immune response

Angiogenesis Growth of new blood vessels

Angioinvasion Growth into or involving vascular channels

Anhidrosis Lack of sweating

Anisocytosis Variation in cell size

Aplastic Characterized by the absence of growth or development, as in aplastic anemia

Apoptosis Programmed cell death

Argyrophilic Silver-staining

Arthropod Animal phylum that includes insects, arachnids, and crustaceans

Array chip (DNA microarray) A solid platform embedded with several thousand microscopic spots, each containing picomoles of a specific DNA probe sequence, that are hybridized to a fluorophore-labeled specimen to detect the relative abundance of particular gene segments

Ashkenazi (Ashkenazim) Jews of central Europe and their descendents; often cited in population-based studies of genetic disease because of their traditionally high rate of endogamy

Athetosis Neurologic disorder characterized by continuous involuntary writhing movements

Atopy Production of immunoglobulin E (IgE) in response to common allergens

Atresia Developmental absence of a patent lumen, as involving the esophagus or biliary tree

Atrophy Decreased cellular volume

Atypia Morphologic aberrance, most often of nuclei

"B" symptoms Fever, night sweats, unintended weight loss

Basaloid Resembling cells found within the basal epithelial layer

Basophilic Preferentially staining blue with hematoxylin

Benign Nonmalignant

Berry aneurysm Focal dilatation of cerebral vasculature that is prone to rupture; patients typically describe the rupture as "the worst headache ever"

Biopsy Removal of individual cells or tissue for histologic evaluation; may involve fine-needle aspiration (FNA), subtotal sampling (incisional), or complete intact removal (excisional)

Blue bloater The typical cyanotic, plethoric appearance of a patient with chronic bronchitis caused by chronic hypoxemia, pulmonary artery vasoconstriction, and right heart failure

Body List of named entities below

BRCA Mutations of tumor suppressor genes (*BRCA1* on chromosome 17q and *BRCA2* on chromosome 13q) are associated with the majority of breast cancers

Calcification Deposition of calcium-containing material that may be within necrotic tissue (dystrophic) or within viable nonosseous tissue (metastatic)

Candida albicans A component of the usual flora within the skin and mucous membranes; potential source of opportunistic infections

Candidiasis Persistent or recurrent superficial infection of the skin or mucous membranes by *Candida* species, most often *C albicans*

Caput medusae Dilation of periumbilical veins often secondary to portal hypertension

Caseous The white cheese-like appearance of necrosis characteristic of tuberculosis in which none of the original histologic architecture is preserved

Cause of death The specific disease state or condition that leads to death (compare to mode and manner of death)

Cavitation Cavity formation, as in pulmonary tuberculosis

Cell injury Alteration in cellular structure or function that may be reversible or irreversible

Cellularity Quantity or condition of cells present within a tissue

Cerebriform Resembling the convolutions of the cerebral cortex

Chemotaxis (chemotactic) Orderly movement of cells either toward (positive) or away from (negative) a specific stimulus

Chloroma An extramedullary focus of malignant myeloblasts; so named for green hue imparted by myeloperoxidase

Chordoid Resembling a chordoma in which clusters and cords of neoplastic cells are present within a myxoid matrix

Chordoma Rare, slowly growing malignant neoplasm arising from the remnants of the notochord

Chylous Turbid white or pale yellow, triglyceride-rich fluid transported from the intestine by lacteals

Ciliary Possessing tail-like projections

Circumscribed Bounded, confined, or limited

Cirrhosis Diffuse hepatocyte injury, nodular regeneration, fibrosis, and architectural disruption characteristic of end-stage liver disease

Chorea Rapid, repetitive involuntary jerks associated with Huntington disease or following rheumatic fever (Sydenham chorea)

Choreoathetosis Movement disorder with combined features of chorea and athetosis

Clear cell Referring to cells with cytoplasmic clearing, usually due to dissolution of cytoplasmic lipid during tissue processing

Collagenous Relating to collagen

Congestion Excess fluid within vascular channels or other passages within a tissue

Condyloma Knob-like or warty growth induced by either epidermotropic human papillomavirus (acuminatum) or secondary syphilis (lata)

Crenation Becoming shriveled with notched or serrated margins

Cubitus valgus Increased carrying angle of the elbow when the arms are placed in the anatomic position; frequently observed in both Turner syndrome and Noonan syndrome

Cystic Characteristic of or containing one or more sacs lined with epithelium; filled with gas, fluid, or semisolid substance

de novo Arising without relation to a prior pathologic process

Decidualization Expansion of and individual lipid accumulation within endometrial cells in preparation for potential implantation and pregnancy

Deformation Congenital anomaly related to mechanical forces (small or abnormal uterus, and oligohydramnios) that restrict or otherwise impede normal growth (club feet or flattened facies)

Desmoplasia A stromal reaction surrounding infiltrating neoplastic cells

Desmopressin Synthetic antidiuretic hormone that also promotes the release of von Willebrand factor from storage sites; effective in cases of type I von Willebrand disease and occasionally type II disease

Diathesis Tissue necrosis, including inflammatory cells, hemolyzed erythrocytes, and degenerated epithelial cells, that is associated with an invasive malignancy

Differentiation Development or presence of cellular morphology specific to a cell line

Diffuse Widespread; opposite of focal

Discoid Coin-shaped or oval, raised lesions classically seen with cutaneous lupus

Disruption Developmental anomaly secondary to destruction of an otherwise normally developing organ or body part (amniotic band syndrome)

Dysplasia Abnormal in form

Dystrophy Progressive degeneration secondary to inadequate metabolism

E-cadherin Calcium-dependent cell-cell adhesion molecule; expression lost by both invasive and in situ lobular carcinoma

Ectatic Having a dilated, tortuous lumen

Ectopic Aberrantly located

Edema Excess fluid within cells or intercellular tissue

Effacement Replacement of normal histologic architecture (as in a lymph node) by a disease process, such as neoplasia

Effusion Pathologic accumulation of fluid in a cavity or tissue

Empyema Purulent fluid within a cavity, usually the pleural space

Endometrioid Resembling endometrial carcinoma

Endophytic Inward growth pattern, (opposite of exophytic)

Eosinophilic Preferentially staining red with eosin

Epithelioid Cellular features that Resemble an epithelial cell, such as epithelioid histiocyte or epithelioid sarcoma

Erythema Redness from capillary dilatation and congestion, often as a sign of inflammation or infection

Erythematous Reddened

Exophthalmos Anterior displacement of the eye associated with Graves disease or an orbital malignancy

Exophytic Outward growth pattern, opposite of endophytic

Extramammary Outside of the mammary gland

Exudate Proteinaceous fluid with an elevated specific gravity that is passed through a tissue, often a result of injury or inflammation

Facies Characteristic facial appearance associated with a particular condition (hyperadrenocorticism, trisomy 21, or Williams syndrome)

Ferruginous bodies Inhaled debris, historically including asbestos, enclosed by iron-containing proteins resulting in small golden-brown nodules within the alveolar septa

Fibrillar Appearance or composition of fibrils

Fibrinoid Resembling fibrin with a homogenously acidophilic appearance

Fibroadenoma Biphasic benign neoplasm of the breast with epithelial and stromal components; the most common benign tumor of the female breast

Fibrosis Presence of fibrous tissue

Fibrous Containing fibroblasts and the strands of connective tissue they produce

Focal Limited to a specific area; opposite of diffuse

Fomite An object, such as personal hygiene items, clothing, or toys, that when handled may transmit pathogens from an infected host

Foveolar Pitted or pit-like

Fusiform Tapered at both ends

Germline Related to gametes and their precursors; mutations within this lineage are transmissible to offspring

GFAP An intermediate filament in glial cells

Giant cell An abnormally enlarged cell, often containing more than one nucleus; modified phagocyte

Glabrous Lacking hair, as on the palmar and plantar surfaces

Gliosis Reactive proliferation of astrocytes following focal injury to the central nervous system, such as with multiple sclerosis or vascular insult

Glycogenated Presence of intracellular carbohydrate-laden vacuoles

Goblet cell Tall columnar cells with intracytoplasmic mucin of a specific type normally scattered along bronchiolar and gastrointestinal epithelium; may be present in cases of intestinal metaplasia secondary to esophageal irritation

Grade The degree of cytologic differentiation and architectural features of a particular tissue

Granulation tissue Highly vascularized tissue with increased fibroblasts and inflammatory cells

Granuloma Nodular inflammatory lesion

Granulomatous Composed of granulomata

Granzyme A constituent of azurophilic granules that induces apoptosis

Grenz zone A narrow band of uninvolved dermis separating a deeper inflammatory or neoplastic infiltrate from normal overlying epidermis

Guttate Drop-like

H&E Hematoxylin and eosin; the routine stain applied to tissue sections

Hamartoma Disordered proliferation of mature tissue

Hapten A low-molecular-weight substance that, although nonimmunogenic by itself, may induce antibody formation when bound to a particular protein or cell

Hemangioma Abnormal vascular proliferation, especially in skin or subcutaneous tissue

Hematogenous Via the bloodstream

Hemoglobin A1C (glycosylated hemoglobin) A form of hemoglobin nonenzymatically and permanently bound with reducing sugars, such as glucose and fructose, in peripheral circulation; used as a measure of average serum glucose during the preceding 2–3 months

Hemoptysis Cough productive of blood or blood-tinged sputum

Hemosiderin Residual yellow-brown pigment from the phagocytic digestion of hematin

Her2/neu Cell surface-bound receptor tyrosine kinase; overexpression is associated with more aggressive forms of breast cancer as well as in gastric and ovarian cancers

Heterotopia Aberrant position of an organ or tissue

Hidradenoma A benign tumor derived from the epithelial cells of sweat glands

Hirsutism Presence of androgen-dependent terminal body hair in an unusual location

Histiocyte Macrophage within a specific tissue, including alveolar macrophages, dermal Langerhans cells, giant cells, and osteoclasts

Human papillomavirus (HPV) A family of DNA viruses that induce mucocutaneous tumors; HPV types 6 and 11 have low oncogenic potential, while types 16 and 18 are associated with higher risk of progression to carcinoma

Hyalin Homogenously eosinophilic and translucent protein formed from cellular degeneration, as with diabetic glomerulosclerosis

Hydrops Excess watery fluid within a tissue or cavity

Hygroma An accumulation of serous fluid within a bursa or cyst

Hyperchromatic Dark or intensely staining chromatin within a nucleus; typically associated with dysplasia or malignancy

Hyperdiploidy Metaphase with more than 46 chromosomes exclusive of 92

Hyperemia Increased local blood flow

Hyperplasia Increased number of normal cells within an enlarged tissue or organ

Hypertrophy Increased size of normal cells

Hypoxemia Deficiency in the concentration of oxygen within arterial blood

Hypoxia Decreased level of oxygen available to a particular region (tissue hypoxia)

Icterus yellow discoloration of skin and mucous membranes

Idiopathic Of unknown etiology

in situ (Latin "in place") Confined to site of origin

Immunofluorescence The application of fluorescent dyes to label antibodies or antigens

Immunophenotype Pattern of antigen expression

Induration Presence of firm tissue

Infarct A necrotic area secondary to arterial or venous insufficiency

Infiltrate An aggregate of cells in higher than usual proportion within a specific tissue

Inflammation Dynamic complex of chemical and cellular responses to injury

Inflammation, acute Characterized by edema, hyperemia, and polymorphonuclear leukocytic infiltrate

Inflammation, chronic Characterized by fibrosis, granulomata, and infiltrates of lymphocytes, plasma cells, and histiocytes

Inflammation, fibrinopurulent Including an exudate with an elevated proportion of fibrin

Intraepithelial Within an epithelial cell layer

Invasion Malignant neoplastic spread through adjacent tissue; may be further classified as either capsular or vascular

Ischemia Decreased perfusion from functional or mechanical blood flow obstruction

Junctional Referring to the interface between epidermis and dermis

Karyolysis Loss of staining affinity by chromatin in cells undergoing swelling

Karyorrhexis Nuclear fragmentation

Keratin pearls Spherical accumulations of keratin that occur when differentiating squamous cells in submucosal nests are unable to slough keratin to a luminal surface

Kernicterus Neurotoxic staining of the basal ganglia, hippocampus, substantia nigra, and brainstem nuclei secondary to severe neonatal hyperbilirubinemia

Koilocytes Enlarged epithelial cells with prominent perinuclear clearing or halo-formation (an artifact of densely packed papillomavirus particles)

Lepidic Scaly or scale-like; often used to describe the growth pattern of bronchoalveolar carcinoma

Leukemia Hematologic malignancy marked by blast proliferation further classified cell lineage (lymphoid, myeloid, erythroid or megakaryocytic) and chronicity (acute or chronic)

Leukoplakia Adherent white plaques on oral cavity associated with chronic mechanical irritation, tobacco use, and HIV infection

Leukopoor Relatively devoid of leukocytes, as in pheresis platelets and plasma products

Lichenoid Band-like lymphohistiocytic inflammation at the epidermal-dermal junction

Lipomatous Similar in appearance to a lipoma

Lipoma Benign neoplasm of adipose tissue

Loculated Consisting of one (uni-) or more (multi-) cavities

Lymphangioma Benign proliferation of lymph vessels commonly within skin or subcutaneous tissue

Lymphoid   Related to lymphocytes or lymphatic tissues

Manner of death   Circumstances surrounding a death, broadly classified as either natural, accident, suicide, homicide, or undetermined

Malformation   A primary anomaly related to organ dysgenesis (esophageal atresia, transposition of the great vessels, or spina bifida)

Malignant   Demonstrating destructive or invasive growth or metastatic spread

Malignant peripheral nerve sheath tumor (MPNST)   Malignant counterpart to neurofibroma and schwannoma composed of spindled cells arrayed in sweeping fascicles among areas of myxoid degeneration; may arise in von Recklinghausen disease (neurofibromatosis type I)

Mast cell (mastocyte)   Cell type with numerous basophilic granules containing vasoactive substances such as heparin and histamine; frequently in connective tissue

Mediators   Vasoactive amines, plasma proteins, arachidonic acid metabolites, platelet-activating factor, cytokines and chemokines, nitric oxide, oxygen-derived free radicals, and neuropeptides

Medullary   Referring to soft tissue (Latin for marrow)

Mesenchymal   Cells that develop into connective tissue, blood vessels, and lymphatic tissue

Mesothelial   Characteristic of the membrane comprising the pleura, pericardium, and peritoneum as well as the tunica vaginalis testis and the tunica serosa uteri

Metaplasia   Cellular development aberrant from the tissue of origin

Metastasis   Spread of neoplastic cells to sites distant from their origin

Microalbuminuria   A form of proteinuria in which small quantities of albumin leak through damaged glomeruli

Micrognathia   Mandibular hypoplasia observed in fetal alcohol syndrome, DiGeorge syndrome, Marfan syndrome, Pierre Robin syndrome, trisomy 13, trisomy 18, Turner syndrome, Treacher Collins syndrome

Microphthalmia   Small eyes associated with fetal alcohol syndrome, trisomy 13, and intrauterine infection (rubella and cytomegalovirus)

Microsatellite instability   Variability in repeated DNA sequences that leads to reduced fidelity during the replication; associated with hereditary nonpolyposis colorectal cancer

Miosis   Pupillary constriction

Moniliasis   Another term for candidiasis

Morule   A focus of oval- or spindle-shaped squamous cells

Mucin   Glycoprotein found normally within goblet cells and other types of specialized epithelium

Müllerian   Referring to the paired ducts that fuse to become the structures of the female reproductive tract – the fallopian tubes, uterus, cervix, and upper two-thirds of the vagina

Multiloculated   Multiple chambers within a cystic structure

Multinodular   Composed of multiple nodules

Myeloid   Related to bone marrow; nonlymphocytic leukocytes

Myxoid   Containing glycosaminoglycans that impart a thinly basophilic appearance with H&E; common to many soft tissue lesions such as myxoid liposarcoma

Necrosis   Tissue death secondary to ischemia, radiation, or toxic injury; variants include coagulative, caseous, gangrenous, and liquefactive

Negative predictive value   The proportion of test subjects correctly diagnosed with a negative result; also defined as true negatives divided by all negatives

Neoplasia   Unregulated, aberrant cell growth

Nuclear-to-cytoplasmic (N:C) ratio   Apparent proportion of nuclear to cytoplasmic volumes which is increased with many types of neoplastic transformation

Opsonophagocytosis   Ingestion of foreign particles or pathogens after coating by either antibodies or complement

Organization   Progressive replacement of inflammatory infiltrate with fibroblasts, granulation tissue, and fibrosis

Os   An opening, as within the cervix

Papillary   Resembling a papilla or similar finger-like projection

Paraneoplastic syndrome   Set of conditions secondary to substances elaborated by a tumor

Pedunculated   Possessing a stalk or stem

Perforin   A constituent of azurophilic granules that opens holes in target cells

Petechia (plural: petechiae)   Focally extravasated erythrocytes often due to platelet disorders, vascular fragility or mechanical forces

Piloid   Hairlike

Pink puffer   The cachetic, barrel-chested appearance of a patient with emphysema

Pleomorphic   Varied in shape

Poikilocytosis   Variation in cell shape

Polymerase chain reaction   Automated, in vitro replication of DNA through repeated cycles of temperature-dependent strand separation, primer attachment, and complementary strand assembly

Positive predictive value   The proportion of test subjects correctly diagnosed with a positive result; also defined as true positives divided by all positives

Protease   Enzyme capable of degrading protein

Pseudorosette   Radial arrangement of cells without a true central lumen and centered instead on small blood vessels

Psoriasiform   Having gross or microscopic characteristics of psoriasis

Ptosis   Loss of tone within the levator palpebrae leading to drooping of the eyelid

Purulent   Containing or pertaining to pus

Pus   Viscous, white or yellow fluid composed of leukocytes, liquified tissue, and cellular debris

Pyknosis   Irreversible chromatin condensation in cells undergoing apoptosis

Reactive   Tissue response to various insults with certain histologic features

Reniform   Shaped like a kidney with a centrally placed indentation

Reticulin (silver or Gomori) stain   Highlights type III collagen-associated protein or procollagen

Rhabdoid   Characteristic of poorly differentiated myocytes with peripherally displaced nuclei and eosinophilic cytoplasm

Rhabdomyosarcoma   Soft tissue malignancy composed of skeletal muscle elements

Rhomboid   Possessing four sides of equal length

Rosette   Radial arrangement of cells about a central lumen or a hub composed of cytoplasmic processes

S-100   A family of low-molecular-weight calcium-binding proteins usually expressed by neural crest-derived cell lines including Schwann cells and melanocytes

Saponification   Alkaline hydrolysis of a triglyceride (fatty acid ester) to glycerol and fatty acid salts observed in acute pancreatitis or ingestion of an alkaline substance (lye)

Sarcomatoid   Resembling a sarcoma, a connective tissue neoplasm

Scirrhous   Hard, knotted

Sclerosis   Densely fibrous connective tissue with little cellularity

Sebaceous   Involving the oil-producing glands of the skin

Sentinel lymph node   The first lymph node or chain of nodes involved by a metastasizing neoplasm

Sequence   A distinct set of anomalies arising secondarily from a single original event or insult, such as the Potter sequence arising from oligohydramnios

Serous   Of or resembling serum, especially lymph

Serpiginous   Wavy, undulant, or serpent-like

Sessile   Flat or without a stalk, as opposed to pedunculated

Sideroblast   An erythroblast in which iron is incompletely incorporated into hemoglobin; individual iron aggregates appear blue with Prussian stain

Signet-ring cell Characterized by a crescentic nucleus peripherally displaced by mucin accumulation; resembling a signet ring

Silver stain See Reticulin stain

Spirochete A bacterium with spiral or worm-like shape; a member of the *Spirochaeta* family

Spongiform Characteristic porous or vacuolated microscopic appearance of cortex infected with one of the transmissible spongiform encephalopathies, including Creutzfeldt-Jakob disease, kuru, fatal familial insomnia, and Gerstmann-Straussler-Scheinker disease

Stage Classification of a tumor based on degree of differentiation, potential responsiveness to treatment, and prognosis

Steatosis Fatty accumulation within hepatocytes seen in various hepatic disorders

Stenosis Narrowing of any luminal structure

Storiform Spindled cells with elongated nuclei radiating from a center

Stroma Supportive tissue

Sustentacular Supportive

Syncytial Characteristic of a syncytium, a large structure formed through the fusion of two or more cells

Syndrome Constellation of findings without a known etiology, as opposed to disease (Goldenhar syndrome)

Telangiectasia Dilation of the small vessels (arterioles, capillaries, or venules) in a spidery configuration with multiple congenital (ataxia-telangiectasia, Osler-Weber-Rendu syndrome, and Sturge-Weber syndrome) and acquired (age-related, postural, and pregnancy) causes

Teratoma Neoplasm derived from more than one germ layer and composed of more than one tissue type

TORCHES An acronym of pathogens that cross the placenta: T: Toxoplasmosis and *Treponema;* O: Other agents (coxsackievirus, *Listeria,* and human parvovirus); R: rubella; C: cytomegalovirus and *Chlamydia;* HE: herpes simplex virus, hepatitis B, HHV4 (ie, Epstein-Barr virus), HHV3 (ie, varicella zoster virus), HIV; S: syphilis

Trabecular Strand-like or resembling a framework

Transformation zone The squamocolumnar junction within the uterine cervix in which dysplasia is most frequently observed

Transudate Abnormal accumulation of fluid with a low protein content and low specific gravity, usually due to hydrostatic or osmotic imbalance; compare to exudate

Trichomoniasis Sexually transmitted infection of *Trichomonas vaginalis*

Trichotillomania Impulse control disorder characterized by repeated hair pulling

Ultrastructural Cellular features observed with the resolution of electron microscopy

Undifferentiated Lacking evidence of cellular lineage; frequently associated with pleomorphic to anaplastic histologic appearance

Villous Possessing the fine hair-like projections present on certain membranous surfaces

Villonodular Characterized by a combined villous and nodular thickening

Window period Time between infection and laboratory detection; most often considered the time to seroconversion with antibody testing

Xanthomatous Composed of yellow, nodular aggregates of lipid-laden histiocytes

Zellballen Alveolar or trabecular pattern observed with paragangliomas, especially pheochromocytoma

II. DISEASES, SIGNS, AND SYNDROMES

Addison disease Hypocortisolism secondary to chronic adrenal insufficiency manifest as orthostatic hypotension and hyperpigmentation

Albers-Schönberg disease (osteopetrosis, marble bone disease) Reduced osteoclastic activity results in decreased bone resorption and markedly increased skeletal density

Albright hereditary osteodystrophy Pseudohypoparathyroidism secondary to an end-organ resistance to the effects of circulating parathyroid hormone

Alport syndrome Rare hereditary defect of collagen type 4 synthesis resulting in thickening and attenuation of the basement membranes; associated with sensorineural deafness, lens displacement, and glomerulonephritis

Alzheimer disease The most common form of dementia; progressive neurodegenerative condition associated with cognitive decline, emotional lability, and eventual withdrawal from social interaction; earlier onset among patient with trisomy 21; histologic findings include neurofibrillary plaques and tangles

Antoni areas The relatively cellular (Antoni A) and hypocellular (Antoni B) areas observed in microscopic sections of schwannoma

Arnold-Chiari syndrome Hypoplasia of the pons or medulla resulting in downward displacement of the medulla, fourth ventricle, and cerebellum into the cervical spinal canal; usually accompanied by myelomeningocele

Askin tumor Primitive neuroectodermal tumor (PNET) within the chest wall

Auer rods Needle-like cytoplasmic inclusions specific to acute promyelocytic leukemia (acute myelogenous leukemia type M3)

Auspitz sign The appearance of punctate hemorrhages follow curettage of parakeratotic scale on patients with psoriasis

Azzopardi phenomenon Presence of the basophilic smudgy nucleic acid rimming blood vessels characteristic of small cell lung carcinoma

Baker cyst A synovial cyst within the popliteal space in the setting of rheumatoid arthritis

Barrett esophagus Metaplasia from normal squamous epithelium to intestinal-type columnar epithelium with goblet cells; considered a premalignant histologic change

Becker muscular dystrophy An X-linked recessive dystrophinopathy that is clinically milder than Duchenne muscular dystrophy; often associated with an exon deletion of the dystrophin (*Xp21*) gene

Beckwith-Wiedemann syndrome Overgrowth disorder characterized by macrosomia (particularly macroglossia), omphalocele, and hypoglycemia

Behçet disease Idiopathic multisystemic inflammation presenting as recurrent oral aphthous ulcers, genital ulcers, and uveitis exclusive of a collagen vascular disease

Bell palsy Facial muscle paralysis due to viral injury to facial nerve

Bence Jones protein A monoclonal immunoglobulin light chain (paraprotein) released by neoplastic plasma cells then renally excreted; also associated with Waldenström macroglobulinemia; detected with urine electrophoresis

Berger disease (IgA nephropathy) Aberrant IgA deposition within the glomerular mesangium; the most common form of glomerulonephritis worldwide and presents as recurrent hematuria associated with intercurrent infection; histologically indistinguishable from Henoch-Schönlein purpura

Bernard-Soulier syndrome Autosomal recessively inherited decrease in glycoprotein Ib/IX/V complex expression on platelets resulting in deficient binding of von Willebrand factor and diminished platelet aggregation; also associated with idiopathic thrombocytopenia

Birbeck granule Membrane-bound organelle with characteristic tennis racket shape and cross-striated internal structure observed in Langerhans cells

Bitot spots Keratin accumulations within the conjunctiva indicative of vitamin A deficiency

Boerhaave syndrome Rare transmural rupture of the esophagus after forceful emesis and ending in potentially massive hemorrhage and death

Bouchard nodes   Osteophytes in the proximal interphalangeal (PIP) joints of the fingers associated with osteoarthritis

Bowen disease   Intraepidermal form of squamous cell carcinoma that presents as an erythematous scaly plaque more frequently in sun-exposed areas of middle aged women

Breslow thickness   Depth of melanoma invasion from the superior aspect of the granular layer or base of superficial ulceration to deepest point of tumor involvement ; tumors less than 1 mm thick are considered low risk while those greater 4 mm are high risk

Brodie abscess   Draining collection of pus secondary to acute osteomyelitis; most frequently involving *Staphylococcus aureus*

Brushfield spots   Pale dapples on the periphery of the irises observed in some cases of trisomy 21 (Down syndrome)

Bruton agammaglobulinemia   A rare X-linked disorder of B-cell maturation characterized by recurrent bacterial infections, especially encapsulated pyogenic organisms

Budd-Chiari syndrome   Triad of abdominal pain, ascites and hepatomegaly secondary to occlusion of either the hepatic vein or inferior vena cava; associated with hypercoagulable states such as polycythemia vera and other myeloproliferative disorders, pregnancy, and abdominal tumors; histologically apparent as centrilobular congestion and necrosis

Burkitt lymphoma   High-grade B-cell malignancy with an endemic (Epstein-Barr virus [EBV]-associated), sporadic form (less often related to EBV), and immunodeficiency-associated forms; on section, scattered macrophages contribute to the often cited but nonspecific "starry sky" pattern; most cases involve a translocation of the *c-myc* oncogene from chromosome 8 to one of the immunoglobulin chain genes on chromosomes 2, 14, or 22

Carney triad   Paraganglioma, pulmonary chondroma, and gastrointestinal stromal tumor (GIST)

Caplan syndrome   Rheumatoid arthritis and pneumoconiosis following chronic inhalation of asbestos, coal dust, or silicates

Chagas disease (American trypanosomiasis)   A biphasic (acute and chronic) parasitic disease resulting from infection by *Trypanosoma cruzi*

Charcot triad   Fever, jaundice, and right upper quadrant pain noted with ascending cholangitis

Chédiak-Higashi syndrome   Rare autosomal recessive, multisystemic disease marked by coagulopathy, hypopigmentation, peripheral neuropathy, and impaired NK-cell function resulting in recurrent infections or lymphoproliferative disorders

Christmas disease (hemophilia B)   X-linked recessive deficiency of factor 9

Churg-Strauss syndrome   Idiopathic granulomatous small-vessel vasculitis

Chvostek sign   Mechanical hyperirritability of peripheral nerves; percussion induces tetany; both Chvostek and Trousseau signs suggest hypocalcemia

Clark level   A measure of melanoma invasion divided into 1 of 5 anatomic layers from epidermal (level 1) to deep fat (level 5)

Codman triangle   Radiographic appearance of new wedge-shaped subperiosteal growth secondary to abscess, osteosarcoma, or Ewing sarcoma

Coombs test (antiglobulin test)   An assessment of immune reaction to red cell antigens; in the direct Coombs test, the presence of immunoglobulin or complement bound to red cells results in agglutination; the indirect Coombs test assesses the presence of specific serum immunoglobulins during incubation with red cells of known antigenicity

Cowden disease (Cowden syndrome or multiple hamartoma syndrome)   Autosomal dominant mutation of the *PTEN* gene (most cases) linked to hamartomatous neoplasms of the skin, mucosa, and central nervous system as well as the gastrointestinal and genitourinary tracts

Crigler-Najjar syndrome   Hereditary deficiency of the glucuronosyltransferase involved with bilirubin excretion resulting in extreme unconjugated hyperbilirubinemia

Crohn disease An inflammatory bowel disease characterized by transmural chronic inflammation with subsequent stricture formation and extension of mesenteric adipose ("creeping fat")

Creutzfeldt-Jakob disease (CJD) Rare, progressive and incurable neurodegenerative disorder; one of several transmissible spongiform encephalopathies, including kuru, fatal familial insomnia, and Gerstmann-Straussler-Scheinker disease, that affect both human and other animals

Curling ulcer Sloughing and ulceration of gastric or duodenal mucosa following profoundly hypovolemic states, particularly with severe burns

Curschmann spirals Twisted strands of mucus, often obtained from tracheal and bronchioalveolar lavages, associated with excess mucus production as in asthma and smoking-related bronchitis

Cushing disease Rare pituitary ACTH-producing tumor that induces adrenal hypersecretion of cortisol

Cushing syndrome Development of moon facies, hirsutism, lipodystrophy (buffalo hump and truncal obesity), and purple striae following prolonged exposure to endogenous or exogenous glucocorticoids; most commonly due to corticosteroid therapy but rarely an ACTH-expressive tumor in the pituitary or adrenal

Dane particle Complete hepadnavirion, the causative DNA virus of hepatitis B

Darier sign The tendency of lesions to become edematous, erythematous, and pruritic when physically stimulated in cases of both urticaria pigmentosa and mastocytoma

De Quervain thyroiditis (subacute granulomatous thyroiditis) Transient granulomatous inflammation clinically manifest as a tender thyroid

Diamond-Blackfan anemia Hereditary red cell aplasia associated with multiple physical anomalies, including craniofacial, thumb, and urogenital abnormalities as well as short stature and developmental delay

DiGeorge syndrome Rare monosomy 22q11 resulting in hypoplasia of the third and fourth pharyngeal pouches with subsequent variable T-cell immune deficiency

Donath Landsteiner antibody IgG autoantibody that binds erythrocytes and fixes complement at cold temperatures and that induces hemolysis at warmer temperatures (biphasic hemolysin); associated with paroxysmal cold hemoglobinuria

Down syndrome (trisomy 21) Characteristic facies (upslanting palpebral fissures and protruding tongue), generalized hypotonia, congenital cardiac anomalies (ventricular septal defects), and variable cognitive impairment secondary to an additional (partial or complete) copy of chromosome 21; associated with an increased risk of leukemia and Alzheimer disease

Dubin-Johnson syndrome Relatively benign familial conjugated hyperbilirubinemia

Duchenne muscular dystrophy An X-linked disorder characterized by progressive skeletal muscle weakness with onset in early childhood

Edwards syndrome (trisomy 18) Whole or partial additional copy of chromosome 18; characterized by developmental delay, micrognathia, cardiac anomalies, renal malformations, and rocker-bottom feet

Ehlers-Danlos syndrome A set of hereditary defects in collagen synthesis resulting in cutaneous hyperextensibility and joint hypermobility

Epstein-Barr virus (EBV) (human herpesvirus 4) Double-stranded DNA virus associated with infectious mononucleosis, Burkitt lymphoma, and nasopharyngeal carcinoma

Erythroplasia of Queyrat Squamous cell carcinoma in situ of the glans penis

Evans syndrome Uncommon combination (either simultaneously or sequentially) of autoimmune hemolytic anemia and idiopathic thrombocytopenic purpura (ITP)

Ewing sarcoma One of several tumors, including primitive neuroectodermal tumor and Askin tumor, arising from neural tissue and associated with fusion of the *EWS* gene (chromosome 22) to the *FLI1* gene (chromosome 11)

Fanconi anemia A hereditary bone marrow failure syndrome also characterized by congenital developmental anomalies (including growth retardation, limb defects, and genitourinary problems) and increased propensity to solid tumors, leukemia, and aplastic anemia

Fanconi syndrome Impaired reabsorption of bicarbonate resulting in type 2 renal tubular acidosis

Felty syndrome Combination of rheumatoid arthritis with chronic neutropenia

Flexner-Wintersteiner rosette Radial pattern of neoplastic cells observed in cases of retinoblastoma

Gardner syndrome A variant of familial adenomatous polyposis with cutaneous manifestations including epidermoid cysts, desmoid tumors (fibromatosis), and other benign tumors

Gaucher cell A macrophage with cytoplasm that resembles crumpled tissue paper due to glucocerebroside accumulation (Gaucher disease)

Gaucher disease An autosomal recessive deficiency of glucocerebrosidase; more common among those of Ashkenazi Jewish descent

Gerstmann-Sträussler-Scheinker disease Type of transmissible spongiform encephalopathy that is rarer and more slowly progressive (usually 5-year course) than Creutzfeldt-Jakob disease

Gilbert syndrome Transient, stress-induced increases in serum unconjugated bilirubin resulting from a mildly reduced activity of a hepatic glucuronosyltransferase

Glanzmann thrombasthenia Rare autosomal recessive absent or dysfunctional glycoprotein IIb/IIIa expression on platelets resulting in impaired aggregation with other platelets and fibrinogen

Goldblatt kidney Hypertension secondary to renovascular compromise, most often from arteriosclerosis

Goodpasture disease (anti-glomerular basement membrane disease) Autoimmune-induced glomerulonephritis and pulmonary hemorrhage; direct immunofluorescence reveals linear immunoglobulin deposition along the glomerular basement membrane and rarely alveolar basement membranes

Gorlin syndrome Autosomal dominant mutation of *PTCH* tumor suppressor gene resulting in a predisposition for basal cell carcinoma, melanoma, breast carcinoma, non-Hodgkin lymphoma, medulloblastoma, meningioma, and ovarian fibroma

Gowers maneuver Use of the hands to raise to a standing position observed in children with proximal muscle weakness, classically with muscular dystrophy

Gram stain The sequential application of crystal violet stain, iodine mordant, and safranin counterstain to differentiate bacterial species

Graves disease Hyperthyroidism with goiter and exophthalmos secondary to autoimmune assault on thyroid-stimulating hormone (TSH) receptors

Guillain-Barré syndrome Acute peripheral neuropathy, frequently presents as an ascending paralysis, that typically follows an infection; elevated cerebrospinal fluid (CSF) protein with normal cellularity (albumino-cytologic dissociation) is noted

Hand-Schüller-Christian triad Lytic bone lesions, diabetes insipidus, and proptosis observed with a subset of Langerhans cell histiocytosis cases

Hamman-Rich syndrome Chronic, progressive idiopathic pulmonary fibrosis

Hashimoto (chronic lymphocytic) thyroiditis Autoimmune destruction of thyroid tissue; most frequent cause of primary hypothyroidism

Heberden nodes Osteophytes in the distal interphalangeal (DIP) joints of the fingers associated with osteoarthritis

Henoch-Schönlein purpura Idiopathic IgA-mediated leukocytoclastic vasculitis often manifest with cutaneous purpura, arthritis, abdominal pain, and nephritis; histologically indistinguishable from other forms of IgA nephropathy

Hirschsprung disease The congenital absence of ganglia in either the Meissner and Auerbach plexi of the large intestine resulting from the migratory arrest of neuroblasts

Hodgkin disease Lymphoma consisting of germinal-center B cells incapable of producing antibodies (Reed-Sternberg or RS cells); characteristic bimodal age distribution

Homer Wright pseudorosettes Neuroblasts clustered about eosinophilic neuropil associated with neuroblastoma, medulloblastoma, pineoblastoma, and primitive neuroectodermal tumor

Horner syndrome (oculosympathetic palsy) Triad of ptosis, miosis, and anhidrosis from a developmental anomaly of or injury to the sympathetic innervation at the level of C8-T4

Huntington disease An autosomal dominant trinucleotide (CAG) expansion within the *huntingtin* gene prompting adult-onset progressive neurodegeneration

Hürthle cells Oncocytic follicular cells within the thyroid displaying cellular enlargement, eosinophilic granular cytoplasm; metaplastic changes observed in both inflammatory and neoplastic processes

Hutchinson freckle Lentigo maligna characterized by atypical melanocytes along the epidermal-dermal junction

Hutchinson sign Herpes zoster infection involving the nasal tip that indicates significant risk to the eye because of the shared enervation by the nasal branch of the nasociliary nerve

Job syndrome (hyperimmunoglobulinemia E) Rare autosomal dominant immunodeficiency with elevated serum levels of IgE, pneumonia, and recurrent skin abscesses (of biblical proportions)

Kaposi sarcoma Dome-shaped vascular lesions originally described in elderly men of Italian, Jewish, or Mediterranean ancestry; also noted in some cases of human herpesvirus 8 and HIV coinfection

Kartagener syndrome (immotile cilia syndrome) Autosomal recessive combination of primary ciliary dyskinesia (resulting in recurrent respiratory infection and reduced fertility) as well as situs inversus

Kawasaki disease (mucocutaneous lymph node disease) Self-limited, idiopathic, multi-organ vasculitis predominately affecting children under the age of 5; coronary artery aneurysms and subsequent myocardial infarction occur in a minority of cases

Kayser-Fleischer rings Darkening of Descemet membrane at the junction of the cornea and sclera observed in many cases of Wilson disease (as below)

Kearns-Sayre syndrome Mitochondrial DNA deletions that typically manifest as progressive ophthalmoplegia, ptosis, and retinal pigmentary degeneration; also associated with myopathy, sensorineural deafness, dementia, and various endocrinopathies

Kimmelstiel-Wilson nodules Hyaline material within the glomerular capillaries (glomerulosclerosis) secondary to nonenzymatic glycosylation among diabetics

Kinyoun stain Substitution of phenol for heat in the Ziehl-Neelsen protocol to alter the cell wall of acid-fast organisms (mycobacteria)

Klatskin tumor Cholangiocarcinoma at the confluence of the right and left hepatic bile ducts

Kleihauer-Betke test An assessment of fetal-maternal hemorrhage performed on Rh-negative mothers of Rh-positive infants to determine the quantity of Rh immunoglobulin required to prevent Rh-related alloimmunization that would threaten future pregnancies

Klinefelter syndrome (XXY syndrome) Variably severe hypogonadism, microorchidism, reduced fertility secondary to sex chromosome aneuploidy

Knudsen hypothesis The proposed requirement that two insults or "hits" inactivate both alleles of a tumor suppressor gene to promote tumorigenesis

Koebner phenomenon The development of lesions in response to physical trauma among patients with psoriasis

Kostmann syndrome Severe static neutropenia that may occasionally progress to either a myelodysplastic syndrome or acute myeloid leukemia

Krukenberg tumor Metastatic signet ring cell carcinoma from the gastrointestinal tract to the ovary

Kulchitsky (enterochromaffin) cells Neuroendocrine cells within the bronchi and gastrointestinal epithelium that produce serotonin; considered the predecessor of small cell carcinoma

Laënnec cirrhosis Alcoholic liver disease

Lambert-Eaton myasthenic syndrome Autoimmune injury to presynaptic voltage-gated calcium channel predominantly associated with small-cell lung cancer; clinical manifestations are similar to myasthenia gravis

Langerhans cell histiocytosis A group of idiopathic proliferative disorders involving epidermal dendritic cells (Langerhans cells) and eosinophils

Leigh disease (subacute necrotizing encephalomyelopathy) Form of rapidly progressive mitochondrial encephalopathy affecting the gray matter seen in children with psychomotor retardation and various movement disorders

Leser-Trélat sign Sudden eruption of multiple seborrheic keratoses suggestive of visceral malignancy

Li-Fraumeni syndrome Rare, autosomal dominant and highly penetrant predisposition to multiple forms of sarcoma, carcinoma, melanoma, and acute leukemias; linked to germline mutations of the p53 tumor suppressor gene

Lichtenberg sign Arborizing pattern noted on the skin following exposure to high intensity current such as lightening

Lines of Zahn Alternating layers of pale fibrin admixed with platelets and darker aggregates of red blood cells; associated with thrombosis at a site rapid blood flow

Lisch nodule Dome-shaped hamartomas of the iris characteristic of neurofibromatosis type 1 (von Recklinghausen disease)

Lynch syndrome Predisposition to hereditary nonpolyposis colorectal cancer as well as malignancies of the brain, skin, ovary, endometrium, and elsewhere along the gastrointestinal tract

Mallory-Weiss tears Longitudinal mucosal lacerations of upper gastrointestinal tract secondary forceful emesis, coughing, or convulsions

Mantoux test Intradermal injection of purified protein derivative (PPD) and assessment of potential induration to screen for exposure to *Mycobacterium tuberculosis*

Marfan disease Autosomal dominant defect in the fibrillin-1 gene leading to a clinically variable set of findings, including tall stature, ectopia lentis, and cardiovascular anomalies such as aortic root dilatation and mitral valve prolapse

May-Hegglin anomaly (or May-Hegglin syndrome) Macrothrombocytopenia due to mutation within the *MYH9* gene on chromosome 22; nonspecifically associated with the presence of Döhle or Amato bodies (2–5 μm within neutrophils and eosinophils; although most patients are asymptomatic, approximately one-quarter have a clinically significant bleeding diathesis

McArdle disease (glycogen storage disease type V) Myophosphorylase deficiency prevents the release of glucose from muscle-entrapped glycogen leading to severe pain with moderate exercise; associated with an increased risk of rhabdomyolysis and renal failure

McLeod phenotype (McLeod neuroacanthocytosis syndrome) Late-onset X-linked multisystem disorder affecting the peripheral and central nervous systems characterized by weakened expression of antigens in the Kell blood group system; occasionally associated with chronic granulomatous disease

Meckel diverticulum Congenital bulge of small intestine resulting from the failure of the embryonic vitelline duct to involute

Meckel-Gruber syndrome Rare autosomal recessive condition marked by the triad of occipital encephalocele, enlarged polycystic kidneys, and polydactyly

Mees lines Transverse pale lines within the fingernail observed with arsenic toxicity

Meigs syndrome The presence of pleural effusion (usually right-sided) and ascites with ovarian neoplasm (fibroma, thecoma, cystadenoma, or granulosa cell tumor)

Muir-Torre syndrome A very rare, predominantly autosomal dominant defect in DNA mismatch repair gene that predisposes patients to carcinoma of the breast, colon, and genitourinary tract as well as skin lesions, including sebaceous adenoma and keratoacanthoma

Munro microabscess The presence of degenerated polymorphonuclear leukocytes in the stratum corneum in patients with psoriasis and seborrheic dermatitis

Niemann-Pick cell A macrophage with finely vacuolated or "foamy" cytoplasm due to sphingomyelin accumulation (Niemann-Pick disease)

Niemann-Pick disease An autosomal recessive sphingomyelinase deficiency resulting in lipid accumulation within the monocyte-macrophage system; more common among those of Ashkenazi Jewish descent

Nikolsky sign The tendency of skin to separate and become eroded with the application of firm, lateral pressure; a nonspecific finding in patients with active blistering

Osler-Weber-Rendu syndrome Autosomal dominant disorder involving abnormal vascular development, particularly hemorrhagic telangiectasia

Paget cells Enlarged epithelial cells with abundant clear cytoplasm and pleomorphic nuclei

Paget disease (osteitis deformans) Idiopathic localized defect of bone remodeling in which excessive osteoclastic activity (lytic phase) is followed by haphazard osteoblastic compensation (mixed then final phases) results in structurally deficient woven bone

Paget disease, extramammary (EMPD) Rare variant of Paget disease arising as a primary cutaneous adenocarcinoma at a site other than the breast

Paget disease, mammary Eczematous condition of the nipple and areolar skin associated with an underlying intraductal carcinoma

Pancoast tumor Pulmonary squamous cell carcinoma involving the branchial plexus producing shoulder pain and muscular atrophy

Papanicolaou (Pap) test Application of a multichromatic staining process (Pap stain) to exfoliated, alcohol-fixed cervical cells to assess for dysplasia, malignancy, and other clinically significant changes within the female lower reproductive tract

Pautrier microabscess The presence of aggregated cerebriform T-cell lymphocytes within the epidermis characteristic of mycosis fungoides

Pelger-Huët anomaly Benign, autosomal dominant mutation of the lamin B receptor gene characterized by the presence of dumbbell-shaped or spectacle-like (*pince nez*) nuclei in granulocytes

Plummer-Vinson syndrome Dysphagia, atrophic glossitis, upper esophageal webs associated with iron-deficiency anemia and koilonychia among patients at increased risk for squamous cell carcinoma

Peutz-Jeghers syndrome Autosomal dominant disorder marked by intestinal hamartomatous polyps and mucocutaneous melanocytic macules clinically notable at the vermilion border; also imparts a higher risk of gastrointestinal tract carcinoma

Pompe disease (glycogenosis type II) Rare, autosomal recessive deficiency of acid maltase resulting in glycogen excess with subsequent multisystemic compromise, particularly myopathy

Pott disease (tuberculous spondylitis) Extrapulmonary extension of mycobacterial infection, usually involving the thoracic spine

Prader-Willi syndrome An abnormality of the methylation imprint within chromosome 15q that manifests clinically with hypotonia and feeding difficulties in early infancy followed by excessive eating and eventual morbid obesity in early childhood

Ramsay Hunt syndrome Facial muscle paralysis, often accompanied by pain, secondary to herpes zoster virus infection of the geniculate ganglion of the facial nerve typically associated with a rash (inflamed vesicles or tiny water-filled bumps in the skin) in or around the ear, and sometimes on the roof of the mouth

Rathke cleft Cystic remnant of between the pars distalis and pars intermedia from which craniopharyngioma develops

Reed-Sternberg cell The neoplastic cell of Hodgkin lymphoma characterized by prominent bi- or multinucleation as well as aberrant expression of CD15 (ordinarily a marker of late granulocytes, monocytes, and activated T cells)

Refetoff syndrome Rare peripheral tissue resistance to thyroid hormone due to one of several mutant forms of thyroid hormone receptor

Reinke crystals Cylindrical or rectangular inclusions pathognomonic of Leydig cell tumors

Reiter syndrome Ocular inflammation (conjunctivitis and uveitis), urethritis, and reactive arthritis following enteric or urogenital infections; associated with human leukocyte antigen (HLA)–B27

Reye syndrome A rare type of acute encephalopathy usually following viral illness (influenza or varicella) in children; earlier associated with aspirin administration resulting in mitochondrial membrane disruption and subsequent inability to incorporate ammonia into urea

Reynold pentad Addition of hypotension and altered mental status to Charcot triad (see above)

Richter transformation (Richter syndrome) Rare evolution of chronic lymphocytic leukemia to diffuse large B cell lymphoma; indicates a poor prognosis

Riedel thyroiditis Rare idiopathic fibrosis of thyroid parenchyma

Rokitansky-Aschoff sinuses Partial invagination of mucosal epithelium into the muscular wall of the gallbladder observed with cholecystitis and cholelithiasis

Romaña sign Swelling of the eyelids following autoinnoculation with infectious insect feces; a sign of acute Chagas disease (as above)

Rosenthal fibers Filamentous eosinophilic aggregates of glial fibrillary acidic protein (GFAP) observed with pilocytic astrocytoma

Schatzki rings Benign mucosal and submucosal rings typically located just proximal to the gastroesophageal junction; may result in intermittent dysphagia

Schirmer test Application of paper strips to the mucous membranes to assess lacrimal function; decreases are observed among patients with Sjögren syndrome

Sézary syndrome (mycosis fungoides) Slowly progressive proliferation of malignant T-lymphocytes within the skin

Sheehan syndrome Postpartum necrosis of the anterior pituitary secondary to hypovolemic shock

Schilling test Assessment of vitamin B12 absorption involving ingestion of radiolabeled vitamin B12; diminished urinary excretion (less than 5% over 24 hours) may be due to either pernicious anemia or malabsorption, whereas increased excretion upon repeat testing with oral intrinsic factor is diagnostic of pernicious anemia secondary to impaired factor production

Sister Mary Joseph nodule Palpable periumbilical induration associated with intra-abdominal and pelvic malignancies

Sjögren syndrome Idiopathic autoimmune destruction of lubricating glands, most often lacrimal and salivary glands, resulting in xerophthalmia, xerostomia, and dysphagia

Stein-Leventhal syndrome Amenorrhea, infertility, and hirsutism in women with enlarged polycystic ovaries enclosed by sclerotic capsules

Stevens-Johnson syndrome Potentially fatal hypersensitivity caused by several medications, viral antigens, and neoplasms leading to epidermal necrosis and subepidermal bulla formation

Sturge-Weber syndrome Congenital neurocutaneous disorder that typically manifests with seizures, glaucoma, and facial port-wine stains

Sweet syndrome An acute febrile neutrophilic dermatosis often associated with hematologic malignancy and autoimmune disease

Takayasu arteritis Idiopathic inflammation of the aortic arch predominantly among young Asian women that manifests clinically with the loss of carotid, radial, or ulnar pulses

Tay-Sachs disease An autosomal recessive defect in hexosaminidase A leading to GM2 ganglioside accumulation with subsequent ganglion cell loss in the cortex and peripheral demyelination; associated with "cherry-red" retinal macula

Tetralogy of Fallot Constellation of ventricular septal defect, pulmonic stenosis, right ventricular hypertrophy, and overriding aorta; an affected heart has boot-shaped (coeur-en-sabot) radiographic appearance

Trousseau sign Muscular contraction distal to transient arterial occlusion (elicited by inflating a sphygmomanometer cuff above systolic blood pressure for several minutes); both Chvostek and Trousseau signs suggest hypocalcemia

Turcot syndrome The combination of familial adenomatous polyposis and central nervous system tumors, typically medulloblastomas and glioblastomas

Turner syndrome Loss of all or part of an X chromosome resulting in short stature, cardiovascular malformations (aortic coarctation or bicuspid aortic valve), gonadal dysgenesis (streak ovaries), and infertility

Tyndall phenomenon Optical effect of incident light on heavily concentrated pigments (melanin) refracted through colloid (skin)

Tzanck cells Cells exhibiting viral cytopathic effects (multinucleation, nuclear enlargement, and clearing with margination of chromatin) associated with herpes viral infection

Upshaw-Schulman syndrome A rare congenital deficiency of ADAMTS-13 that results in thrombotic thrombocytopenic purpura

Verocay bodies Ovoid structures composed of compact pairs of well-aligned nuclei enclosing a central fibrillary area; characteristic of schwannoma

Virchow node (Troisier sign) Supraclavicular lymphadenopathy considered pathognomonic of gastric carcinoma

Virchow triad Stasis, altered coagulability of the blood, and vessel wall damage that increase the risk of thrombosis

von Gierke disease (glycogen storage disease type I) Glucose-6-phosphatase deficiency hobbles the hepatic export of glucose resulting in hepatomegaly and recurrent fasting hypoglycemia

von Hippel disease Retinal capillary hemangioma

von Hippel-Lindau disease Hemangioma or hemangioblastoma within the central nervous system in addition to visceral adenomas (particularly renal cell carcinoma); hereditary forms are associated with mutations of the *VHL* tumor suppressor gene on chromosome 3

von Recklinghausen disease (neurofibromatosis type 1 or peripheral neurofibromatosis) An autosomal dominant mutation of *neurofibromin* gene on chromosome 17 characterized by variable dysplasia of ectodermally and mesodermally derived tissues; associated with café au lait macules, Lisch nodules, soft cutaneous neurofibromas, and pheochromocytoma

von Recklinghausen disease of bone (osteitis fibrosa cystica) Bone loss secondary to hyperparathyroidism (both primary and secondary) characterized by osteoclast-lined cystic spaces filled by vascular fibrous stroma and hemorrhage (brown tumors); predisposes patients to microfracture

von Willebrand disease A set of common hereditary bleeding disorders arising from abnormalities, either quantitative or qualitative, of von Willebrand factor; individual cases range from asymptomatic to severe hemophilia

von Willebrand factor A large multimeric glycoprotein involved in both primary (platelet adhesion) and secondary (factor VIII carrier) hemostasis

Waldenstrom macroglobinemia (hyperglobulinemic purpura) Idiopathic proliferation of IgM-producing lymphoid cells

Wallerian degeneration Axonal and nerve sheath degeneration distal to nerve transection

Waterhouse-Friderichsen syndrome Fulminant meningococcemia induces massive hemorrhage into the adrenal glands with subsequent adrenocortical insufficiency

Wegener granulomatosis Small-vessel vasculitis involving the upper respiratory tract, lungs, and kidneys; associated with c-ANCA (antineutrophil cytoplasmic antibody-cytoplasmic pattern)

Wernicke-Korsakoff syndrome Thiamine deficiency-induced cerebellar degeneration and hemorrhage into mamillary bodies presenting as ataxia, ophthalmoplegia, and short-term memory loss

Whipple disease Malabsorption, arthropathy, or neurologic symptoms due to intestinal, joint, and central nervous system infection by *Tropheryma whippelii* (a gram-positive actinomycete)

Whipple triad Criteria that suggest a pancreatic insulinoma: 1) signs and symptoms (tachycardia, tremor, altered mental status) that are likely secondary to hypoglycemia; 2) measured hypoglycemia (serum glucose <50 mg/dL); 3) symptomatic relief with glucose administration

Wickham striae Delicate white lines on the papules and plaques of lichen planus

Wilms tumor (nephroblastoma) The most common pediatric abdominal malignancy; composed of epithelial, blastemal, and stromal elements

Wilson disease (hepatolenticular degeneration) Autosomal recessive disorder of copper accumulation that presents in adolescents and young adults

Wiskott-Aldrich syndrome Rare X-linked recessive combined immune deficiency characterized by recurrent infections, thrombocytopenia with functionally impaired platelets, and eczema

Zenker diverticulum Posterior herniation of esophageal mucosa between the cricopharyngeus and inferior pharyngeal constrictor muscles frequently resulting in dysphagia, aspiration, and regurgitation

Ziehl-Neelsen stain The sequential application of heat or steam, basic fuchsin stain, an acid-alcohol decolorizer, then a methylene blue counterstain to reveal acid-fast organisms such as *Mycobacteria*

Zollinger-Ellison syndrome The presence of intractable ulcers secondary to a gastrin-secreting tumor (gastrinoma) of either the pancreas or duodenum; a component of multiple endocrine neoplasia type I (MEN I) in a fourth of all cases of Zollinger-Ellison syndrome

III. BODIES

Call-Exner body An accumulation of densely staining material within granulosa cells in maturing ovarian follicles; associated with ovarian tumors of granulosal origin

Councilman bodies Eosinophilic cytoplasmic inclusions within dying hepatocytes

Döhle body Basophilic staining agglutinated ribosomes within the cytoplasm of neutrophils; associated with inflammation and increased granulocytopoiesis

Heinz (Ehrlich, Heinz-Ehrlich) body Irregularly-shaped granules of denatured hemoglobin, visible with crystal violet, within the erythrocytes; non-specifically associated with thalassemic hemolytic anemia as well as oxidant sensitivity, especially to primaquin, in patients with glucose-6-phosphate dehydrogenase (G6PD) deficiency

Howell-Jolly body Rounded remnants of erythrocytic nuclear chromatin; associated with hemolytic anemia, megaloblastic anemia, and after splenectomy

Mallory body (Mallory hyaline) Eosinophilic, intracellular accumulations of cytokeratin filaments nonspecifically associated for alcohol-induced hepatic damage

Michaelis-Gutmann body Macrophage with basophilic calcified, iron-encrusted lysosomes associated with malakoplakia

Pappenheimer body Iron aggregates within the mitochondria and ribosomes of erythrocytes; associated with severe anemias and thalassemias

Pick bodies Argyrophilic (silver staining) spherical inclusions composed of disarrayed tau proteins, alpha-synuclein, and apolipoprotein E primarily within neurons of patients with frontal lobar dementias

Psammoma body A concentrically laminated calcification most often observed with papillary thyroid carcinoma, papillary renal cell carcinoma, serous papillary ovarian adenocarcinoma (cystadenocarcinoma), endometrial adenocarcinomas, meningioma, and mesothelioma

Schiller-Duval body An aggregate of germ cells surrounding a central blood vessel, resembling a glomerulus; observed in yolk sac tumors

Weibel-Palade body Rod-shaped intracytoplasmic microtubular bundle, specific to vascular endothelium, that contains von Willebrand factor

INDEX

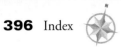

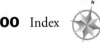